R 2B Viva

urvival Guide

Final FRCR 2B Viva

A Survival Guide

Edited by

Kiat Tsong Tan
Attending Radiologist, Queen Elizabeth Hospital,
Charlottetown, Prince Edward Island, Canada

John Curtis
Consultant Radiologist, University Hospital Aintree,
Liverpool, UK

Jessie Aw
Neuroradiology Fellow, University of Chicago,
Chicago, IL, USA

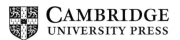

CAMBRIDGE
UNIVERSITY PRESS

University Printing House, Cambridge CB2 8BS, United Kingdom

One Liberty Plaza, 20th Floor, New York, NY 10006, USA

477 Williamstown Road, Port Melbourne, VIC 3207, Australia

314-321, 3rd Floor, Plot 3, Splendor Forum, Jasola District Centre, New Delhi - 110025, India

79 Anson Road, #06 -04/06, Singapore 079906

Cambridge University Press is part of the University of Cambridge.

It furthers the University's mission by disseminating knowledge in the pursuit of
education, learning and research at the highest international levels of excellence.

www.cambridge.org
Information on this title: www.cambridge.org/9780521183079

© Cambridge University Press 2012

First published 2012
Reprinted 2020

Printed in the United Kingdom by TJ International Ltd. Padstow Cornwall

A catalogue record for this publication is available from the British Library

ISBN 978-0-521-18307-9 Paperback

Library of Congress Cataloging in Publication data
Final FRCR 2B viva : a survival guide / [edited by] Kiat Tsong Tan, John Curtis, Jessie Aw.
    p. ; cm.
  Final FRCR twoB viva
  Includes bibliographical references and index.
  ISBN 978-0-521-18307-9 (pbk.)
  I. Tan, Kiat Tsong.   II. Curtis, John (John Michael)   III. Aw, Jessie.   IV. Title: Final
  FRCR twoB viva.
  [DNLM: 1. Radiography – Case Reports.   2. Radiography – Examination
  Questions. WN 18.2]
  616.07'57–dc23
  2011028340

For my parents, Tan Boon Keng and Ng Liew
KTT
For Juliet and Matthew
JC
For my parents, Khin Khin Cho and Sein Hwat, and to all my family,
Jac, Rich, Hannah, Izzy and Nat
JA

Contents

Contents

Cases

1. Cardiothoracic and vascular radiology

Cardiothoracic radiology

3. Musculoskeletal radiology

4. Neuroradiology

5. Genitourinary and breast radiology

Genitourinary radiology

Breast radiology

6. Paediatric radiology

7. Nuclear medicine

Contributors

Jessie Aw MRCP FRCR
Neuroradiology Fellow, University of Chicago, Chicago, IL, USA

Han Wei Aw-Yeang MRCP FRCR
Consultant Radiologist, Wirral University Teaching Hospital NHS Foundation Trust, Arrowe Park Hospital, Upton, UK

John Curtis DMRD FRCP FRCR
Consultant Radiologist, University Hospital Aintree, Liverpool, UK

Patricia Dunlop MD FRCPC
Attending Radiologist, Sunnybrook Health Sciences Centre Department of Medical Imaging, Toronto, Ontario, Canada

Richard Hopkins MRCP FRCR
Consultant Radiologist, Cheltenham General Hospital, Cheltenham, UK

Iain D. Lyburn MRCP FRCR
Consultant Radiologist, Cheltenham General Hospital, Cheltenham, UK

Richard J. T. Owen MRCP FRCR
Associate Professor, Radiology and Diagnostic Imaging, University of Alberta, Edmonton, Canada

Rachana Shukla FRCR
Consultant Radiologist, Royal Gwent Hospital, Newport, UK

Rekha Siripurapu MRCP FRCR
Consultant Radiologist, Salford Royal NHS Foundation Trust, Salford, UK

Kiat T. Tan MD MRCP FRCR FRCPC
Attending Radiologist, Queen Elizabeth Hospital, Charlottetown, Prince Edward Island, Canada

Foreword

This wonderful book has brought together radiologists in Britain, Australia and North America with a passion for education and talent for condensing key information into a succinct and useful format. The focus of the book is the preparation of radiologists in training for the final oral examination of their professional career and provides the trainees with a series of viva examination-type cases that comprehensively review most of what the competent radiology graduate needs to know. The book is an enjoyable read and, for the examination candidate, it provides an opportunity to confirm what is known and understood and which areas may require some additional attention as the examination approaches.

The images are high quality and representative of both common and important unusual conditions. The text for each case is presented as one would approach the subject in the viva examination, with description followed by crucial clinical questions and a brief discussion with suggestions for further reading. Experts in the sub-specialty fields of clinical radiology and education in diagnostic imaging have been involved in the development of each section.

In addition to the examination candidate, the material is very suitable for those of us who are longer in the tooth and may be seeking continuing medical education through a non-confrontational method of self-evaluation. The material is applicable to radiologists anywhere in the world. The content is based on up-to-date reviews with many fine examples of conventional imaging and presentation of state-of-the-art cross-sectional studies that illustrate the timeless principles of diagnostic radiology.

I highly recommend this book to any candidate presenting themselves for Royal College or board examination on any continent. I also strongly encourage practising radiologists that are past this challenge to consider this excellent opportunity for self-assessment that will provide some direction for further improvement with the assurance that it will be equally educational and more enjoyable than repeating the test on both sides of the pond.

Dr Robert GW Lambert, MB BCh, FRCR, FRCPC, Professor and Chair,
Department of Radiology and Diagnostic Imaging, University of Alberta

Preface

The inspiration for this book came from the legendary *An Aid to the MRCP Short Cases* by Ryder, Freeman and Mir. It was the single most helpful text when I (KTT) was preparing for the incredibly stressful MRCP exam many moons ago (I'm showing my age!). This was the book that was the foundation for the way I present my cases, and it has been tried and tested in both the FRCR and its close cousin the FRCPC.

It was therefore surprising to find no equivalent book designed for the FRCR on the market. Radiology is the most visual of the medical specialities. The basis of our practice is to be able to spot the abnormality and to communicate our findings effectively. This is basically what the FRCR 2B viva and equivalent exams worldwide are designed to assess. Indeed, to paraphrase a well-known physician, the FRCR is designed to teach as much as it is to test.

The core of this book consists of 263 cases that are typical of the FRCR viva. For each case, a presentation (a model answer) is provided to act as a 'template'. There are many styles of case presentation, and this is reflected in the writing of the various chapter authors, all of whom have sat for and passed the FRCR exam (or the FRCPC).

Finally, facts that are clinically important but not readily available in common textbooks, or which could add the 'wow factor' during your exam presentation, are included in this text. We trust that in addition to helping you with the exam, this might also make a difference to your day-to-day practice.

Introduction

The FRCR viva, together with its sibling, the rapid reporting session, is responsible for the majority of failures in the exam. Like all postgraduate exams, the key to passing the viva is to play the game wisely and to know what to expect.

Pre-preparation
Before preparing for the viva, read the exam guidelines published by the Royal College of Radiologists. Many candidates are unaware of what to expect at the exam until just before the exam. Do not be one of them.

Reporting
This book is a good starting point. Look at the images. Present the cases to yourself (or even better, a study partner). Working 'templates' to generate a radiology report are given below.

The ideal situation
1. Pause for a couple of seconds to look at the film and think before talking.
2. 'This is a [type of radiological investigation] of a [male/female] [adult/child/infant/newborn].' (*This gives you a couple more seconds to look at the film and think.*)
3. 'The investigation shows [findings]. The diagnosis/differential diagnoses is/are ...' (Give a *maximum* of 3–4.)
4. 'I would like to ...' (Tell them what you wish to do to confirm your diagnosis or your further management plan.)
5. Answer any questions.
6. Film comes down.

Of course, things are often more complicated. If you see no obvious abnormality, try the following:

1 and 2 as above.
3. Go through the imaging systematically, while presenting the normal findings. For example, on a chest x-ray, say 'There are no obvious lung abnormalities. I will now look at the review areas carefully ...'
4. Most of the time, you will see the abnormality. Continue as above. If not, ask for additional history (which might prompt the examiner to help you) and look at the film again.
5. If you can see the abnormality but do not know what it is, describe it and give a list of possible differential diagnoses.
6. If appropriate, you could suggest further investigation based on the patient's presenting complaint (although this can be risky strategy). For example, if you cannot see an abnormality in the chest x-ray of someone with progressive shortness of breath, you may try to get the examiner to show you a CT by suggesting that this is what you would do in your clinical practice. However, do not use this trick more than a couple of times, and do not suggest an outlandish or non-indicated test.

6. If you *really* cannot see the abnormality, cut your losses and say you cannot see it and try to move on (if the examiner lets you). It is better to score badly on one image and make up for it on later images than fail the session completely by not moving on.

Other preparation

1. Be proactive. Organize formal FRCR viva sessions with your consultants.
2. Go through the local film collection with a study partner. Practise reporting the images found in major textbooks. As a rule, diseases found in Grainger & Allison and Sutton are considered fair game for the viva.
3. Have a book of lists like Chapman & Nakielny or Dähnert to come up with a reasonable list of differential diagnoses.
4. Go on at least one course. There are countless FRCR courses on offer in the UK and abroad. These courses may seem expensive, but they are certainly cheaper than having to resit the exam. This advice is especially true for candidates from outside the UK.
5. Do not ignore the other components of the exam. The key to passing the long cases is time management, and for the rapid reporting it is getting at least 27/30 correct. Practice is crucial to passing these two components.
6. Do not lose track of the fact that revising for this exam will make you a better radiologist.

Things to do during the exam

1. Be polite to everyone. Smile. Greet the examiner and thank them at the end.
2. Dress appropriately. This means a dark suit, a tie (for men) and long skirt/trousers for women. Not only will the examiners take you more seriously if you look the part, you will feel more confident. (Before your exam, perhaps you can tell yourself that although you're the one being examined, at least your suit is of a better cut than those of the examiners – a great confidence booster!)
3. Talk clearly.
4. Follow instructions.
5. Think before you speak.
6. Always listen to the examiner. They are trying to pass you. If they ask a question like 'Are you sure?', it is not to trip you up but because the answer you gave is not the one they expected.
7. Remember that examiners could be impassive, friendly or somewhere in between. The examiner's affect does not really reflect your performance.
8. Remember that you might actually know more than the examiner (*great confidence booster*). You have just spent months preparing for this exam and are at the peak of your powers. The examiner may be a subspecialist who passed the exams in 1980 and is showing you films outside his/her subspecialist area.
9. Remember to play it safe. Only say and do what you would reasonably do in real life. If asked to describe a procedure that you do not do, always start by saying you do not do it yourself before giving the description. If asked about small radiological minutiae that you do not know anything about, either say you do not know or say you will look it up on PubMed or Google, or in the local medical library.
10. If you get asked about something completely esoteric – e.g. 'Can you elaborate on what you mean by a true FISP MRI sequence?' – it often means that you are doing well.

Things not to do during the exam

1. Smoke before the viva (unless you can make absolutely sure that you do not smell of cigarettes).
2. Chew gum.
3. Go to pieces if a case goes badly – a.k.a. 'the downward spiral syndrome' (see scenarios below). Even when things appear to be going wrong, it is still possible to pass the exam.
4. Argue with the examiner. You will lose.
5. Regurgitate the 10 differential diagnoses given in Dähnert. If the examiner wishes to hear more than the 3–4 differentials, he/she will ask you for it.
6. Answer a question you do not know the answer to. It could lead to a bottomless pit of further questions on the subject. It is often better to say you do not know and move on.
7. 'Kill' the patient. The examiners are here to make sure you are a safe general radiologist.

The following two scenarios are 'fly on the wall' accounts of actual FRCR vivas.

Scenario 1

EXAMINER1: Hello Dr _____, I'm Dr _____ and this is Dr _____. Please have a seat.

CANDIDATE: Hello. Pleased to meet you.

EXAMINER1: I will start. Please report this investigation. (*Puts up a pelvic x-ray*)

CANDIDATE: This is a pelvic x-ray of a male patient. There are multiple lucencies with well-defined mildly sclerotic borders in the proximal right femur. The lesions have a narrow zone of transition. The areas of lucency appear to have a 'ground-glass appearance'. The diagnosis is fibrous dysplasia. (*Expecting the film to go down, which it doesn't*)

EXAMINER1: Anything else?

CANDIDATE: Oh … There is a pathological fracture through the femur. (*Starting to feel stressed*)

EXAMINER1: (*Removes film*) This infant has abdominal pain. (*Puts up paediatric abdominal x-ray*)

CANDIDATE: This is a paediatric abdominal radiograph. There is gross dilatation of the stomach and the duodenum. The distal small bowel and colon are not dilated. The diagnosis is consistent with proximal small bowel obstruction, for which the differential diagnoses are wide. An upper GI barium study would be useful for further investigation.

EXAMINER1: Exactly … (*Puts up small bowel FT*)

CANDIDATE: The barium study shows a corkscrew appearance of the proximal small bowel. (*Suddenly realises he cannot remember the diagnosis associated with corkscrew small bowel. Starts getting more stressed*) There is complete proximal small bowel obstruction. The patient requires a surgical referral.

EXAMINER1: What causes of paediatric proximal small bowel obstruction do you know of?

CANDIDATE: Annular pancreas, small bowel hypoplasia/atresia. I cannot remember the exact cause of a corkscrew small bowel …

EXAMINER1: (*Smiles*) … Calm down. (*Takes film down and puts up a CXR*)

CANDIDATE: Oh … the previous case was malrotation.

EXAMINER1: (*Smiles*) … OK. Look at this chest radiograph.

CANDIDATE: This is a PA chest radiograph of an adult patient. The NG tube tip is above the diaphragm and pointing towards the left. This needs to be repositioned and a repeat chest radiograph obtained. The heart is enlarged. There are a couple of linear lines in the lung bases, which could suggest heart failure.

EXAMINER1: I would actually call those linear atelectasis … Where do you think the NG tube is?

CANDIDATE: It is above the diaphragm and could be in either the distal oesophagus or the left brochial tree.

EXAMINER1: Look again and tell me where it is.

CANDIDATE: It's in the left lower lobe bronchus.

EXAMINER1: (*Film comes down*) Relax … (*Shows another CXR*)

CANDIDATE: This is a PA chest radiograph of an adult female. There is upper lobe blood diversion. There are linear shadows in both lower zones. The heart is enlarged. The diagnosis is … (*Pauses*)

EXAMINER1: Tell me the diagnosis.

CANDIDATE: Heart failure.

EXAMINER1: (*Smiles. Film comes down*)

At this point, the candidate started to relax a bit more and the rest of the viva passed smoothly. The candidate went on to pass the exam.

Scenario 2

CANDIDATE: Good morning.

EXAMINER1: Hello, I'm Dr _____.

EXAMINER2: And I'm Dr _____. Please have a seat.

CANDIDATE: Thank you.

EXAMINER1: I will start. (*Puts up a CXR*)

CANDIDATE: This is an AP radiograph of an adult. There is obscuration of the retrocardiac left hemidiaphragm, along with a triangular left retrocardiac shadow. There is no associated volume loss. No pleural effusion. The findings are consistent with left lower lobe consolidation, most likely due to pneumonia. I would like to confirm this with a history.

EXAMINER1: Patient has a fever and raised white cell count. What else would you recommend?

CANDIDATE: Treat with antibiotics and chest x-ray follow-up in 4 weeks.

EXAMINER1: (*Film comes down*) This man has abdominal pain. (*Puts up a CT scan*)

CANDIDATE: This is a CT scan of an adult male. There are multiple cavitating lymph nodes in the retroperitoneum and porta hepatis. The pancreas is abnormal with a heterogeneous mass in the pancreatic head. The findings are consistent with a pancreatic tumour with lymph node spread. No intraperitoneal free fluid. The liver, adrenals and kidneys are normal. I would like to look at the lung windows to look for pulmonary spread. The patient will need to be discussed at the MDT for further management.

EXAMINER1: (*Film comes down*) This patient has abdominal pain. (*Puts up an AXR*)

CANDIDATE: There is gross large and small bowel dilatation. Hernial orifices appear normal. No radiological evidence of surgery. Findings are consistent with large bowel obstruction of uncertain cause. A history would be helpful. Further investigation by CT or barium enema can be arranged, as guided by clinical history. (*Expecting to be shown more investigations*)

EXAMINER1: What else does this film show?

CANDIDATE: There is no obvious free gas but I will confirm this by obtaining an erect chest radiograph …

EXAMINER1: Are you sure there is no free gas?

CANDIDATE: (*Starting to sweat*) Uh … there is no lucency over the liver. Rigler's sign is negative. No obvious triangular gas shadows … I don't see any free gas.

EXAMINER1: Look again.

CANDIDATE: The falciform ligament is evident, consistent with free gas … I will inform the surgeons about this finding. (*Sweating even more*)

EXAMINER1: (*Film comes down*) Tell me about this foot. (*Puts up radiographs of the left foot*)

CANDIDATE: I cannot see any obvious abnormality … There are no fractures …

The film showed a subtle Lisfranc fracture dislocation, which the candidate eventually got. The rest of the viva continued to go badly and the candidate failed the examination. Unlike in the first scenario, the examiners were impassive throughout the viva.

The take-home messages from these two scenarios are:
1. Have a system when reporting and stick to it no matter how stressed or confident you are.
2. Missing radiological findings does not necessarily mean failure.

Cardiothoracic Case 1

KIAT T. TAN AND PATRICIA DUNLOP

Clinical history
No history.

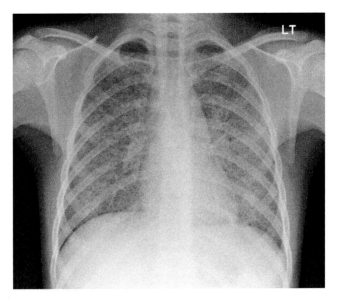

Figure 1.1

Model answer
This is a good-quality frontal chest radiograph of a young patient (Figure 1.1). There are multiple small well-defined nodules that are around 1–2 mm in diameter, spread evenly throughout both lungs with no zonal predominance. No calcification and no pleural effusion. The heart and mediastinal contours are within normal limits. No bony abnormality. The two main differential diagnoses in this case would be infection (such as miliary tuberculosis, fungal and viral pneumonia) or metastatic disease. Less common differential diagnoses would include pneumoconiosis (such as silicosis and coal worker's pneumoconiosis) or atypical sarcoidosis. I would want to look at previous chest radiographs to look for evidence of prior TB or lung nodules and speak to the clinician to obtain a full history as well as to discuss further management. Further investigations may include bronchoscopy with acid- and alcohol-fast bacilli (AAFB)/ cultures and CT chest/abdomen/pelvis to look for multiorgan involvement.

Questions
1. **How do you define miliary shadowing?**
   Multiple small (less than 1–2 mm) nodular shadows scattered evenly throughout the lungs.
2. **What are the typical causes of malignant miliary shadows?**
   Thyroid and renal cancer.

3. **Is miliary TB seen in primary or post-primary tuberculosis?**
   Both.

Key points
- Miliary nodules are named after their resemblance to millet seeds. It is due to spread of the free organisms in the blood rather than infected thrombi (as occurs with septic emboli).
- Miliary disease complicates up to 3% of cases of tuberculosis.
- The vast majority of patients have multiorgan involvement.

Further reading
Jeong YJ, Lee KS. Pulmonary tuberculosis: up-to-date imaging and management. *AJR Am J Roentgenol* 2008; **191**: 834–44.

Miller WT. Chest radiographic evaluation of diffuse infiltrative lung disease: review of a dying art. *Eur J Radiol* 2002; **44**: 182–97.

Tables of differential diagnosis. In Fraser RS, Müller NL, Colman N, Paré PD, eds., *Fraser and Paré's Diagnosis of Diseases of the Chest*, 4th edn. Philadelphia, PA: Saunders, 1999; 3144–9.

Cardiothoracic Case 2

KIAT T. TAN AND PATRICIA DUNLOP

Clinical history
Chest pain.

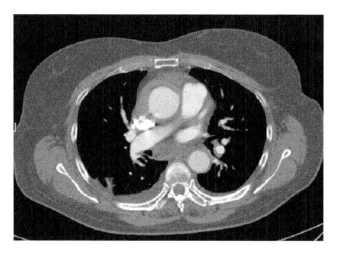

Figure 1.2

Model answer
This is a single image from a contrast-enhanced CT scan of the chest (Figure 1.2). The ascending aorta is dilated and the aortic wall is thickened and of high attenuation. Bilateral pleural effusions and a pericardial effusion are present. The findings

are strongly suggestive of a type A intramural haematoma (IMH). I would like to review the images on a workstation to assess the size and density of the pericardial and pleural effusions as well as the extent of aortic involvement. If possible, I would also like to view the pre-contrast and delayed scans to assess for the degree of contrast enhancement. The presence or absence of concurrent aortic dissection, atherosclerosis and aortic valve involvement should be determined. The cardiothoracic surgeons and cardiologists need to be informed immediately of this finding, as a type A intramural haematoma can progress to frank aortic dissection and/or rupture.

Questions

1. **What is an intramural haematoma?**
   Haematoma within the aortic wall with no intimal flap, intimal tear or direct communication of flow with the lumen.
2. **What is the aetiology?**
   Bleeding from vasa vasorum, penetrating atherosclerotic ulcer.
3. **How do you classify thoracic aortic intramural haematomas?**
   According to the Stanford system, in which an intramural haematoma involving the ascending aorta is classified as type A, and, regardless of the extent, all others are type B.
4. **What are the adverse radiological features associated with intramural haematoma?**
   Adverse features include maximal diameter, thickness of the haematoma, presence of aortic ulceration and location in the ascending aorta. Type A IMH has an early mortality rate of up to 55% if treated medically alone.

Key points

- IMH is part of a spectrum of aortic diseases that include aortic dissection and penetrating aortic ulcer.
- Ideal investigation is by triple-phase ECG-gated CT scan (pre-contrast, arterial phase, delayed phase).

Further reading

Lee YK, Seo JB, Jang YM, *et al*. Acute and chronic complications of aortic intramural hematoma on follow-up computed tomography: incidence and predictor analysis. *J Comput Assist Tomogr* 2007; **31**: 435–40.

Macura KJ, Corl FM, Fishman EK, Bluemke DA. Pathogenesis in acute aortic syndromes: aortic dissection, intramural hematoma, and penetrating atherosclerotic aortic ulcer. *AJR Am J Roentgenol* 2003; **181**: 309–16.

Nienaber CA, Richartz BM, Rehders T, Ince T, Petzsch M. Aortic intramural haematoma: natural history and predictive factors for complications. *Heart* 2004; **90**: 372–4.

Cardiothoracic Case 3

KIAT T. TAN AND PATRICIA DUNLOP

Clinical history
Shortness of breath.

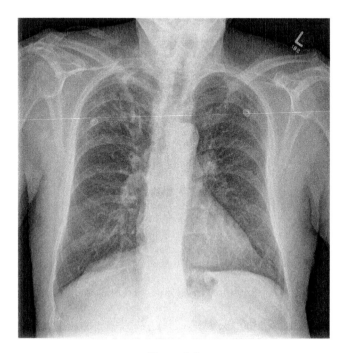

Figure 1.3

Model answer
This is a frontal chest radiograph of an adult (Figure 1.3). The right upper lobe bronchi are thick-walled and dilated. This sign is often referred to as 'tramline' opacities. A 'signet ring' shadow is seen adjacent to the right hilum. There is also a tubular opacity in a right apical bronchus due to mucus plugging (ancillary finding). Less severe changes are present in the left upper lobe bronchi. The finding of bronchial dilatation is consistent with bronchiectasis.

Possible underlying causes of the bronchiectasis include infection (such as tuberculosis, viral pneumonia, aspiration), genetic susceptibility (such as cystic fibrosis, alpha-1-antitrypsin deficiency), immunological deficiencies, defects of mucociliary clearance (which could be congenital, such as in Kartagener's syndrome, or acquired, such as those occurring with aspirated foreign bodies and slow-growing tumours) and immunological (as in cases of allergic bronchopulmonary aspergillosis or rheumatoid disease).

Potential complications of bronchiectasis include recurrent infections, deteriorating pulmonary function, cor pulmonale and haemoptysis (sometimes torrential).

The patient should have an HRCT to assess the severity and distribution of disease. He or she should also be referred to the chest physician for assessment and follow-up.

Questions

1. **What is the definition of bronchiectasis?**
   Abnormal, permanent dilatation of the bronchi, usually associated with inflammation.
2. **What are the HRCT findings of bronchiectasis?**
   - Bronchial lumen diameter greater than accompanying artery (bronchoarterial ratio > 1): high sensitivity, low specificity.
   - Absence of bronchial tapering (seen on longitudinal sections through bronchi).
   - Presence of a visible bronchus within 1 cm of the pleura or mediastinum.
3. **What are the morphological types of bronchiectasis?**
   Classically, bronchiectasis has been classified on morphology into cylindrical (less severe), cystic and varicose (more severe). Cylindrical bronchiectasis refers to disease where there are thick-walled dilated bronchi that have regular diameters. In cystic bronchiectasis, the bronchi are grossly dilated with a 'ballooned' appearance. Varicose bronchiectasis refers to disease that contains interspersed bronchial dilatation and constriction.

Key points

- A widespread pattern of bronchial dilatation affecting both lungs is an indication of systemic disease, such as cystic fibrosis, immunodeficiency states and alpha-1-antitrypsin deficiency. Localized bronchiectasis is usually caused by a focal lesion, e.g. infection and obstruction.
- Certain diseases also tend to affect particular parts of the lung. For example, in tuberculosis bronchiectasis involves mainly the upper lobes, whereas *Mycobacterium avium-intracellulare* (MAI) in non-immunocompromised individuals tends to involve most of the lungs without a predilection for a specific lobe(s). It has been stated that bronchiectasis with a middle lobe and lingular prominence is seen in elderly women with the non-classic form of MAI infection, 'Lady Windermere syndrome'.
- Cystic fibrosis has an upper lobe predominance, and allergic bronchopulmonary aspergillosis a central and upper lung zone predominance.
- Localized bronchiectasis may be surgically curable, but disease with a diffuse pattern is not.

Further reading

Hansell DM. Bronchiectasis. *Radiol Clin North Am* 1998; **36**: 107–28.

Koh WJ, Lee KS, Kwon OJ, *et al*. Bilateral bronchiectasis and bronchiolitis at thin-section CT: diagnostic implications in nontuberculous mycobacterial pulmonary infection. *Radiology* 2005; **235**: 282–8.

Primack SL, Logan PM, Hartman TE, Lee KS, Müller NL. Pulmonary tuberculosis and Mycobacterium avium-intracellulare: a comparison of CT findings. *Radiology* 1995; **194**: 413–17.

Reich JM, Johnson RE. Mycobacterium avium complex pulmonary disease presenting as an isolated lingular or middle lobe pattern: the Lady Windermere syndrome. *Chest* 1992; **101**: 1605–9.

Cardiothoracic Case 4

KIAT T. TAN AND PATRICIA DUNLOP

Clinical history
Acutely unwell.

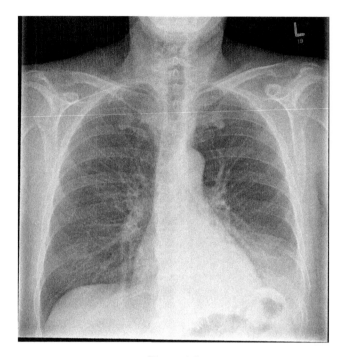

Figure 1.4

Model answer

This frontal chest radiograph of an adult (Figure 1.4) shows airspace opacification in the left lower lung zone with obscuration of the left hemidiaphragm and lower lobe vessels. The left heart border is well visualized and there is a triangular area of opacification behind the heart. There are no air bronchograms. No volume loss. There is an associated left pleural effusion.

The findings are consistent with left lower lobe consolidation, which is most commonly the result of infection. Community-acquired lobar pneumonia is most often caused by *Streptococcus pneumoniae*; less common causative organisms include *Klebsiella pneumoniae, Legionella pneumophila, Haemophilus influenzae* and *Mycobacterium tuberculosis*. The patient should have sputum cultures and should be commenced on antibiotics. The patient should have a repeat chest radiograph in 3–4 weeks to assess regression and eventual resolution of consolidation.

Questions
1. **Why should the patient have a repeat chest radiograph?**
   To assess for resolution of airspace changes, to assess for complications and to re-evaluate the effusion. Failure of resolution could indicate inappropriate antibiotic

therapy, development of a complication (such as abscess, empyema), underlying disease (such as lung cancer or immunodeficiency states) or another diagnosis.

2. **Why is the consolidation limited to one lobe in lobar pneumonia?**
   Bacteria spread directly between alveoli (i.e. via the pores of Kohn and small airways). The spread of infection is thus limited by the lung fissures.

Key points

- Slowly resolving pneumonia refers to disease that fails to demonstrate radiological improvement of at least 50% in two weeks or completely by four weeks.
- Alveolar shadowing that fails to respond to antibiotics may be due to cryptogenic organizing pneumonia (COP), drug reaction, eosinophilic pneumonia, neoplasm (lymphoma, bronchoalveolar carcinoma), vasculitis (haemorrhage), fat (lipoid pneumonia) due to aspiration, radiation pneumonitis and resistant microorganisms.

Further reading

Goodman P. Pulmonary infection in adults. In Adam A, Dixon AK, eds., *Grainger and Allison's Diagnostic Radiology*, 5th edn. London: Churchill Livingstone, 2008 (ebook).

Rome L, Murali G, Lippmann M. Nonresolving pneumonia and mimics of pneumonia. *Med Clin North Am* 2001; **85**: 1511–30.

Cardiothoracic Case 5

KIAT T. TAN AND PATRICIA DUNLOP

Clinical history
26-year-old with history of previous tuberculosis.

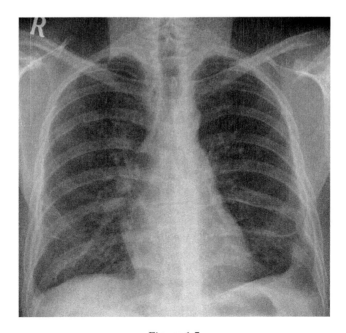

Figure 1.5

Model answer

This is a frontal chest radiograph of a skeletally mature person (Figure 1.5). There are linear shadows in both lung bases, which could be consistent with either scarring or atelectasis. Blunting of costophrenic angles is consistent with either small pleural effusions or thickening. The findings are in keeping with the previous history of tuberculosis. Reactivation tuberculosis can only be excluded if these findings are unchanged for over six months, and I would like to review previous radiographs to confirm stability.

There is right-sided inferior rib notching affecting the fifth to eighth ribs. The remaining ribs are spared. The aortic knuckle is left-sided. The heart is left-sided and there is no cardiac enlargement. The findings are suggestive of aortic coarctation involving the origin of the left subclavian artery. Either a CT or MR thoracic aortogram should be performed for further characterization of the aorta. If coarctation is diagnosed, the patient will require either an echocardiogram or a cardiac MR to determine the presence of left ventricular hypertrophy and/or a bicuspid aortic valve.

Questions

1. **What causes the rib notching in aortic coarctation?**

   In aortic coarctation there is obstruction of blood flow to the lower body. A potential collateral pathway involves the flow of blood through the internal mammary arteries into the intercostal vessels and retrogradely into the aorta. Enlarged intercostal arteries can press against adjacent ribs, causing a notch to form over time. Rib notching can resolve after treatment of the coarctation.

2. **What is the significance of unilateral versus bilateral rib notching in coarctation?**

   Unilateral right-sided rib notching indicates the presence of coarctation at or proximal to the origin of the left subclavian artery. Bilateral rib notching would be consistent with coarctation distal to the left subclavian artery (assuming a normal aortic arch branching pattern). Unilateral left rib notching due to aortic coarctation is extremely rare, as this would require coarctation to occur between the origin of the left subclavian and an aberrant right subclavian artery.

Key points

- Superior rib notching, which may or may not be associated with inferior rib notching, can occur in diseases that cause excessive bone resorption or defective bone formation. These include connective tissue diseases (rheumatoid arthritis), osteogenesis imperfecta, local pressure (for example, from neural tumours as in neurofibromatosis) and hyperparathyroidism.
- Inferior rib notching is much more common. The causes include arterial collaterals (for example, in aortic coarctation and Takayasu's arteritis), venous collaterals (for example, in vena cava obstruction), neurogenic tumours (in neurofibromatosis) and hyperparathyroidism.
- Unilateral right-sided third to eighth rib notching, with sparing of the remaining ribs (as in this case), is almost always due to aortic coarctation.

Further reading

Guttentag AR, Salwen JK. Keep your eyes on the ribs: the spectrum of normal variants and diseases that involves the ribs. *Radiographics* 1999; **19**: 1125–42.

Pemberton J, Sahn DJ. Imaging of the aorta. *Int J Cardiol* 2004; **97** (Suppl 1): 53–60.

Cardiothoracic Case 6

KIAT T. TAN AND PATRICIA DUNLOP

Clinical history

35-year-old man presenting with a stroke.

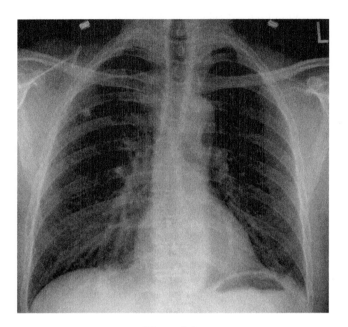

Figure 1.6a

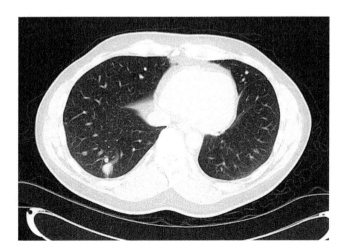

Figure 1.6b

Model answer

This is a frontal chest radiograph of a skeletally mature individual (Figure 1.6a). There is a small lung nodule projected over the right diaphragmatic recess. A branch of the pulmonary artery that leads into this lesion appears larger than anticipated. No other pulmonary lesions are evident. Heart and mediastinal contours are normal. In light of the clinical history, the findings would suggest a pulmonary arteriovenous malformation (AVM). A contrast-enhanced CT scan is required to confirm this.

The one image from a CT scan (Figure 1.6b) shows a right lower lobe nodule supplied by a dilated feeding vessel. This is the characteristic appearance of a lung AVM. I would like to review the imaging of the rest of the lungs as well as the images from the mediastinal windows to detect the presence of other AVMs. I would also like to review his previous brain imaging to find out if his stroke is related to an intracerebral AVM. In the absence of intracerebral AVMs, the most likely cause of the patient's neurological symptoms would be from embolization via his pulmonary AVM.

I would like to find out from the clinician if this patient has hereditary haemorrhagic telangiectasia. If so, the patient and his family may require genetic testing.

Questions

1. **How are pulmonary AVMs treated?**
   Pulmonary AVMs should be embolized (preferably by an interventional radiologist!). Surgical resection is reserved for the small minority of patients for whom embolization is contraindicated. Embolization has an immediate success rate of nearly 100% and a long-term success rate of over 80%. Antibiotic cover to prevent cerebral abscesses for certain medical procedures should be continued even after successful embolization of AVMs. The patient should have a CT scan one year after successful AVM embolization and then every 3–5 years.

2. **What causes pulmonary AVMs?**
   Hereditary haemorrhagic telangiectasia (HHT), hepatopulmonary syndrome, post congenital cyanotic heart disease surgery and idiopathic AVM.

Key points

- HHT (Osler–Weber–Rendu syndrome) is an autosomal dominant disease.
- It is associated with epistaxis, cutaneous telangiectasia, AVMs in various organs.
- Patients with HHT can present with haemorrhage, or with symptoms/complications of shunting in virtually any organ system. Commonly affected organs include the brain, gastrointestinal tract and lungs. High-output cardiac failure and pulmonary hypertension are also complications.
- Genetic testing of related individuals may be indicated.
- A suspected AVM should *not* be biopsied.

Notes

The patient in this case had HHT and multiple pulmonary AVMs, which required multiple visits for embolization.

Further reading

Faughnan ME, Granton JT, Young LH. The pulmonary vascular complications of hereditary haemorrhagic telangiectasia. *Eur Respir J* 2009; **33**: 1186–94.

Pelage JP, El-Hajjam M, Lagrange C, *et al*. Pulmonary artery interventions: an overview. *Radiographics* 2005; **25**: 1653–67.

Cardiothoracic Case 7

KIAT T. TAN AND PATRICIA DUNLOP

Clinical history
No history.

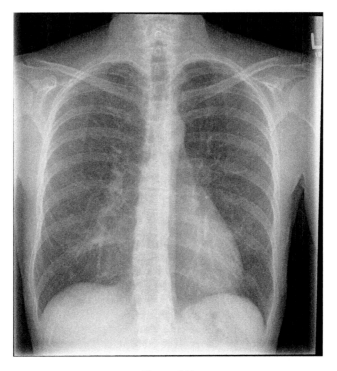

Figure 1.7

Model answer
There is blurring of the right heart border with apparent opacification of the right cardiophrenic angle (Figure 1.7). The posterior ribs are quite horizontal and some are angled superiorly. This is in contrast to the gentle downward angulation of ribs seen on a normal chest radiograph. The findings are consistent with pectus excavatum. No other significant pathology.

Questions
1. **What is pectus excavatum?**
   The sternum is depressed into the chest, resulting in a concave appearance of the anterior chest wall.
2. **Does pectus excavatum result in clinical symptoms?**
   Most patients are asymptomatic, although the deformity may be associated with a decrease in cardiopulmonary reserve. Most morbidity is psychological, due to the cosmetic effect of the deformity.

Key points

- Pectus excavatum is often an isolated finding. However, it can be associated with Marfan's syndrome.
- A lateral chest radiograph is confirmatory, but all attempts should be made to establish this diagnosis clinically.

Further reading

Williams AM, Crabbe DC. Pectus deformities of the anterior chest wall. *Paediatr Respir Rev* 2003; **4**: 237–42.

Cardiothoracic Case 8

KIAT T. TAN AND PATRICIA DUNLOP

Clinical history

? Myocardial infarction. Patient is haemodynamically stable at present. Report the chest radiograph first.

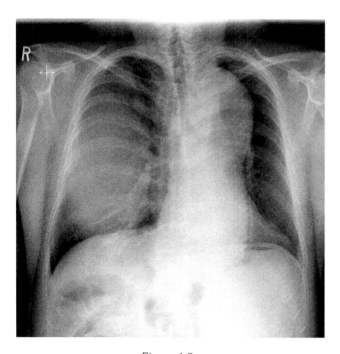

Figure 1.8a

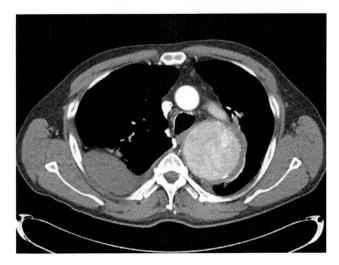

Figure 1.8b

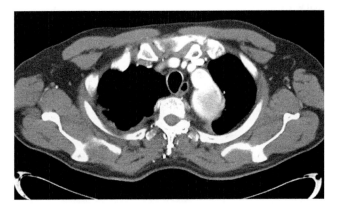

Figure 1.8c

Model answer

This is a frontal chest radiograph of a skeletally mature patient (Figure 1.8a). There is gross enlargement of the thoracic aorta. Large oval opacification extending from the right mid zone to the base without obscuration of the vessels. Left lung is clear. Findings are consistent with either a leaking aortic aneurysm or a leaking thoracic aortic dissection. I would contact the admitting clinician and the local interventional radiologist as well as the cardiothoracic surgeons. The patient will require urgent intervention. I will also arrange an urgent CT scan of the chest.

Selected images from a CT scan of the chest (Figures 1.8b, 1.8c) confirm the presence of a large descending thoracic aortic aneurysm with a moderate right haemothorax and small left haemothorax. The aneurysm appears to arise distal to the origin of the left subclavian artery, although I would want to review the CT scan on a workstation to confirm this finding. I would also want to find out the distal extent of the aneurysm.

Questions

1. **How should the CT scan be performed?**

   Non-enhanced and enhanced scans from the neck to the femoral heads should be obtained. Timing of the bolus is key (bolus trigger, high rate 4–5 ml/s). If available, prospective ECG gating may be used to evaluate the ascending thoracic aorta and proximal coronary arteries. Prospective ECG gating only results in a minimal (if any) increase in overall radiation dose but requires a well-trained radiographer (or radiologist!).

2. **How would a CT scan be helpful? Shouldn't the patient have immediate surgery?**
The CT scan aids delineation of anatomy in the haemodynamically stable patient. The cardiothoracic surgeons would want to know the extent of the aneurysm, whether it involves the branches of the arch and the ascending aorta and if there is aortic valve disease/compromise. If the aneurysm arises at or beyond the origin of the left subclavian, it could potentially be amenable to endovascular stenting, thus sparing the patient an open repair. Obviously, if the patient is haemodynamically unstable, an immediate thoracotomy may be his only chance for survival.

Key points
- Incidence of thoracic aortic aneurysms is increasing, possibly due to increasing use of cross-sectional imaging.
- Non-ruptured thoracic aortic aneurysms should be surgically treated when they have a diameter of 5.5 cm or more in uncomplicated cases. Patients with Marfan's syndrome, bicuspid aortic valve or a family history of aortic aneurysms should be treated when the aneurysm size reaches 5 cm.
- Elective endovascular treatment of thoracic aortic aneurysm is a promising treatment modality but there is a lack of convincing evidence of its long-term efficacy.

Notes
This patient had successful endovascular treatment of his disease by an interventional radiologist. He was discharged from hospital shortly afterwards.

Further reading
Agarwal PP, Chughtai A, Matzinger FR, Kazerooni EA. Multidetector CT of thoracic aortic aneurysms. *Radiographics* 2009; **29**: 537–52.
Castañer E, Andreu M, Gallardo X, *et al*. CT in nontraumatic acute thoracic aortic disease: typical and atypical features and complications. *Radiographics* 2003; **23**: S93–110.
Yoo SM, Lee HY, White CS. MDCT evaluation of acute aortic syndrome. *Radiol Clin North Am* 2010; **48**: 67–83.

Cardiothoracic Case 9

KIAT T. TAN AND PATRICIA DUNLOP

Clinical history
Progressive shortness of breath over months.

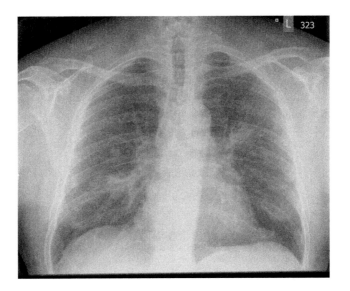

Figure 1.9a

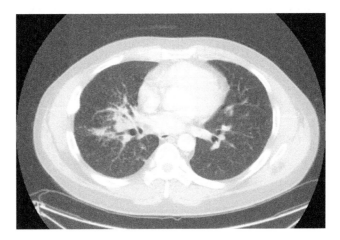

Figure 1.9b

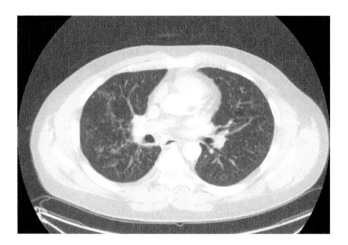

Figure 1.9c

Model answer
This is a frontal chest radiograph of a skeletally mature adult (Figure 1.9a). A bilateral reticulonodular pattern is noted, most marked in the perihilar regions, with relative sparing of the lower lung zones. There are areas of more confluent opacification within the right mid, left upper and left lower lung zones. Both hila are prominent. The findings would be most likely due to stage II sarcoidosis, although tuberculosis, silicosis and lymphangitis carcinomatosa are in the differential diagnosis.

The two lung window images from the CT scan (Figures 1.9b, 1.9c) show multiple small perifissural, subpleural and peribronchovascular nodules. Areas of beading and irregular thickening can be seen along the bronchovascular bundles. No enlarged lymph nodes are seen on these selected images. The findings are consistent with sarcoidosis. I would want to review the entire CT scan to assess the extent of disease, the presence of lymphadenopathy and the presence of fibrosis.

I would like to discuss the case with the clinician, and a referral to a chest physician is required. A search for other foci of disease should be performed. Pulmonary function tests should be performed. The serum angiotensin converting enzyme should be measured. The combination of the histological finding of non-caseating granuloma and the absence of acid- and alcohol-fast bacilli (AAFB) on biopsy samples is the gold standard for the diagnosis of sarcoidosis.

Questions
1. **How do you stage sarcoidosis on the chest radiograph?**
   Stage 0: no radiological abnormality
   Stage 1: bilateral hilar lymphadenopathy
   Stage 2: bilateral hilar lymphadenopathy with parenchymal involvement
   Stage 3: parenchymal involvement with no lymphadenopathy
   Stage 4: pulmonary fibrosis
2. **What is the purpose of staging sarcoidosis on the radiograph? Does this staging apply to the CT findings?**
   It helps predict outcome: stage 1 disease is associated with 55–90% resolution, stage 2 disease with 40–70%, stage 3 with 10–20%, stage 4 with 0%. The staging does not apply to the CT findings.
3. **How do you make the diagnosis of sarcoidosis?**
   Diagnosis is clinical and radiological with pathological confirmation (non-caseating granulomas). In many cases, a confident diagnosis can be made with classic imaging and clinical findings without the need for biopsy.

Key points

- Sarcoidosis is a multisystem disorder of unknown aetiology, and virtually all organs can be affected by the disease. The commonest cause of death is from lung disease. Cardiac involvement is also an important cause of mortality.
- It is commoner in males and blacks.
- Hilar and mediastinal lymphadenopathy is common.
- Sarcoidosis (pulmonary and skeletal) is a great mimic of other conditions and is commonly encountered in the FRCR. Classic pulmonary sarcoidosis is described above.
- Skeletal sarcoidosis can present as: (a) well-defined well-corticated lytic lesions; (b) lace-like bony destruction; (c) acro-osteolysis; (d) subperiosteal resorption (similar to hyperparathyroidism).

Further reading

Koyama T, Ueda H, Togashi K, *et al.* Radiologic manifestations of sarcoidosis in various organs. *Radiographics* 2004; **24**: 87–104.

Statement on Sarcoidosis. Joint Statement of the American Thoracic Society (ATS), the European Respiratory Society (ERS) and the World Association of Sarcoidosis and Other Granulomatous Disorders (WASOG) adopted by the ATS Board of Directors and by the ERS Executive Committee, February 1999. *Am J Respir Crit Care Med* 1999; **160**: 736–55.

Travis WD, Colby TV, eds. *Atlas of Nontumor Pathology: Non-Neoplastic Disorders of the Lower Respiratory Tract.* Washington DC: American Registry of Pathology and the Armed Forces Institute of Pathology, 2002; 123.

Cardiothoracic Case 10

KIAT T. TAN AND PATRICIA DUNLOP

Clinical history

Elderly lady with infective endocarditis. Post insertion of PICC line for parenteral antibiotics.

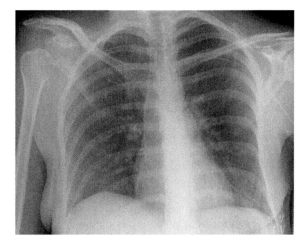

Figure 1.10

Model answer

This is a frontal chest radiograph of an adult female (Figure 1.10). The PICC line tip is projected over the right atrium. The patient should ideally have the line withdrawn under fluoroscopic guidance so that its tip lies at the cavoatrial junction. Lungs are clear. Heart and mediastinal contours are normal. There is inferior subluxation of the right humeral head. An ill-defined region of lucency is seen in the inferomedial aspect of the humeral head. There is an apparent bony fragment within the joint. The findings would be suggestive of an inflammatory process in the right glenohumeral joint. With the history of infective endocarditis, septic arthritis is a major consideration. Reactive arthritis or other inflammatory arthritides are differential diagnoses. I would like to look at previous imaging of the chest and shoulder. The patient should have a joint aspirate and x-ray examination of the shoulder.

Questions

1. **What is the treatment of septic arthritis?**

   The treatment of septic arthritis in this lady is with parenteral antibiotics, which she is already receiving for her endocarditis. Aspiration of joint fluid is necessary both for symptom relief and for removal of infected joint fluid. The radiologist is often called upon to aspirate the joint.

Key points

- Septic arthritis is a medical emergency that can rapidly destroy a joint.
- The radiograph can be normal in early disease.
- Remember to look at the extrathoracic structures as well!

Notes

The diagnosis was missed on the initial chest radiograph. The diagnosis was only made a few weeks later when the patient was re-presented with gross shoulder destruction.

Further reading

Lossos IS, Yossepowitch O, Kandel L, Yardeni D, Arber N. Septic arthritis of the glenohumeral joint: a report of 11 cases and review of the literature. *Medicine (Baltimore)* 1998; **77**: 177–87.

Cardiothoracic Case 11

KIAT T. TAN AND PATRICIA DUNLOP

Clinical history

No history.

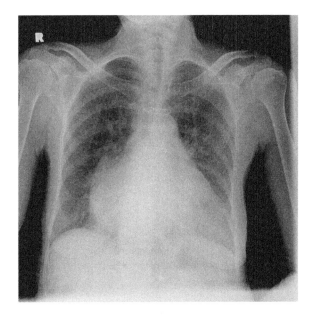

Figure 1.11a

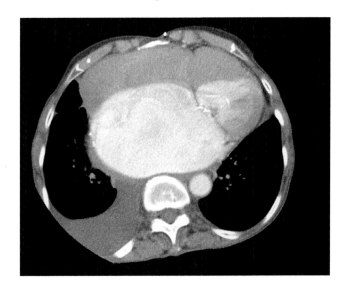

Figure 1.11b

Model answer

This is a frontal chest radiograph of a skeletally mature individual (Figure 1.11a). Previous median sternotomy is noted. Wires are intact. There are prominent pulmonary veins. No airspace opacification. The carina is splayed and the heart is grossly enlarged. No pleural effusions.

The single image from an ungated CT scan (Figure 1.11b) shows gross left atrial enlargement with a relatively normal-sized left ventricle. There is mitral valve thickening and calcification. The right heart chambers are relatively normal. A moderate right pleural effusion is present.

The radiological findings are consistent with mitral stenosis, with pressure overload of the left atrium and pulmonary venous hypertension. The patient will need further assessment by echocardiography. A referral to a cardiologist or cardiothoracic surgeon is required for further management.

Questions

1. **How does one differentiate between mitral stenosis and mitral regurgitation on an ungated CT scan?**
   Mitral stenosis results in left atrial enlargement while sparing the left ventricle. Mitral regurgitation causes both chambers of the left heart to dilate.

2. **What are the other secondary signs of mitral stenosis in the lungs?**
   Small calcified pulmonary nodules can develop in long-standing mitral stenosis. Pulmonary haemosiderosis can develop as a result of tiny recurrent haemorrhages due to venous hypertension. These are seen as punctate opacities in both lungs.

Key points

- Rheumatic fever is the commonest cause of mitral stenosis in adults. Other causes include congenital mitral stenosis and severe mitral annular calcification.
- The degree of calcification is proportional to disease severity in valvular heart disease. Heart valve calcification seen on plain film should always be investigated, as should severe calcification on CT.

Further reading

Chandrashekhar Y, Westaby S, Narula J. Mitral stenosis. *Lancet* 2009; **374**: 1271–83.

Cardiothoracic Case 12

KIAT T. TAN AND PATRICIA DUNLOP

Clinical history
Shortness of breath.

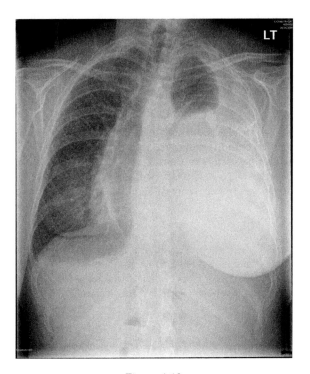

Figure 1.12

Modal answer
Frontal chest radiograph of an adult (Figure 1.12). Left subclavian line in situ with the tip satisfactorily placed at the cavoatrial junction. Some linear opacification at the right lower zone, most likely the result of compressive atelectasis. There is a large left pleural effusion that is displacing the mediastinal contents to the right and causing subtotal collapse of the left lung. Tiny right pleural effusion. There has been a previous right mastectomy with axillary dissection. No bony destruction.

The findings are strongly suggestive of a malignant left pleural effusion that is under tension. In this case, this is most likely due to breast cancer. The patient will need a therapeutic thoracentesis, with samples sent to cytology, biochemistry and microbiology. A contrast-enhanced CT scan of the chest and abdomen will be required for staging of disease.

Questions
1. **Can you think of any other cause for a pleural effusion in this patient?**
   Insertion of the left subclavian line could have resulted in a haemothorax. However, this should be obvious clinically, as a haemothorax of this size would

have resulted in cardiovascular compromise. In addition, the thoracentesis would provide a definitive diagnosis.
2. **What are other causes of massive pleural effusions?**
   Cirrhosis and, less likely, infection or congestive heart failure.
3. **Does the size of the malignant effusion affect prognosis?**
   Massive malignant effusions have been shown to be associated with worse survival independent of age and histological subgroup when compared to smaller malignant effusions.

Key points
- Mastectomy + pleural effusion = malignant effusion unless proven otherwise (especially in the exam setting).
- Although the risk is usually greatest in the first three years post treatment, malignant pleural effusion can occur many years after the initial 'curative' therapy.

Further reading
Jimenez D, Diaz G, Gil D, *et al.* Etiology and prognostic significance of massive pleural effusions. *Respir Med* 2005; **99**: 1183–7.
Jung JI, Kim HH, Park SH, *et al.* Thoracic manifestations of breast cancer and its therapy. *Radiographics* 2004; **24**: 1269–85.
Matthay RA, Coppage L, Shaw C, Filderman AE. Malignancies metastatic to the pleura. *Invest Radiol* 1990; **25**: 601–19.

Cardiothoracic Case 13

KIAT T. TAN AND PATRICIA DUNLOP

Clinical history
Tired all the time. Report the chest radiograph first.

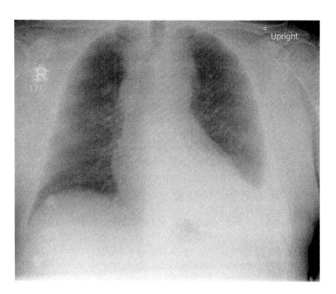

Figure 1.13a

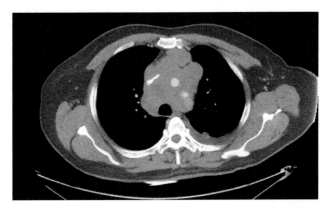

Figure 1.13b

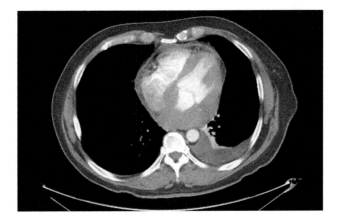

Figure 1.13c

Model answer

This is a frontal chest radiograph of a skeletally mature individual (Figure 1.13a). The superior mediastinum is widened, with a lobulated contour. The right paratracheal stripe is grossly thickened. The aortic arch remains visible. There is a triangular opacity in the left retrocardiac region with depression of the left mainstem bronchus and hilum consistent with volume loss in the left lower lobe. Small left pleural effusion is present. The differential diagnoses of a lobulated superior mediastinal mass include lymph node enlargement (such as due to lymphoma, metastatic disease and tuberculosis), thymoma, thyroid pathology and germ-cell tumour. This patient will require a CT scan of the neck, chest, abdomen and pelvis.

The two selected images from the CT scan (Figures 1.13b, 1.13c) confirm the presence of a superior mediastinal mass. This mass encases the great vessels and extends inferiorly to affect the heart. The atrial septum is grossly thickened. There are small left pleural and pericardial effusions. The findings are most likely due to lymphoma, with secondary cardiac involvement. I would like to review the images on a workstation to assess the extent of the mass as well as the degree of cardiac involvement. A biopsy is essential for diagnosis. The patient should have an echocardiogram and/or a cardiac MRI to assess heart function. A baseline ECG should be obtained. I would like to discuss the case with the clinician and the oncologist.

Questions

1. **How do you stage lymphoma?**

   Both Hodgkin's and non-Hodgkin's lymphoma are staged using the Ann Arbor (Cotswold revision) criteria:

   Stage 1: involvement of single lymph node region or organ

   Stage 2: two or more lymph node regions/organs on the same side of the diaphragm

   Stage 3: tumour on both sides of the diaphragm

   Stage 4: non-lymphatic organ spread

2. **Why is a biopsy crucial in lymphoma?**

   It is difficult, if not impossible, to distinguish between Hodgkin's and non-Hodgkin's lymphoma using imaging alone. In addition, non-Hodgkin's lymphoma is a heterogeneous group of diseases and tissue diagnosis is essential for treatment planning and prognostication.

3. **What is the role of PET imaging?**

   Evaluation of metabolic activity, response to therapy and detection of treatment failure or recurrence.

Key points

- Treated lymphoma is a cause of lymph node calcification, which may have the egg-shell configuration.
- Hodgkin's disease is potentially curable and tends to have a better prognosis. Survival from both Hodgkin's and non-Hodgkin's lymphoma has been increasing due to better treatment.
- Lymphoma can be associated with paraneoplastic syndromes.

Further reading

Ha CS, Medeiros LJ, Charnsangavej C, Crump M, Gospodarowicz MK. Lymphoma. *Radiographics* 2006; **26**: 607–20.

Lister TA, Crowther D, Sutcliffe SB, *et al.* Report of a committee convened to discuss the evaluation and staging of patients with Hodgkin's disease: Cotswolds meeting. *J Clin Oncol* 1989; **7**: 1630–6.

Moog F, Bangerter M, Diederichs CG, *et al.* Extranodal malignant lymphoma: detection with FDG PET versus CT. *Radiology* 1998; **206**: 475–81.

Cardiothoracic Case 14

KIAT T. TAN AND PATRICIA DUNLOP

Clinical history

HIV-positive. Presents with malaise and dry cough for a week. Please report the chest radiograph first.

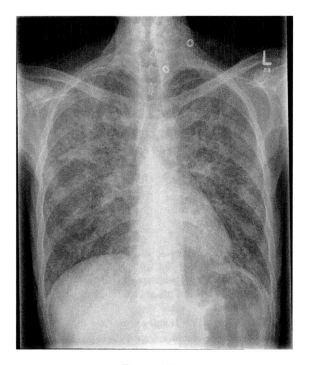

Figure 1.14a

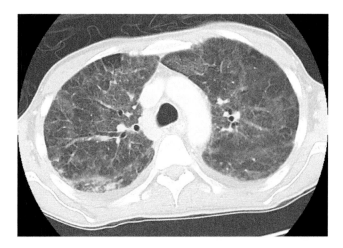

Figure 1.14b

Model answer

This is a frontal chest radiograph of a skeletally mature individual (Figure 1.14a). There is widespread reticular opacification, most prominent in the perihilar regions and patchy airspace opacification. No pleural effusion. Heart size is normal.

In view of the history of HIV infection and clinical symptoms, the major differential diagnosis would be an infectious process, the most likely of which would be *Pneumocystis jirovecii* (formerly *carinii*). Other infections that could cause this picture include CMV and bronchiolitis with bronchopneumonia. Non-infectious differential diagnoses would include pulmonary oedema, adult respiratory distress syndrome and haemorrhage.

I would inquire about the CD4 count and arrange for a CT scan of the chest.

The patient will need referral to the appropriate HIV specialist, measurement of lactate dehydrogenase (sensitivity of > 90%) and sputum induction/bronchoalveolar lavage for organism isolation.

The single image from the CT scan (Figure 1.14b) shows widespread bilateral ground-glass opacification with some lobular areas of sparing, which results in a geographic appearance, often referred to as 'mosaic attenuation'. Some focal areas of consolidation and interlobular septal thickening are also noted. In the presence of the appropriate history, this appearance is consistent with *P. jirovecii* infection. I would like to review the rest of the imaging to look for other features of *Pneumocystis*, including cysts and fibrosis.

Questions

1. **Would you expect to find lymphadenopathy in *Pneumocystis* pneumonia?**
   Lymph node enlargement, pleural effusions and lung nodules are uncommon in *Pneumocystis* pneumonia (although they have been described). The presence of any/all of these findings should prompt a search for alternative or coexisting pathology, such as mycobacterial infection and lymphoma.
2. **Does a normal CT scan exclude *Pneumocystis* pneumonia?**
   Yes. A normal CT scan has been shown to have a 100% sensitivity and 100% negative predictive value in diagnosing *Pneumocystis* pneumonia.

Key points

- *Pneumocystis jirovecii* pneumonia normally has a perihilar or lower lung zone predominance.
- *Pneumocystis* pathology in patients on inhaled pentamidine prophylaxis tends to present with upper lobe disease. This group of patients is also at increased risk of pneumothorax. Pneumatoceles may complicate *Pneumocystis* disease, and they tend to occur in the upper lobes. They are more likely to occur in those receiving inhaled pentamidine.
- Systemic *Pneumocystis* infection may affect those on pentamidine prophylaxis or severely depleted CD4 counts. It is **possible** to have systemic *Pneumocystis* disease *without* pulmonary involvement.

Further reading

Chaffey MH, Klein JS, Gamsu G, Blanc P, Golden JA. Radiographic distribution of *Pneumocystis carinii* pneumonia in patients with AIDS treated with prophylactic inhaled pentamidine. *Radiology* 1990; **175**: 715–19.

Gruden JF, Huang L, Turner J, *et al.* High-resolution CT in the evaluation of clinically suspected *Pneumocystis carinii* pneumonia in AIDS patients with normal, equivocal, or nonspecific radiographic findings. *AJR Am J Roentgenol* 1997; **169**: 967–75.

Hidalgo A, Falco V, Mauleon S, *et al.* Accuracy of high-resolution CT in distinguishing between *Pneumocystis carinii* pneumonia and non-*Pneumocystis carinii* pneumonia in AIDS patients. *Eur Radiol* 2003; **13**: 1179–84.

Cardiothoracic Case 15

KIAT T. TAN AND PATRICIA DUNLOP

Clinical history
40-year-old male heavy smoker. History of increasing shortness of breath over the past year, non-productive cough. Report the chest radiograph first.

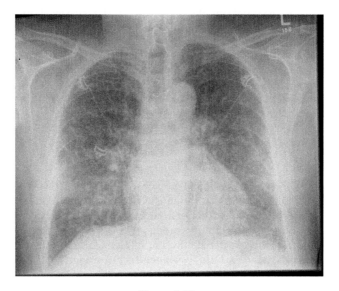

Figure 1.15a

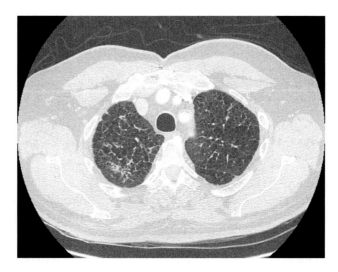

Figure 1.15b

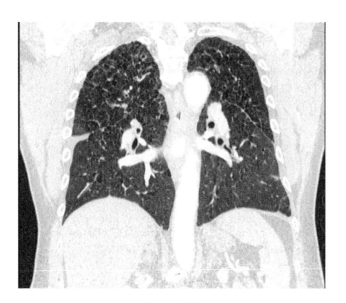

Figure 1.15c

Model answer

This is a frontal chest radiograph of an adult patient (Figure 1.15a). Previous median sternotomy is noted. There is bilateral symmetrical reticulo-nodular opacification, with relative sparing of the lung bases. The lung volumes are well preserved, given the amount of interstitial opacification. No pleural effusions. No Kerley B lines. No pneumothorax. Heart size is within normal limits. Bones appear normal.

The findings could be due to interstitial lung disease, such as pulmonary oedema on a background of emphysema or Langerhans cell histiocytosis (LCH). Hypersensitivity pneumonitis is a differential diagnosis. Pulmonary fibrosis of the usual interstitial pneumonitis (UIP) type is less likely, given the distribution and pre-served lung volume. I would want to know whether or not the findings are acute or chronic by comparing with older studies, and I would want to arrange an HRCT for further investigation.

The two lung window images from the HRCT examination (Figures 1.15b, 1.15c) demonstrate the presence of cysts of varying sizes and wall thickness. Small cavitat-ing nodules are present. There is sparing of the lung bases.

The findings are consistent with LCH. I would like to discuss the case with the chest physicians. The patient will require pulmonary function testing, which typic-ally demonstrates a reduced diffusing capacity for carbon monoxide (DLCO) (pre-sent in 60–90% of cases). In severe cases there is restrictive, obstructive and mixed pulmonary function abnormalities. Bronchoalveolar lavage showing raised macro-phage counts and presence of Langerhans cells may support the diagnosis. Definitive diagnosis is made by VATS biopsy showing Langerhans granulomas.

Questions

1. **How do you distinguish between LCH and idiopathic pulmonary fibrosis (IPF)?**

   Severe forms of LCH can resemble idiopathic pulmonary fibrosis. LCH is more severe in the upper lobes and tends to affect the central and peripheral lung regions, while there is relative sparing of the lung bases. Conversely, IPF tends to involve the periphery and the bases.

2. **What is the clinical presentation?**
   Symptoms include dyspnoea, non-productive cough, chest pain, fatigue, weight loss and fever. Haemoptysis or finger clubbing are rare. 25% are asymptomatic. 10–16% present with pneumothorax.
3. **How do imaging findings vary with chronicity of disease?**
   Early stages: 1–10 mm nodules are seen with upper to mid lung zone predominance.
   Later stages: development of cystic spaces in the same distribution.
   Advanced stages: innumerable cysts and fibrosis, with upper lung zone predominance involving the central and peripheral lung zones.

Key points

- Langerhans cell histiocytosis can present in three distinct but overlapping syndromes. LCH affecting mainly the bones is found principally in infants and young children. Multisystem (multiorgan involvement) LCH is a serious condition found predominantly in infants. The pulmonary (single-organ) form of LCH is usually seen in adult smokers.
- In LCH the disease begins with the development of Langerhans granulomas centred on bronchioles, which are seen as nodules on HRCT. These nodules, which are of differing shapes and sizes, enlarge and cavitate. The cavitating lesions become progressively more thin-walled as the disease progresses. HRCT of late-stage disease shows multiple thin-walled cysts, which can be difficult to differentiate from those of lymphangioleiomyomatosis.
- Treatment
  - Medical: cessation of smoking, chemo +/– steroids.
  - Surgical: pneumothorax may require pleurodesis. If end stage, may develop pulmonary hypertension, and lung or heart/lung transplant may be considered.

Further reading

Abbott GF, Rosado-de-Christenson ML, Franks TJ, Frazier AA, Galvin JR. From the archives of the AFIP: pulmonary Langerhans cell histiocytosis. *Radiographics* 2004; **24**: 821–41.

Vassallo R, Ryu JH, Colby TV, Hartman T, Limper AH. Pulmonary Langerhans'-cell histiocytosis. *N Engl J Med* 2000; **342**: 1969–78.

Vassallo R, Ryu JH, Schroeder DR, Decker PA, Limper AH. Clinical outcomes of pulmonary Langerhans'-cell histiocytosis in adults. *N Engl J Med* 2002; **346**: 484–90.

Cardiothoracic Case 16

KIAT T. TAN AND PATRICIA DUNLOP

Clinical history
79-year-old man with progressive shortness of breath.

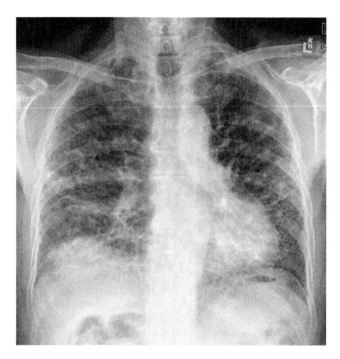

Figure 1.16a

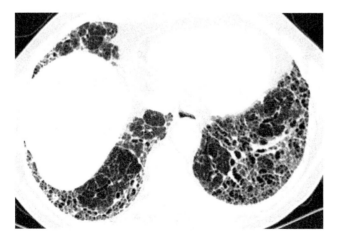

Figure 1.16b

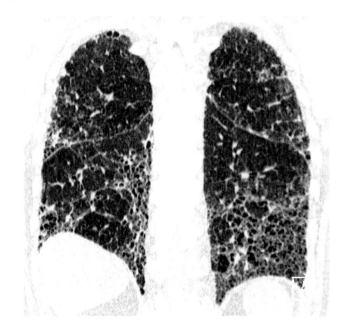

Figure 1.16c

Model answer

This is a frontal chest radiograph of an adult (Figure 1.16a). The chest radiograph demonstrates low lung volumes and a subpleural reticular pattern involving the entire lung with a basal predominance. The heart and mediastinal contours are within normal limits. The findings are consistent with pulmonary fibrosis due to the histological pattern of usual interstitial pneumonitis (UIP). I would like to arrange a high-resolution CT of the chest for further characterization of the disease.

These are two selected images from an HRCT examination (Figures 1.16b, 1.16c). CT images demonstrate a symmetrical, predominantly subpleural pattern of reticulation with intralobular septal thickening, traction bronchiectasis and bronchiolectasis as well as severe subpleural honeycombing. Small amounts of ground glass in areas of architectural distortion. The findings are present in all lung zones, increasing in severity in a caudal direction. There is relative sparing of the central lung. The CT findings are in keeping with the histological diagnosis of UIP.

The histological pattern of UIP can be due to idiopathic pulmonary fibrosis (IPF), connective tissue disease (in particular rheumatoid arthritis), asbestosis or drug reaction. Idiopathic pulmonary fibrosis is essentially a diagnosis of exclusion.

I would review the rest of the imaging to look for pleural plaques, which may indicate asbestos exposure, as well as evidence of inflammatory joint disease. The presence of a dense liver may be seen with amiodarone therapy and may provide a link to the underlying cause of fibrosis. I would discuss the case with the clinician, as further clinical history would be invaluable. The patient will need to be referred to the chest physicians. Pulmonary function tests, which typically show a restrictive pattern with limited diffusion, should be ordered.

Questions

1. **What are the strongest predictors of UIP on high-resolution CT?**
   Lower lung zone honeycombing (odds ratio 5.36) in association with upper lung reticulation (odds ratio 6.28).

2. **What is the difference between idiopathic pulmonary fibrosis and usual inter-stitial pneumonitis?**
IPF is a diagnosis made clinically, with radiological and pathological support. UIP is the *histological* pattern of disease seen in IPF. UIP is also seen in the lung fibrosis associated with connective tissue disorders (such as rheumatoid arthritis) and asbestosis.

3. **Can you think of a few drugs that could cause this appearance?**
Nitrofurantoin, cyclophosphamide, methotrexate and amiodarone (look for the dense liver).

Key points

- The definitive diagnosis of idiopathic pulmonary fibrosis can only be made by a combination of clinical, imaging and/or surgical–histopathological features. A highly probable diagnosis of IPF can be made without a lung biopsy if the clinical and radiological features fulfil four major criteria and at least three minor criteria.
- The major criteria are:
  1. pulmonary function tests demonstrating a restrictive physiology with impaired gas exchange
  2. basal reticular opacities with minimal ground-glass opacification
  3. transbronchial lung biopsy or bronchoalveolar lavage results do not support alternative diagnoses
  4. exclusion of other diagnoses.
- Minor criteria are:
  1. age > 50 years
  2. bibasal inspiratory crackles
  3. unexplained breathlessness on exertion
  4. duration > 3 months.
- UIP can be complicated by infection and lung tumour.
- UIP can be associated with enlarged mediastinal lymph nodes. The presence of these does not necessarily indicate the development of complications.

Further reading

American Thoracic Society, European Respiratory Society. American Thoracic Society/European Respiratory Society International Multidisciplinary Consensus Classification of the Idiopathic Interstitial Pneumonias. This joint statement of the American Thoracic Society (ATS), and the European Respiratory Society (ERS) was adopted by the ATS board of directors, June 2001 and by the ERS Executive Committee, June 2001. *Am J Respir Crit Care Med* 2002; **165**: 277–304. [Published correction appears in *Am J Respir Crit Care Med* 2002; **166**: 426.]
Lynch DA, Godwin DJ, Safrin S, *et al.* High-resolution computed tomography in idiopathic pulmonary fibrosis: diagnosis and prognosis. *Am J Respir Crit Care Med* 2005; **172**: 488–93.
Mueller-Mang C, Grosse C, Schmid K, Stiebellehner L, Bankier AA. What every radiologist should know about idiopathic interstitial pneumonias. *Radiographics* 2007; **27**: 595–615.

Images courtesy of Dr Nestor Müller, Vancouver General Hospital.

Cardiothoracic Case 17

KIAT T. TAN AND PATRICIA DUNLOP

Clinical history

45-year-old male non-smoker with history of rheumatoid arthritis, six-month history of cough and mild shortness of breath.

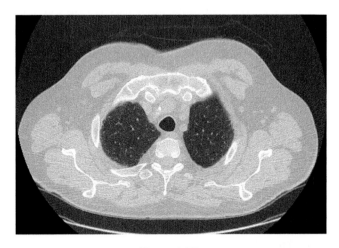

Figure 1.17a

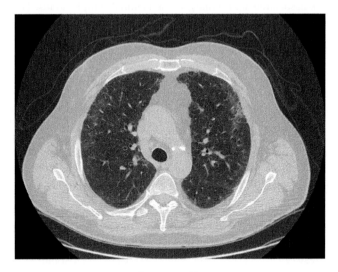

Figure 1.17b

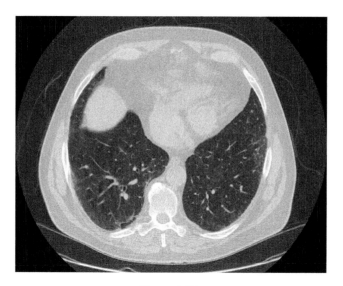

Figure 1.17c

Model answer

These are three lung window images from a CT scan of an adult male (Figures 1.17a–1.17c). There are areas of ground-glass opacification, most prominent in the mid to lower zones with sparing of the apices. These changes affect both central and peripheral lung regions. Reticulation is seen most prominently in the upper lobes, with less severe involvement of the lower lobes. Bronchiolectatic changes are present in both upper lobes. The changes are bilateral and relatively symmetrical. No consolidation, central bronchiectasis, cysts or lung nodules. The radiological findings are non-specific and the differential diagnoses would include non-specific interstitial pneumonitis (NSIP), desquamative interstitial pneumonitis (DIP) and hypersensitivity pneumonitis (HP). However, given the clinical history, NSIP is the most likely diagnosis. Usual interstitial pneumonitis (UIP) is unlikely, as the radiological features are extremely atypical for this diagnosis.

I would like to review the rest of the imaging on a workstation to further assess disease extent and distribution. The patient will need to be referred to the chest physicians for bronchoscopy/bronchoalveolar lavage. Lung biopsy may be necessary if the diagnosis remains unclear.

Questions

1. **Why do you say that NSIP is the most likely diagnosis, as opposed to DIP and hypersensitivity pneumonitis?**
   NSIP is radiologically similar to DIP. However, DIP is rare in non-smokers. Hypersensitivity pneumonitis presents with mid to lower zone ground-glass opacification and, in long-standing cases, upper lobe fibrosis. The six-month history of cough and shortness of breath are atypical of hypersensitivity pneumonitis. Finally, NSIP is associated with collagen vascular diseases.

2. **Why is this not a UIP pattern of disease?**
   There is prominent ground-glass opacification, no honeycombing, and lung changes which affect both peripheral and central portions of lung. These are not typical features of UIP (*see also Case 16*).

3. **How would bronchoalveolar lavage help?**
   BAL shows increased macrophage count in DIP and lymphocytosis in both NSIP and hypersensivity pneumonitis.

Key points

- NSIP affects individuals between 40 and 50 years of age and is associated with collagen vascular disease. It presents with *non-specific* clinical features. It is the second most common cause of interstitial pneumonitis.
- HRCT features are *non-specific* and typically include ground-glass changes, reticulation and traction bronchiectasis. The changes are typically symmetrical and affect the lower lung zones, usually with relative subpleural sparing. Honeycombing and consolidation may be present.
- Diagnosis of NSIP is made by a combination of clinical, imaging and histological features. Diagnosis of NSIP should always be accompanied by a hunt for predisposing factors, as treatment of these can result in marked improvement. For example, a dilated oesophagus suggests that NSIP is due to scleroderma.

Further reading

American Thoracic Society, European Respiratory Society. American Thoracic Society/European Respiratory Society International Multidisciplinary Consensus Classification of the Idiopathic Interstitial Pneumonias. This joint statement of the American Thoracic Society (ATS), and the European Respiratory Society (ERS) was adopted by the ATS board of directors, June 2001 and by the ERS Executive Committee, June 2001. *Am J Respir Crit Care Med* 2002; **165**: 277–304. [Published correction appears in *Am J Respir Crit Care Med* 2002; **166**: 426.]

Kligerman SJ, Groshong S, Brown KK, Lynch DA. Nonspecific interstitial pneumonia: radiologic, clinical, and pathologic considerations. *Radiographics* 2009; **29**: 73–87.

Cardiothoracic Case 18

KIAT T. TAN AND PATRICIA DUNLOP

Clinical history

56-year-old former IV drug abuser with left lung transplant three years ago. Report the chest radiograph first.

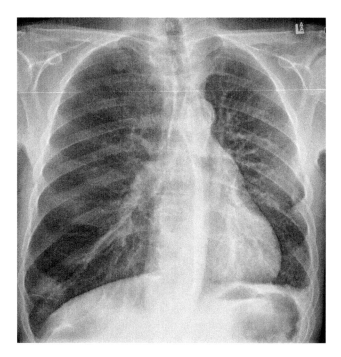

Figure 1.18a

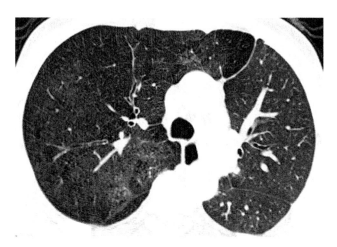

Figure 1.18b

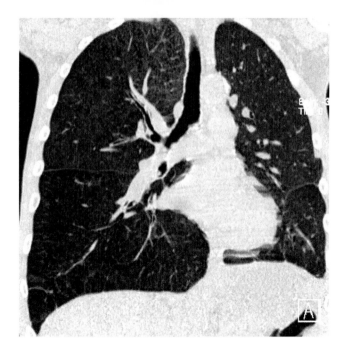

Figure 1.18c

Model answer

This is a frontal chest radiograph of an adult (Figure 1.18a). There is significant hyperinflation of the right lung with leftward shift of the mediastinum. The linear line projected to the left of the mediastinum represents the anterior junction line due to the extensive hyperinflation. There are linear opacities in the right mid to lower lung zones and left retrocardiac region that are most consistent with atelectasis/scarring. Focal linear opacity and cystic change are noted at the right lateral costophrenic angle. There are subtle fine nodular opacities thoughout both lungs, most clearly seen on the right. Post-surgical changes are noted in the left lateral sixth and seventh ribs. There is blunting of the left costophrenic angle. No adenopathy noted. The pulmonary arteries are enlarged. The findings could be due to talcosis, with recurrence in the transplanted lung. Pulmonary hypertension is present. A clinical history and chest CT would be useful in elucidating the exact cause of the patient's problem.

These are two images from a CT scan of the chest (Figures 1.18b, 1.18c). There is panlobular and centrilobular emphysema in the right lung. There is a fine nodular pattern in both lungs. No lymphadenopathy. The main pulmonary artery is enlarged and its branches are larger than the accompanying bronchi, consistent with pulmonary hypertension. The patient requires an echocardiogram for further characterization of cardiac function and pulmonary arterial pressure. The findings are most likely due to talcosis. Other differential diagnoses include silicosis, coal worker's pneumoconiosis and alveolar microlithiasis.

Questions

1. **What is the origin of the talc?**
   Talc is often a component of oral medications. Alternatively, it could be added during the 'cutting' of street drugs. When these drugs are injected, the insoluble talc lodges in the pulmonary circulation.
2. **Does the lung damage stop after the cessation of IV drug abuse?**
   The disease may progress (similar to silicosis).

3. **What are the physiological effects of talcosis?**

The lodging of talc in the pulmonary arterioles/capillaries may result in pulmonary hypertension. The material may also migrate into the pulmonary interstitium, eliciting an inflammatory response that leads to fibrosis. The inflammatory nodules can become confluent, leading to areas of consolidation which are of high attenuation on CT.

4. **Which laboratory test is diagnostic of talcosis?**

The presence of plate-like strongly birefringent crystals on microscopy is the gold standard for diagnosis.

Key points

- Talcosis could be due to either injected or inhaled talc (hydrated magnesium silicate).
- Talc may be inhaled with silica or asbestos, in which case the clinical/imaging characteristics of the latter may predominate.
- Inhalation talcosis is associated with reticulo-nodular opacification and large confluent opacities.
- Injection talcosis typically causes emphysema, ground-glass and nodular opacities. Large conglomerate masses may also occur.

Further reading

Marchiori E, Lourenço S, Gasparetto TD, *et al*. Pulmonary talcosis: imaging findings. *Lung* 2010; **188**: 165–71.

Nguyen ET, Silva CI, Souza CA, Müller NL. Pulmonary complications of illicit drug use: differential diagnosis based on CT findings. *J Thorac Imaging* 2007; **22**: 199–206.

Fraser RS, Colman N, Müller NL, Paré PD. Embolic and thrombotic diseases of the lungs. In Fraser RS, Colman N, Müller NL, Paré PD, eds., *Synopsis of Diseases of the Chest*. Philadelphia, PA: Elsevier Saunders, 2005; 542–80.

Paré JP, Cote G, Fraser RS. Long-term follow-up of drug abusers with intravenous talcosis. *Am Rev Respir Dis* 1989; **139**: 233–41.

Cardiothoracic Case 19

KIAT T. TAN AND PATRICIA DUNLOP

Clinical history
'Unwell in emergency department.'

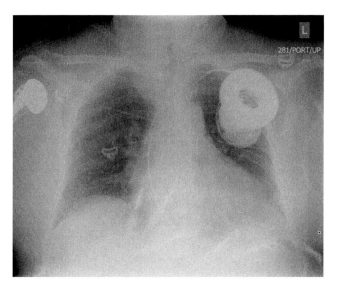

Figure 1.19

Model answer
This is a frontal chest radiograph of a skeletally mature patient (Figure 1.19). The patient has a dual-chamber implantable defibrillator. Both defibrillator leads have become displaced, with the atrial lead projected over the SVC and the ventricular lead projected over the atrium. A round metallic opacity with a lucent centre is seen over the defibrillator box, most likely representing a magnet to deactivate the defibrillator that is discharging indiscriminately. The heart is enlarged. No acute lung lesion or signs of pulmonary oedema. Right shoulder replacement is noted.

The patient needs to be monitored in the coronary care unit. An external defibrillator/pacer should be on standby. The patient will need urgent review by the cardiologist for replacement of the defibrillator leads. A repeat chest radiograph with frontal and lateral views should be obtained after defibrillator lead replacement. The patient should be advised not to twiddle with the box.

Questions
1. **How do you tell the difference between an implantable defibrillator and a conventional pacemaker?**
   The ICD leads have focally thickened portions while conventional pacemaker leads are of uniform thickness.
2. **Where should the tips of the defibrillator leads be located?**
   For single-chamber ICDs, in the right ventricular wall. Dual-chamber ICDs, right atrial and right ventricular walls. Biventricular pacemaker defibrillators (three leads), right atrial and right ventricular walls as well as coronary sinus.

Key points

- When examining the pacemaker on the chest radiograph, make sure that the leads are plugged into the box, not fractured (a 'kink' may indicate subtle fracture) and in the correct position.
- Look out for pneumo- or haemothorax in post-pacemaker insertion chest radiographs.

Further reading

Burney K, Burchard F, Papouchado M, Wilde P. Cardiac pacing systems and implantable cardiac defibrillators (ICDs): a radiological perspective of equipment, anatomy and complications. *Clin Radiol* 2004; **59**: 699–708.

Cardiothoracic Case 20

KIAT T. TAN AND PATRICIA DUNLOP

Clinical history

Long-standing painful right arm in a 35-year-old tennis coach.

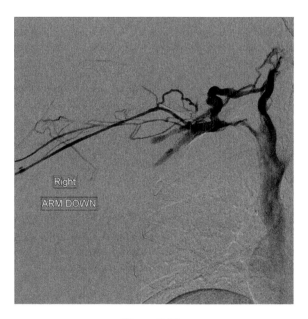

Figure 1.20a

Further reading
Verschakalen JA. The chest wall, pleura, and diaphragm. In Adam A, Dixon AK, eds., *Grainger and Allison's Diagnostic Radiology*, 5th edn. London: Churchill Livingstone, 2008 (ebook).

Cardiothoracic Case 22

KIAT T. TAN AND PATRICIA DUNLOP

Clinical history
Shortness of breath.

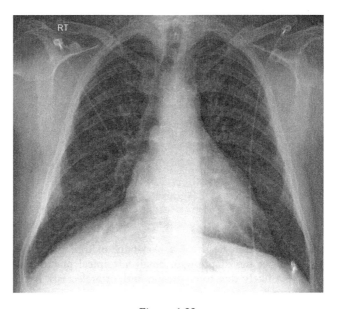

Figure 1.22

Model answer
This is a frontal chest radiograph of a skeletally mature patient (Figure 1.22). There has been previous coronary artery bypass grafting. There are prominent interstitial lines, including the presence of Kerley B lines. The pulmonary veins are prominent, with upper lobe blood diversion and indistinctness of the vessels. Bronchial wall thickening is present. No pleural effusion. Heart size is towards the upper limit of normal. The findings are consistent with interstitial pulmonary oedema due to fluid overload secondary to heart failure.

The lungs are hyperinflated, which may suggest underlying COPD. There is right tracheal deviation at the thoracic inlet, which is most likely due to unfolded/ dilated vasculature. The differential would include thyroid enlargement and lymphadenopathy.

Healed left clavicle fracture is noted. I will inform the clinicians regarding the chest radiograph findings. The patient will require a repeat chest radiograph after appropriate diuretic treatment and an echocardiogram.

Questions

1. What are Kerley B lines?

These are short parallel lines in the lung periphery, perpendicular to the pleura and continuous with it, resembling rungs on a ladder. They represent thickened interlobular septa. They are most commonly seen in fluid overload (e.g. in heart failure and renal disease), although other pulmonary interstitial processes, such as idiopathic pulmonary fibrosis and lymphangitis carcinomatosa, can also result in their presence.

2. What are the features of heart failure?

The earliest finding is upper lobe blood diversion, followed by interstitial oedema. Leakage of fluid into the alveoli results in overt airspace opacification. 'Overspill' of fluid from the interlobular septa into the space between lung and visceral pleura gives rise to the so-called 'lamellar' pleural effusion.

Key points

- Pulmonary oedema can be due to heart failure even in the presence of a 'normal' echocardiogram, as assessment of diastolic function can be difficult on echocardiography (this requires tissue Doppler studies, not available in all centres).
- Renal disease is a much-overlooked cause of fluid overload when reporting chest radiographs.

Further reading

Fraser RS, Müller NL, Colman N, Paré PD. Pulmonary edema. In *Fraser and Paré's Diagnosis of Diseases of the Chest*, 4th edn. Philadelphia, PA: Saunders, 1999; 441–4.

Gluecker T, Capasso P, Schnyder P, *et al*. Clinical and radiologic features of pulmonary edema. *Radiographics* 1999; **19**: 1507–31.

Peddu P, Desai SR. Airspace disease. In Adam A, Dixon AK, eds., *Grainger and Allison's Diagnostic Radiology*, 5th edn. London: Churchill Livingstone, 2008 (ebook).

Cardiothoracic Case 23

KIAT T. TAN AND PATRICIA DUNLOP

Clinical history

25-year-old lawyer feeling tired all the time. Report the chest radiograph first.

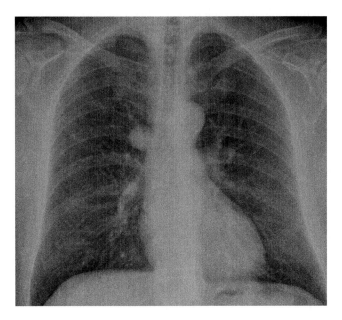

Figure 1.23a

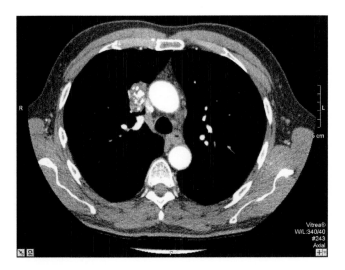

Figure 1.23b

Model answer

This is a frontal chest radiograph of a skeletally mature individual (Figure 1.23a). There is a large round and well-defined solitary nodule in the right suprahilar region. The nodule appears to contain some coarse calcifications. The lungs are otherwise clear. Heart and mediastinal contours are normal. The findings are suggestive of a pulmonary hamartoma, although bronchial carcinoid is a differential diagnosis, especially in a central lesion. A CT is suggested to confirm the presence of fat and popcorn-like calcifications which are diagnostic of pulmonary hamartoma.

The CT scan (Figure 1.23b) shows the well-defined nodule within the anterior segment of the right upper lobe adjacent to the mediastinum. The lesion contains coarse 'popcorn' calcification and fat. Findings are diagnostic of a pulmonary hamartoma. No further investigation is required.

Questions

1. **What is a pulmonary hamartoma?**
   A tumour-like malformation made up of disorganized tissues that are normally present in the organ in which they are found. Pulmonary hamartomas are composed mainly of adipose tissue and cartilage.
2. **Is the presence of fat diagnostic of hamartomas?**
   The presence of fat is diagnostic of hamartomas in lesions that are less than 2.5 cm in diameter.

Key points

- Popcorn calcification is diagnostic of pulmonary hamartomas.
- Non-fatty non-calcified hamartomas cannot be differentiated from pulmonary neoplasms.
- Endobronchial hamartomas can cause bronchial obstruction and haemoptysis.
- Carney's triad is a condition in which pulmonary hamartomas are associated with gastric epithelioid leiomyosarcoma and functioning extra-adrenal paragangliomas. This is a rare syndrome, occurring mainly in women under the age of 35.

Further reading

Müller NL, Fraser RS, Colman NC, Paré PD. *Radiologic Diagnosis of Diseases of the Chest*. Philadelphia, PA: Saunders, 2001; 240.

Padley S, MacDonald SL. Pulmonary neoplasms. In Adam A, Dixon AK, eds., *Grainger and Allison's Diagnostic Radiology*, 5th edn. London: Churchill Livingstone, 2008 (ebook).

Cardiothoracic Case 24

KIAT T. TAN AND PATRICIA DUNLOP

Clinical history
Feeling unwell.

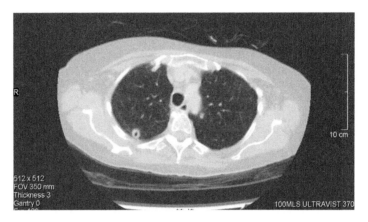

Figure 1.24a

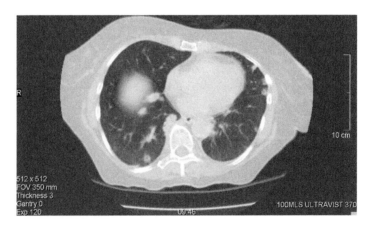

Figure 1.24b

Model answer
These are two selected images from a CT scan (Figures 1.24a, 1.24b). There are multiple nodules of varying sizes in both lungs. Some of these nodules are cavitating. The differential diagnoses include staphylococcal infection (usually acute), septic emboli from endocarditis, tuberculosis (usually chronic), fungal, metastatic tumour, and inflammatory (e.g. Wegener's granulomatosis). I would want to review the images on the workstation to look for associated findings such as lymphadenopathy,

involvement of other organs and other lung findings. I would like to find out more about the clinical history and presentation from the clinician. Other investigations should be based on the clinical history.

Questions

1. **Which tumours typically metastasize to the lung?**
   Breast, kidney, lung, GI tract, sarcomas and testicular tumours.
2. **Which metastatic tumours most often cavitate?**
   Approximately 5% of metastatic lesions cavitate. Typical pulmonary metastases that cavitate include squamous cell carcinoma (primarily from the head/neck and cervix), adenocarcinomas (which are usually from the GI tract) and sarcoma, especially osteogenic ones.
3. **What are the other chest manifestations of Wegener's granulomatosis?**
   Pulmonary haemorrhage, consolidation, ground-glass opacification and tracheo-bronchial thickening and stenosis, pleural effusions.

Key points

- Wegener's granulomatosis is a multisystem autoimmune condition that most commonly affects the lungs and kidneys.
- Wegener's is characterized by a positive c-ANCA.
- Wegener's most commonly affects the lungs and kidneys, although virtually every other organ system can be affected.
- If given a plain film of multiple cavitating nodules, give above differential diagnosis and get a CT scan of the chest.

Notes

The cavitating nodules in this particular patient were due to Wegener's granulomatosis, but it is impossible to distinguish this condition from the other differential diagnoses based on imaging alone.

Further reading

Castañer E, Alguersuari A, Gallardo X, *et al*. When to suspect pulmonary vasculitis: radiologic and clinical clues. *Radiographics* 2010; **30**: 33–53.

Murfitt J, Robinson P, Whitehouse R, *et al*. The normal chest: methods of investigation and differential diagnosis. In Sutton D, ed., *Textbook of Radiology and Imaging*, 7th edn. London: Elsevier, 2003; 1–57.

Cardiothoracic Case 26

KIAT T. TAN AND PATRICIA DUNLOP

Clinical history

74-year-old man. No history. Report the chest radiograph first.

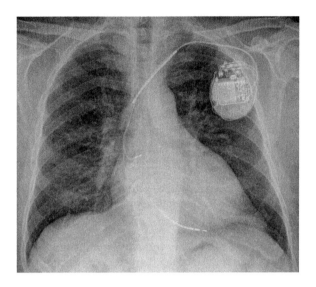

Figure 1.26a

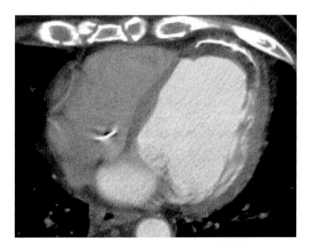

Figure 1.26b

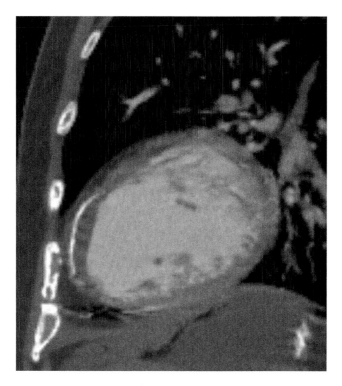

Figure 1.26c

Model answer

This is a frontal chest radiograph of a skeletally mature patient (Figure 1.26a). There is an ICD with atrial and ventricular leads in good position. There is prominence of the pulmonary veins, consistent with pulmonary venous hypertension. No evidence of overt pulmonary oedema. There is a thin curvilinear dense opacity projected over the apex of the heart. This is most consistent with myocardial calcification, although pericardial calcification is a less likely possibility. The patient requires an echocardiogram. Myocardial calcification is most often due to previous infarction with left ventricular aneurysm formation. Pericardial calcification is associated with previous pericarditis (especially tuberculous) and haemopericardium.

I am presented with axial and sagittal images from a contrast-enhanced CT (Figures 1.26b, 1.26c). These confirm the presence of left ventricular apical calcification. There is an adjacent smooth curvilinear filling defect along the wall suggestive of thrombus formation. Although the study is not gated, the left ventricle appears dilated, with thinning of apex and anterior septum. Assuming normal coronary anatomy, the culprit vessel is most likely the left anterior descending artery. The patient requires an echocardiogram for assessment of left ventricular structure and function.

Questions

1. **What is the clinical significance of a left ventricular aneurysm?**

   Left ventricular aneurysms can be asymptomatic, act as foci for arrhythmias or cause heart failure. Acute LV thrombus can result in distal embolization. Chronic LV thrombus is much less likely to embolize.

2. **How do you differentiate between pericardial and myocardial calcification on plain radiography?**

   Pericardial calcification tends to occur over the atrioventricular groove and right ventricle, while myocardial calcification tends to affect the left ventricular apex.

However, differentiating the two can be difficult, especially when the left ventricular aneurysm is not well seen.

3. **How do you differentiate between pericardial and myocardial calcification on CT?**
This is straightforward on a contrast-enhanced study, where myocardial calcification can be seen to be continuous with the myocardium. Differentiating between the two can be difficult without intravenous contrast; generally, the presence of calcification deep to the subpericardial fat is indicative of myocardial calcification, while calcification superficial to it is pericardial. Myocardial calcification can also be seen to be separate from the thin rim of pericardial fluid.

Key points

- Cardiac calcification can be classified according to the structure affected. These are: (1) coronary arteries; (2) pericardium; (3) myocardium; (4) heart valves; (5) endocardium. It is important to differentiate between these, as they give rise to different clinical manifestations.
- A left ventricular aneurysm is defined as the part of the left ventricle that demonstrates both abnormal *diastolic* and *systolic* bulging. This is distinct from akinesia or dyskinesia, where there is only *systolic* bulging.
- When identified, a left ventricular aneurysm should be differentiated from a left ventricular pseudoaneurysm. The former can often be left alone (especially if asymptomatic) while the latter is a medical emergency that must be treated surgically. Pseudoaneurysms have a thin neck and there may be evidence of a defect in the myocardium (this may not be obvious, because of thrombus formation). They are often found in the lateral and posterior LV walls. A left ventricular aneurysm has a wide neck and is often found in apical and anterior walls.

Further reading

MacDonald SL, Padley S. The mediastinum, including the pericardium. In Adam A, Dixon AK, eds., *Grainger and Allison's Diagnostic Radiology*, 5th edn. London: Churchill Livingstone, 2008 (ebook).

MacGregor JH, Chen JT, Chiles C, et al. The radiographic distinction between pericardial and myocardial calcifications. *AJR Am J Roentgenol* 1987; **148**: 675–7.

Cardiothoracic Case 27

KIAT T. TAN AND PATRICIA DUNLOP

Clinical history
Shortness of breath.

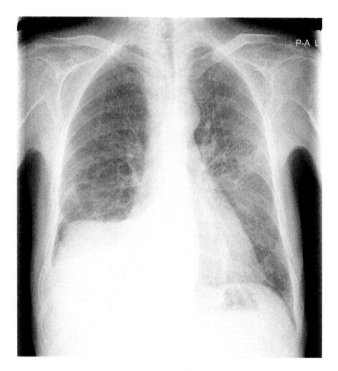

Figure 1.27

Model answer
This is a PA chest radiograph of a skeletally mature patient (Figure 1.27). The cardio-pericardial silhouette is slightly enlarged with prominent upper lobe pulmonary veins and peribronchial cuffing. There is bilateral perihilar hazy opacity and an ill-defined opacity in the left mid lung zone. There is apparent elevation of the right hemidiaphragm with lateral shift of the diaphragmatic hump. There is passive atel-ectasis of the underlying right lower lung zone. A small amount of fluid is noted in the minor fissure. These findings are most likely due to pulmonary oedema with a right subpulmonic effusion. Also noted are healed left rib fractures and deformity of the proximal humeri.

I would like to obtain a decubitus view of the chest to confirm the presence of a subpulmonic effusion. The patient will require an echocardiogram to assess cardiac function. A repeat chest radiograph should be obtained after appropriate treatment to assess resolution of the abnormalities.

Questions
1. What is a subpulmonic effusion?

The term refers to the situation where fluid is situated between the inferior surface of the lower lobe and diaphragm, mimicking a raised hemidiaphragm, often referred to as a 'pseudodiaphragmatic contour'.

Further reading

Fraser RS, Müller NL, Colman N, Paré PD. Pleural abnormalities. In *Fraser and Paré's Diagnosis of Diseases of the Chest*, 4th edn. Philadelphia, PA: Saunders, 1999; 566–71.

Rubens MB, Padley SG. The pleura. In Sutton D, ed., *Textbook of Radiology and Imaging*, 7th edn. London: Elsevier, 2003; 87–107.

Cardiothoracic Case 28

KIAT T. TAN AND PATRICIA DUNLOP

Clinical history
Chest infection. Report the chest radiograph first.

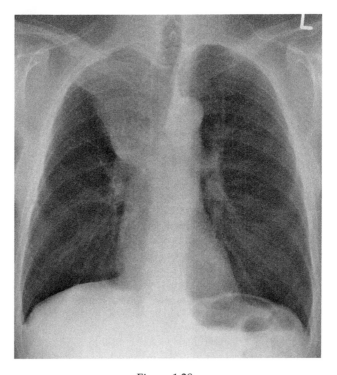

Figure 1.28a

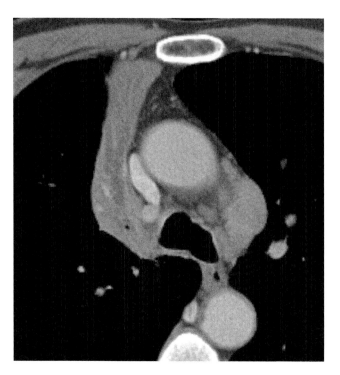

Figure 1.28b

Model answer

This is a PA chest radiograph of a skeletally mature male (Figure 1.28a). There is opacification of the right apex, associated with loss of volume with elevation of the minor fissure and right tracheal deviation. No air bronchograms are seen within the opacity. Increased density is seen in the lower right paratracheal region and hilum. The lower border of the opacity forms an inverted 'S'. These findings are consistent with the S sign of Golden, which is classically ascribed to right upper lobe collapse as a result of tumour. No evidence of secondary pulmonary nodules. No lymphadenopathy. No pleural effusion. There is no bony destruction.

The single axial CT mediastinal window image (Figure 1.28b) demonstrates the collapsed right upper lobe adjacent to the mediastinum. The linear low-density opacity within the collapsed lobe is consistent with inspissated mucus/obstructive pneumonitis. There are enlarged para-aortic nodes. The findings are most likely to be due to lung tumour with mediastinal lymph node spread.

I would like to review the remainder of the mediastinal and lung window images to further assist in the staging of this carcinoma. The patient will need a referral to the chest physicians and bronchoscopy.

Questions

1. **What forms the Golden S sign?**
   The upper concavity is formed by the edge of the collapsed lobe while the more medial convexity is due to the obstructing tumour. Although classically described in the right upper lobe, the sign can sometimes be observed in other lobes.
2. **What is the importance of the lack of air bronchograms?**
   This finding indicates complete airway obstruction. Therefore, this sign is virtually pathognomonic of endobronchial obstruction, which may be due to foreign body, mucus plugging or tumour.

Key points
- The right upper lobe tends to collapse towards the mediastinum, giving rise to an inverted triangular opacity with the apex pointing towards the mediastinum (in contrast to the left upper lobe, which collapses towards the anterior chest wall).

Further reading
Copley SJ. Pulmonary lobar collapse: essential considerations. In Adam A, Dixon AK, eds., *Grainger and Allison's Diagnostic Radiology*, 5th edn. London: Churchill Livingstone, 2008 (ebook).

Fraser RS, Müller NL, Colman N, Paré PD. Pulmonary carcinoma. In *Fraser and Paré's Diagnosis of Diseases of the Chest*, 4th edn. Philadelphia, PA: Saunders, 1999; 1121.

Images courtesy of Dr Harry Shulman, Sunnybrook Health Sciences Centre, Toronto.

Cardiothoracic Case 29

KIAT T. TAN AND PATRICIA DUNLOP

Clinical history
28-year-old female, non-smoker, presents with flushing for several weeks and recent fever.

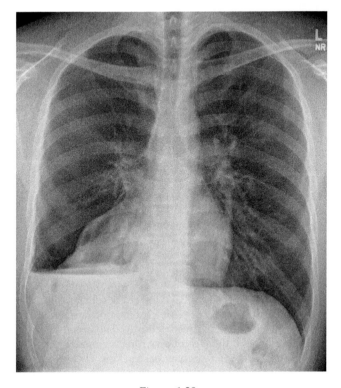

Figure 1.29a

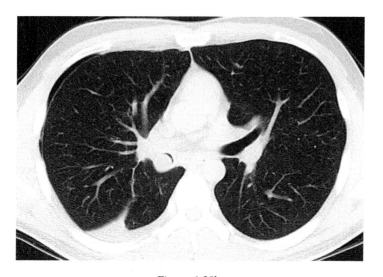

Figure 1.29b

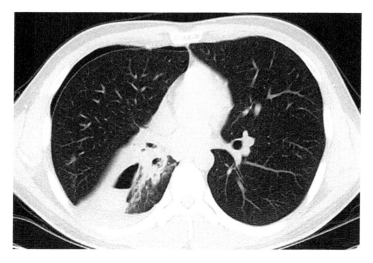

Figure 1.29c

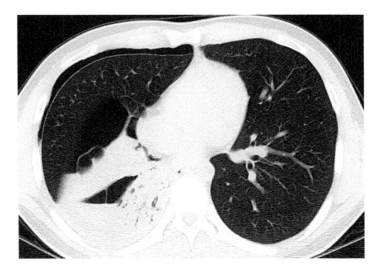

Figure 1.29d

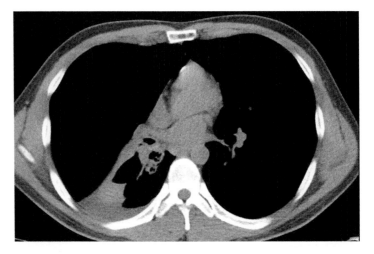

Figure 1.29e

Model answer

This is a PA chest radiograph of a skeletally mature individual (Figure 1.29a). A right hydropneumothorax is present. There is consolidation as well as air bronchograms within the right lower lobe. Two well-defined lucencies in the right lower lobe are consistent with bullae or pneumatoceles. The left lung is clear. No evidence of lymphadenopathy.

The consolidation is most likely infective in nature. The hydropneumothorax may be due to a ruptured bulla or development of a bronchopleural fistula. The most likely diagnosis in this young female patient is an endobronchial process, i.e. carcinoid tumour with post-obstructive pneumonitis and subsequent infection. The differential would include a foreign body or congenital abnormality of the airway with superimposed infection.

I have been provided with axial CT images of the chest (Figures 1.29b–1.29e) which demonstrate a well-defined soft tissue lesion in the right bronchus intermedius with debris within the right middle lobe bronchus and dilated lower lobe bronchi. Right

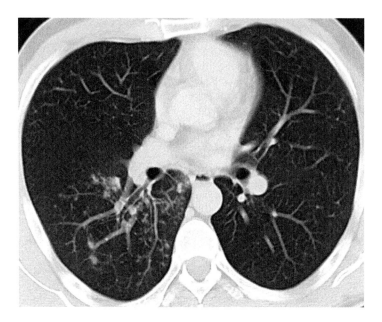

Figure 1.30b

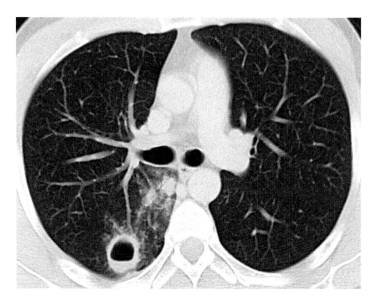

Figure 1.30c

Model answer

This is a frontal chest radiograph of a skeletally mature individual (Figure 1.30a). A cavity is seen projected over the right hilar region along with multiple nodular opacities in the right mid zone. No lymphadenopathy. No pleural effusions. No bony lesions.

The findings are most consistent with reactivation tuberculosis. The radiological differential diagnoses include other infections (such as fungal infection and lung abscess), inflammatory disorders such as Wegener's granulomatosis and lung cancer. The patient requires a chest CT for further characterization of disease, sputum culture (for AAFB and MC&S) and a Mantoux test. The referring clinician needs to be informed of the findings immediately, as the patient will require isolation for TB. Serial radiographic follow-up is required.

These are two axial images from a CT scan (Figures 1.30b, 1.30c). There is a thin-walled cavity with an air–fluid level within the superior segment of the right lower lobe with adjacent tree-in-bud opacities and nodular areas of consolidation. I would want to review the remainder of the images to assess the extent of infection and to look for adenopathy and pleural effusion. The findings would be in keeping with infection, with reactivation tuberculosis being the most likely cause.

Questions

1. **What do you understand by the terms primary and post-primary tuberculosis?**
   Primary tuberculosis refers to the disease which develops after the initial exposure. Post-primary tuberculosis refers to disease which develops as a result of reactivation of previous infection or reinfection. Many patients who are initially exposed to tuberculosis do not have any radiological abnormalities.
2. **Are the clinical, pathological and radiological manifestations of primary and post-primary tuberculosis different?**
   The clinical features of tuberculosis depend on the immune status of the infected individual. Children and the immunosuppressed develop the primary pattern of infection, whereas immunocompetent adults tend to have the post-primary pattern of disease. However, there is considerable overlap between the two patterns and the treatment of both is identical.
3. **What are the signs of active infection on CT?**
   Centrilobular nodules or tree-in-bud pattern suggest active disease. The consolidation and tree-in-bud opacities can resolve after several months. Chronic findings include bronchovascular distortion, fibrosis, emphysema and bronchiectasis. Cavitation can be seen in active and inactive disease.
4. **Can you exclude active tuberculosis on a single radiograph?**
   No. The diagnosis of 'old tuberculosis' can only be made if there is no change in the radiographic appearance over six months or more.

Key points

- If the patient is acutely unwell, the most likely differential diagnoses of cavitating pulmonary lesions are cavitating bronchopneumonia (e.g. staphylococcal/fungal) and inflammatory disease (e.g. Wegener's granulomatosis).
- Radiological findings of primary TB in children are adenopathy (90–95%) and consolidation (70%). Pleural effusions are less common in children (5–10%). In adults, primary TB tends to present with consolidation (90%). Adults are less likely to have adenopathy (10–30%).
- Post-primary TB tends to present with focal/patchy consolidation or reticulonodular opacities in the apical and posterior segments of the upper lobes or superior segments of the lower lobes, cavitation (20–45%), lymph node enlargement (5–10%) and pleural effusion (15–25%).
- The tree-in-bud appearance in the setting of pulmonary infection is an indication of spread of disease via the small airways.

Further reading

Goodman PC. Pulmonary infection in adults. In Adam A, Dixon AK, eds., *Grainger and Allison's Diagnostic Radiology*, 5th edn. London: Churchill Livingstone, 2008 (ebook).

Im JG, Itoh H, Shim YS, *et al*. Pulmonary tuberculosis: CT findings. Early active disease and sequential change with antituberculous therapy. *Radiology* 1993; **186**: 653–60.

Cardiothoracic Case 31

KIAT T. TAN, PATRICIA DUNLOP AND JOHN CURTIS

Clinical history

66-year-old woman presents with a one-month history of cough and shortness of breath. Remote history of oesophageal surgery for benign disease. Report the chest radiographs first (PA followed by lateral).

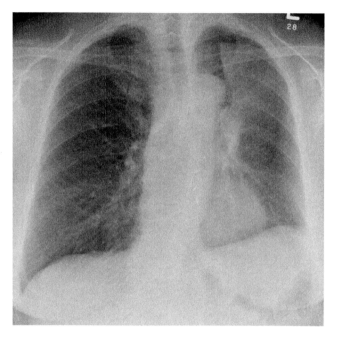

Figure 1.31a

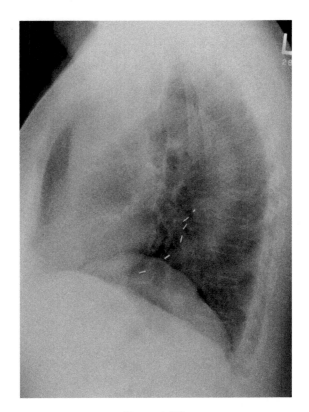

Figure 1.31b

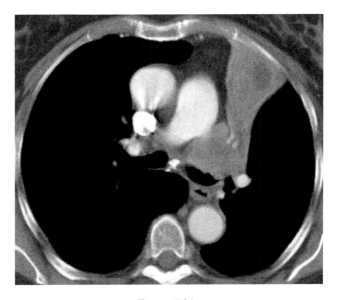

Figure 1.31c

Model answer

This is a PA chest radiograph of a skeletally mature individual (Figure 1.31a). A veil-like opacity is projected over the left hemithorax. There is loss of the normally sharp outline of the left heart border. A well-demarcated lucency is projected over the left apex and extends along the mediastinum to the level of the left hilum. There is evidence of volume loss within the left hemithorax, with elevation of the left hemidiaphragm and leftward shift of the mediastinum. The left hilum is prominent. The radiological findings are consistent with left upper lobe collapse. The right lung is clear. Surgical clips are noted mid-thorax, consistent with the prior oesophageal surgery. I would like to review a lateral radiograph for confirmation.

The lateral radiograph (Figure 1.31b) shows no bony destruction. It confirms the left upper lobe collapse and hyperexpansion of the left lower lobe with anterior displacement of the major fissure. The retrosternal lucency represents the hyperinflated right lung crossing the midline.

I would like to discuss the case with the referring clinician. The left upper lobe collapse is most likely due to lobar bronchial obstruction, which in this case is suspicious for neoplasm. If more acute, the left upper lobe collapse could be due to secretions or inhaled foreign body. I would like a CT exam to further characterize the aetiology of the collapse and to stage the presumed carcinoma.

This is a mediastinal window image from a thoracic CT scan (Figure 1.31c). There is a left hilar mass, which is obstructing the origin of the left upper lobe bronchus. There is resultant collapse of the left upper lobe. A focal hypoattenuating lesion can be seen within the collapsed upper lobe, which may represent a neoplasm (with resultant left hilar adenopathy) or a focal area of necrosis (for example, from post-obstructive abscess). There is also evidence of old granulomatous disease. I would like to review the remainder of the images to stage this neoplasm and refer the patient for bronchoscopy.

Questions

1. **Why does left upper lobe collapse present with a veil-like opacity over the hemithorax?**
   The left lung tends to collapse anteriorly to lie against the anterior chest wall. The left lower lobe overinflates to fill in the space.
2. **What is the focal lucency at the left apex and along the mediastinum?**
   This represents the overinflated left superior lower lobe segment, termed the 'Luftsichel' sign (which means air crescent). As the superior segment is pulled forward, its medial margin abuts the aorta, thereby making the aortic arch and descending aorta visible on the chest radiograph.

Key points

- In adults, neoplasms commonly cause lobar collapse. In children, lobar collapse is commonly caused by inhaled foreign bodies, asthma or mucous plugs, but only rarely by neoplasms.
- In any case of lobar collapse, always keep looking at the chest radiograph searching for bony involvement, other pulmonary lesions and complications of any treatment.
- Even if there is no bony destruction, look for it and give a commentary to the examiners to inform them that you are looking!
- Always suggest further imaging, which should include staging the tumour – staging CT of the lung.

Further reading

Fraser RS, Müller NL, Colman N, Paré PD. Atelectasis. In *Fraser and Paré's Diagnosis of Diseases of the Chest*, 4th edn. Philadelphia, PA: Saunders, 1999; 543–9.

Murfitt J, Robinson PJ, Whitehouse RW, *et al*. The normal chest: methods of investigation and differential diagnosis. In Sutton D, ed., *Textbook of Radiology and Imaging*, 7th edn. London: Elsevier, 2003; 1–57.

Images courtesy of Dr Harry Shulman, Sunnybrook Health Sciences Centre, Toronto.

Cardiothoracic Case 32

KIAT T. TAN AND PATRICIA DUNLOP

Clinical history
Earache.

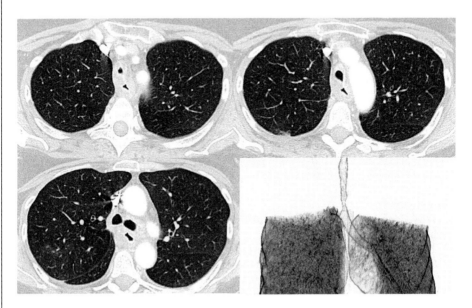

Figure 1.32

Model answer
These are three selected axial CT lung window images and one 3D reconstruction image of an adult (Figure 1.32). There are centrilobular nodules, areas with a tree-in-bud appearance and subtle ground-glass opacity seen predominantly in the right upper lobe. These could correspond to inspissated secretions and/or infection.

The tracheal wall is thickened with irregular luminal stenosis just cranial to the carina. The anterior and lateral walls are thickened, with sparing of the posterior wall. The diagnosis is relapsing polychondritis. I would want to review the images on a workstation to look for evidence of calcification in the cartilage, which is another sign of relapsing polychondritis. I would also like to elucidate other sites of involvement, paying particular attention to the manubriosternal and costochondral joints. An expiration scan may provide useful information as to the degree of airway compromise, as loss of the cartilage leads to increased collapsibility (tracheomalacia). I would like to discuss the case with the referring clinician, and the patient will need an urgent respiratory opinion, as airway compromise is a significant risk. He/she will also need a full haematological, immunological and cardiopulmonary workup.

Questions
1. **Do you have a differential diagnosis?**
   Wegener's granulomatosis is a possible differential diagnosis for patients with earache and tracheomalacia. Tuberculosis should be considered in patients with

perichondritis and radiological evidence of infection. However, the anterior and lateral tracheal wall thickening with posterior wall sparing is virtually pathognomonic of relapsing polychondritis.

2. **How is relapsing polychondritis diagnosed?**
   When three or more of the following are present: non-erosive seronegative inflammatory polyarthritis; bilateral auricular chondritis; eye inflammation; vestibular impairment; nasal chondritis; tracheobronchial chondritis.

3. **What is this patient at risk of developing?**
   Asphyxiation due to tracheal collapse/stenosis. Tracheostomy is the best method to preserve the airway in this patient. Intubation is extremely hazardous in patients with relapsing polychondritis.

Key points

- Although predominantly an autoimmune disease of cartilage, relapsing polychondritis can affect virtually every organ in the body. Central nervous system symptoms, aortitis and renal damage are potential complications.
- Relapsing polychondritis is treated with systemic steroids and immunosuppressive therapy.

Further reading

Müller NL, Silva CI. *Imaging of the Chest*. Philadelphia, PA: Saunders, 2008; 1009–12.

Prince JS, Duhamel DR, Levin DL, Harrell JH, Friedman PJ. Nonneoplastic lesions of the tracheobronchial wall: radiologic findings with bronchoscopic correlation. *Radiographics* 2002; **22**: S215–30.

Cardiothoracic Case 33

KIAT T. TAN AND PATRICIA DUNLOP

Clinical history

No history.

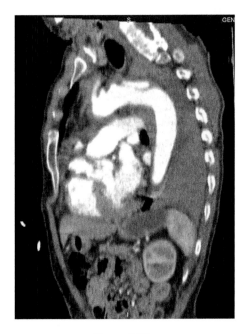

Figure 1.33a

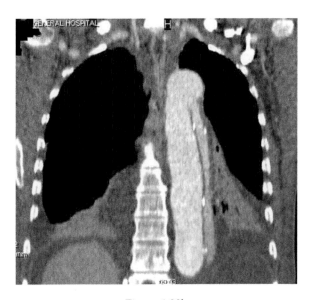

Figure 1.33b

Model answer

These are one image from a coronal section and another from the sagittal section of a CT thoracic aortogram (Figures 1.33a, 1.33b). The aorta has two apparent lumens, the so-called 'double-barrelled' appearance. The abnormality commences at the aortic arch, just distal to the origin of the left subclavian artery. It extends into the abdominal aorta, although the distal end is not visualized. The larger of the two lumens is continuous with the normal proximal aorta. The smaller of the two lumens is on the left and appears slightly less dense, with visible hypoattenuating strands. There is calcification in both the medial and lateral walls of the smaller lumen. There are bilateral pleural effusions, which are of high attenuation. Passive basal pulmonary atelectasis noted. The findings are consistent with a leaking Stanford type B aortic dissection, with the false lumen being smaller.

I would want to review the images on a workstation to assess the distal limit of the dissection. In addition, I would want to find out if the blood supply to any of the visceral organs has been compromised by the dissection. I would contact the referring clinician immediately, as the patient will need urgent surgical/endovascular intervention. Endovascular intervention is a possibility, and I would also speak to my interventional radiology colleagues.

Questions

1. **How do you tell which is the true lumen?**

   The presence of 'cobwebs' or hypoattenuating strands is a characteristic of the false lumen. The true lumen can be seen to be in continuity with the proximal normal aorta. The true lumen tends to be of higher attenuation on the arterial-phase scan because of higher blood flow (although it can be darker on delayed-phase imaging, due to faster washout). The true lumen is often anteromedial and tends to be smaller than the false lumen (*although the latter is not true in this particular case*). The presence of a beak sign is indicative of the false lumen.

2. **Why is differentiating the true from the false lumen important?**

   It is extremely important for the planning of endovascular treatment of aortic dissection and its complications, whether by stenting or by fenestration. Obviously, the stent-graft should be placed in the true lumen!

Key points

- Operative treatment is indicated for patients with type A dissection. Patients with type B dissection should be operated on acutely if there is: (a) evidence of rupture/leak; (b) ischaemic compromise of vital organs; (c) acute enlargement of aorta; or (d) failure to control hypertension/clinical symptoms on medical management.
- Endovascular treatments of aortic dissection include stenting and fenestration (i.e. creating a hole in the dissection flap to maintain organ perfusion).

Further reading

Castaner E, Andreu M, Gallardo X, *et al.* CT in nontraumatic acute thoracic aortic disease: typical and atypical features and complications. *Radiographics* 2003; **23**: S93–110.

Cardiothoracic Case 34

KIAT T. TAN AND PATRICIA DUNLOP

Clinical history

75-year-old male with shortness of breath and history of adenocarcinoma of the lung diagnosed two years ago. Report the chest radiograph first.

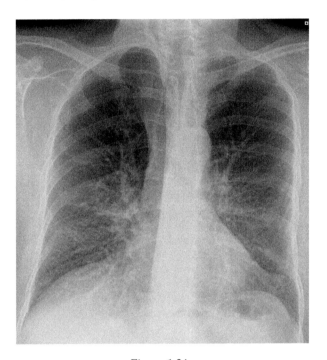

Figure 1.34a

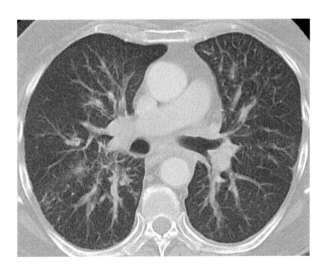

Figure 1.34b

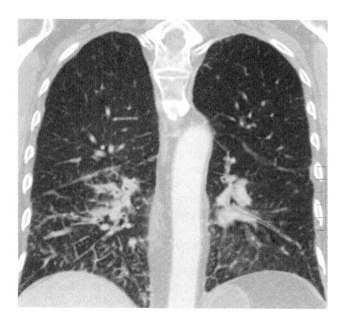

Figure 1.34c

Model answer

This is a frontal chest radiograph of a skeletally mature individual (Figure 1.34a). There is a coarse reticulonodular pattern in the mid to lower zones bilaterally, with asymmetrical peribronchial cuffing. Some patchy airspace opacification is seen in the right infrahilar region. Cardiac silhouette is not enlarged and there is no pleural effusion. There is fluid/thickening along the right minor fissure. With the history of a previous lung cancer, the most likely diagnosis is lymphangitis carcinomatosa. The differential diagnoses would include atypical infection, pulmonary oedema and interstitial fibrosis.

Axial and coronal lung windows of a CT thorax study have been provided (Figures 1.34b, 1.34c). There is bilateral asymmetrical interlobular septal thickening with no architectural distortion. A few secondary pulmonary lobules within the affected lobes are unaffected. There is nodular thickening along fissures and in the subpleural regions. Peribronchial cuffing is present and most prominent in areas of interlobular septal thickening. Given the history of previous malignancy, the findings are consistent with lymphangitis carcinomatosa.

I would like to look at the rest of the imaging on a workstation to find other evidence of metastasis, such as bone destruction and lymphadenopathy. I would also like to discuss the case with the referring clinician.

Questions

1. **Are the chest radiographic and CT lung findings diagnostic of lymphangitis carcinomatosa?**

   The differential for bilateral interlobular septal thickening with nodularity along the fissures would include lymphoma, lymphangitic disease and sarcoidosis. Lymphangitis carcinomatosa is the most likely diagnosis in patients with a history of cancer. Secondary signs that would point towards a diagnosis of lymphangitis carcinomatosa include lymphadenopathy, lung nodules and other evidence of malignancy.

2. **What are the most common primary tumours that cause lymphangitis carcinomatosis?**
Breast, lung, gastrointestinal, pancreas, prostate.

Key points
- Interstitial thickening (+ nodularity) + relevant history of malignancy = lymphangitis carcinomatosa until proven otherwise.
- Lymphangitis carcinomatosa can be caused by one of two pathological pathways: (a) initial haematogenous spread of tumour to the lung. The pulmonary lymphatic channels are subsequently invaded by these tumour cells; (b) direct lymphatic spread of tumour cells from affected hilar nodes, lung tissue or pleura. Central hilar lymphadenopathy can cause obstruction to the return of lymph fluid, leading to smooth interlobular septal thickening.
- Prognosis is usually poor, with most patients succumbing within weeks to months. However, there can sometimes be a dramatic response to treatment.

Further reading
Müller NL, Silva CIS. *Imaging of the Chest.* Philadelphia, PA: Saunders, 2008; 568–79.
Padley S, MacDonald SL. Pulmonary neoplasms. In Adam A, Dixon AK, eds., *Grainger and Allison's Diagnostic Radiology*, 5th edn. London: Churchill Livingstone, 2008 (ebook).

Cardiothoracic Case 35

KIAT T. TAN AND PATRICIA DUNLOP

Clinical history
62-year-old man with chest pain. Report the chest radiograph first.

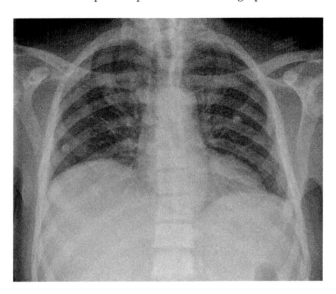

Figure 1.35a

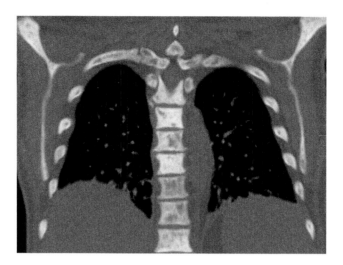

Figure 1.35b

Model answer

This is a PA chest radiograph of a skeletally mature individual (Figure 1.35a). Multiple ribs are sclerotic, as are many vertebral bodies. Lungs are clear. Heart and mediastinal contours are within normal limits. The findings are most likely due to metastatic prostate cancer. Differential diagnoses include renal osteodystrophy, fluorosis and myelofibrosis.

The single coronal reformat image (Figure 1.35b) confirms the extensive sclerotic lesions involving the ribs, spine and scapula. I would like to obtain a history of prostate cancer from either the patient or the referring clinician. Possible further investigations include sampling the prostate-specific antigen (PSA) levels, getting a radioisotope bone scan and/or imaging/biopsying the prostate.

Questions

1. **What metastatic diseases most likely cause generalized sclerosis of the bone?**
   Prostate cancer in men and breast cancer in women are most often associated with sclerotic bony metastases. Other tumours that cause sclerotic bony metastases include osteosarcomas, adenocarcinomas, carcinoid, bladder tumours and lymphoma.
2. **What are the complications of skeletal metastases?**
   Fracture and bone marrow failure due to replacement by tumour cells.
3. **Can interventional radiological techniques help?**
   If the patient's symptoms can be localized to a particular area, focal tumour ablation and/or cement injection may help symptoms. However, these techniques are of limited use in widespread bony disease.

Key points

- Patients with diffuse sclerotic bony lesions often have a 'superscan' on radioisotope bone scans. This is defined as the loss of renal uptake, and it could be the only manifestation of disease on the radioisotope study (a differential diagnosis of 'superscan' is renal failure).
- Watch out for the symmetrical and diffuse lesions.

Further reading

Stoker DJ, Saifuddin A. Bone tumours (2): malignant lesions. In Adam A, Dixon AK, eds., *Grainger and Allison's Diagnostic Radiology*, 5th edn. London: Churchill Livingstone, 2008 (ebook).

Cardiothoracic Case 36

KIAT T. TAN AND PATRICIA DUNLOP

Clinical history
40-year-old homeless man found collapsed.

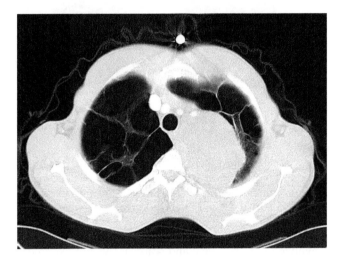

Figure 1.36a

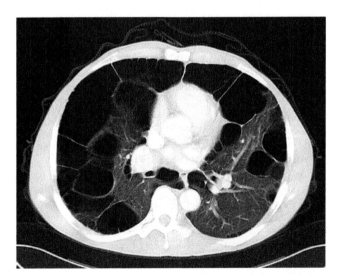

Figure 1.36b

Model answer
These are two selected axial lung window images from a CT scan of the chest (Figure 1.36a, 1.36b). Bilateral widespread bullous changes are noted, extending from the apex to at least the level of the mid-chest. A well-demarcated left apical lung mass is seen

posterior to and indenting the left subclavian artery. The findings are most consistent with a primary lung cancer with a background of bullous emphysema, most likely related to heavy smoking. In view of the severity of the radiological emphysematous bullous changes in a relatively young person, the possibility of either crack cocaine or marijuana abuse should also be considered. The differential for this appearance would be bullous disease associated with neurofibromatosis, or, less likely, cystic lung disease. I would like to review the remainder of the images to evaluate the rest of the lung parenchyma. I would like to further evaluate the left apical lesion to confirm its solid nature and to exclude a vascular cause.

This patient will need to be referred to the chest physicians. Formal pulmonary function testing should be arranged. Should this represent a lung mass a biopsy to confirm cell type should be considered. However, this is likely to be hazardous in view of the adjacent bullae and should preferably be done with appropriate resuscitation/chest drain equipment on standby.

Questions

1. **You mentioned crack cocaine and bullous emphysema. What are the other lung complications of abusing cocaine?**
   In addition to 'precocious emphysema', cocaine abuse can cause a range of lung disease, including (but not limited to) the following: acute respiratory distress syndrome, asthma, talcosis, allergic reactions, lung fibrosis, bronchiolitis, pulmonary oedema, pulmonary hypertension and haemorrhage.
2. **Can smoking illicit drugs cause lung cancer?**
   Yes. Smoking cocaine/marijuana has a carcinogenic effect, which is additive to the effect of tobacco.

Key points

- The prevalence of cocaine abuse is increasing.
- The pulmonary complications of cocaine abuse are extensive and encompass a whole range of imaging findings.
- Remember to look at adjacent structures even when presented only with lung windows.

Notes

This patient smoked tobacco, crack and marijuana since he was 12.

Further reading

Johnson MK, Smith RP, Morrison D, Laszlo G, White RJ. Large lung bullae in marijuana smokers. *Thorax* 2000; **55**: 340–2.

Restreppo CS, Carrillo JA, Martinez S, *et al*. Pulmonary complications from cocaine and cocaine-based substances: Imaging manifestations. *Radiographics* 2007; **27**: 941–56.

Cardiothoracic Case 37

KIAT T. TAN AND PATRICIA DUNLOP

Clinical history
61-year-old male. Report the chest radiograph first.

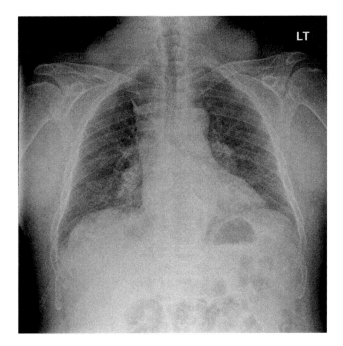

Figure 1.37a

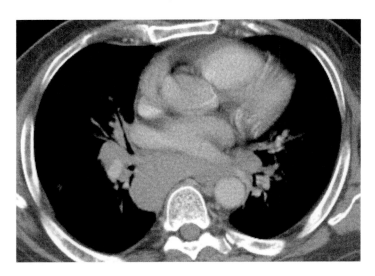

Figure 1.37b

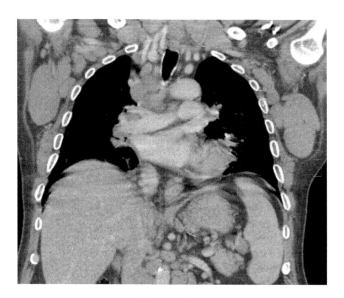

Figure 1.37c

Model answer

I have been provided with a frontal chest radiograph of a skeletally mature individual (Figure 1.37a). There is some increased opacification at the lung bases, which may be due to bronchovascular crowding or atelectasis. Increased density and convexity is seen in the right paratracheal, subcarinal and hilar regions. Cardiac silhouette is normal. There are bilateral nodular soft tissue densities in the supraclavicular and axillary regions. The findings would be consistent with extensive lymphadenopathy. The differential diagnoses for bilateral hilar and *axillary and supraclavicular* lymphadenopathy include: lymphoma/leukaemia (usually chronic lymphatic leukaemia), metastasis, infection (e.g. TB, EBV, CMV) and, less likely, sarcoidosis. Sarcoidosis does not typically cause such gross supraclavicular and axillary lymphadenopathy.

The selected axial and coronal mediastinal images from a thoracic CT examination (Figures 1.37b, 1.37c) confirm significant supraclavicular, bilateral axillary, prevascular, paratracheal, perihilar and subcarinal adenopathy. There are enlarged coeliac axis lymph nodes. No splenic enlargement. I will discuss the case with the clinician. Management is guided by the clinical/laboratory picture, and further investigations may include a CT scan of the abdomen, bronchoscopy, and biopsy of lymph nodes and bone marrow.

Questions

1. **You have mentioned the differential diagnoses for bilateral hilar lymph node enlargement. What are the differential diagnoses for unilateral hilar lymph node enlargement?**

Tuberculosis, lung cancer, lymphoma.

Key points

• A film showing hilar lymphadenopathy is commonly used in the FRCR viva.

Notes

This patient had chronic lymphatic leukaemia.

Further reading

Murfitt J, Robinson PJ, Whitehouse RW, *et al.* The normal chest: methods of investigation and differential diagnosis. In Sutton D, ed., *Textbook of Radiology and Imaging*, 7th edn. London: Elsevier, 2003; 1–57.

Cardiothoracic Case 38

KIAT T. TAN AND PATRICIA DUNLOP

Clinical history
66-year-old man with chronic illness presents with fever. Report the chest radiograph first.

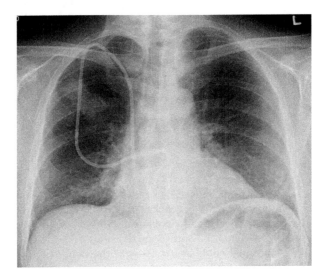

Figure 1.38a

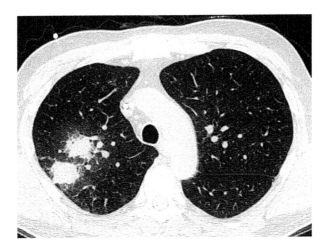

Figure 1.38b

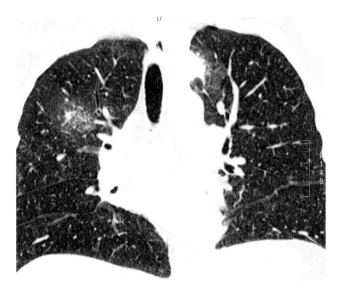

Figure 1.38c

Model answer

This is a single AP portable chest radiograph (Figure 1.38a). A tunnelled central venous catheter is noted, with its tip projected over the right atrium. There is ill-defined opacification in the right upper lung zone and the medial aspect of the left apex. The heart is not enlarged. There are no pleural effusions or osseous lesions. The differential diagnoses would include infection (such as bronchopneumonia and fungal) and inflammatory diseases such as Wegener's granulomatosis. Neoplastic disease is a consideration, although these do not typically present with fever. I would like to discuss the case with the referring clinicians and inquire about the patient's immune status and underlying chronic condition. Depending on clinical history, further imaging by CT may be useful for further characterization of disease.

These are two lung window images from a CT scan of the chest (Figures 1.38b, 1.38c). There are nodular opacities in both upper lobes. Ill-defined ground-glass opacification can be seen extending from the nodules into adjacent lung tissue. If the patient is immunocompromised, the findings would be strongly suggestive of angioinvasive aspergillosis. In the immunocompetent patient, the differential diagnoses include infection, Wegener's granulomatosis, haemorrhagic metastases or cryptogenic organizing pneumonia.

I would like to review the CT scan on a workstation to look for other lesions. I will communicate the results urgently to the referring clinician, as the patient will require immediate antifungal therapy if he is immunocompromised.

Questions

1. **What are the forms of *Aspergillus* lung disease that you know of?**
   Lung disease can present in five ways and is influenced by the immune status of the patient: (a) aspergilloma, (b) allergic bronchopulmonary aspergillosis, (c) semi-invasive aspergillosis, (d) airway invasive aspergillosis, (e) angioinvasive aspergillosis.

2. **What causes the characteristic ground-glass opacification of angioinvasive pulmonary aspergillosis?**
   Haemorrhagic infarction of lung tissue due to fungal infiltration.

3. **What is the prognosis?**
   Angioinvasive pulmonary aspergillosis carries a high mortality (at least 40%), even if treated.

Key points

- *Aspergillus* is a genus of fungus found in the environment. *Aspergillus fumigatus* is the most usual cause of human disease.
  - **Saprophytic infection** (aspergilloma). The fungus colonizes a pre-existing lung cavity or dilated airway. Radiologically, this disease is characterized by a mobile mass outlined by air within a cavity ('air-crescent sign').
  - **Allergic bronchopulmonary aspergillosis**. This disease represents a hypersensitivity reaction in response to *Aspergillus* colonization of the airways. The patient often has a history of asthma. If untreated, the disease leads to bronchiectasis. CT demonstrates predominantly central bronchiectasis with mucoid impaction.
  - **Semi-invasive aspergillosis** (chronic necrotizing aspergillosis). This is a rare form of aspergillosis and occurs in chronically ill patients (e.g. patients on corticosteroids, diabetics). Radiography often shows slowly progressive lobar consolidation, bronchial scarring, pulmonary nodularity and pleural thickening. The pulmonary lesions can cavitate. The disease is difficult to distinguish from tuberculosis clinically and radiologically.
  - **Airway invasive aspergillosis** tends to affect immunocompromised patients. The fungus invades the airway basement membrane. It can cause tracheobronchitis, bronchiolitis or bronchopneumonia, with a corresponding radiographic pattern.
  - **Angioinvasive aspergillosis** occurs in severely immunocompromised patients. The infection is due to invasion of blood vessels resulting in infarction and necrosis. Initially presents as ill-defined, nodular areas of consolidation which on CT has a ground-glass halo. When patients mount an immune response these areas will cavitate, and an air-crescent sign will be seen just like that seen in aspergillomas in immunocompetent individuals.
- Early angioinvasive pulmonary aspergillosis often only manifests as ill-defined nodular areas of consolidation, and on CT you will see the surrounding ground-glass halo. Cavitation in the immunosuppressed is a late sign as the patient mounts an immune response (recovery stage).

Further reading

Franquet T, Müller NL, Gimenez A, *et al*. Spectrum of pulmonary aspergillosis: histologic, clinical, and radiologic findings. *Radiographics* 2001; **21**: 825–37.

Kenney HH, Agrons GA, Shin JS. Best cases from the AFIP. Invasive pulmonary aspergillosis: radiologic and pathologic findings. *Radiographics* 2002; **22**: 1507–10.

Images courtesy of Dr Nestor Müller, Vancouver General Hospital.

Cardiothoracic Case 39

KIAT T. TAN AND PATRICIA DUNLOP

Clinical history
25-year-old male involved in road traffic collision. In extremis. Shock.

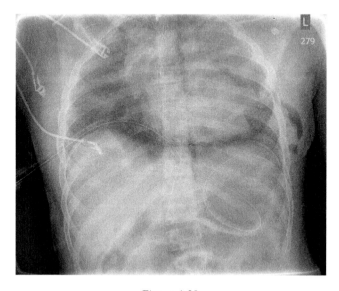

Figure 1.39

Model answer
This is a frontal chest radiograph of a skeletally mature patient (Figure 1.39). The right central-line tip is projected over the right innominate vein and is kinked as it crosses the first rib. This line will need to be replaced. The NG tube is appropriately placed. There is a large-bore tube that extends from the lower right chest, with its side-hole over the mediastinum and tip over the epigastrium.

There is a moderate left pneumothorax. A large pneumopericardium is present. Associated pneumomediastinum is also present. Subcutaneous gas is seen in the left lower chest. There is airspace opacification in both lungs, which is more prominent on the left. The differential diagnoses for this finding are wide, and include lung contusion, fluid overload and aspiration. In severe trauma it is worth considering head injuries, which may be implicated in the development of 'neurogenic' pulmonary oedema. There is widening of the superior mediastinum and the aortic arch is indistinct, which may suggest traumatic aortic injury. No rib fractures.

The radiological findings could be consistent with tension pneumopericardium. The right-sided large-bore tube may be either a malpositioned chest drain or a pericardial drain. Appropriate clinical information would be important in this situation. Clinical findings of tension pneumopericardium include raised JVP, pulsus paradoxus and cardiogenic shock. I will liaise with the clinician to determine if the patient should have immediate pericardial drainage. When the tension pneumopericardium has been treated, the patient will need a CT scan to assess the severity of chest injury as well as to detect occult injury. Particular attention should be paid to the aorta.

Questions
1. **What is tension pneumopericardium?**
   Compression of the heart by air in the pericardium, resulting in poor cardiac filling (similar to cardiac tamponade).
2. **How is it treated?**
   Immediate pericardial drainage.

Key points
- Tension pneumopericardium is uncommon but is associated with 50% mortality.
- Tension pneumopericardium is usually due to trauma. Other causes include infection by gas-forming organisms, fistulation between a hollow viscus and the pericardium and tracking of gas along the mediastinum with subsequent dissection into the pericardium.

Further reading
Hutchison SJ. *Pericardial Diseases: Clinical Imaging Atlas.* Philadelphia, PA: Elsevier, 2009.

Cardiothoracic Case 40

KIAT T. TAN AND PATRICIA DUNLOP

Clinical history
69-year-old man. Report the chest radiograph first.

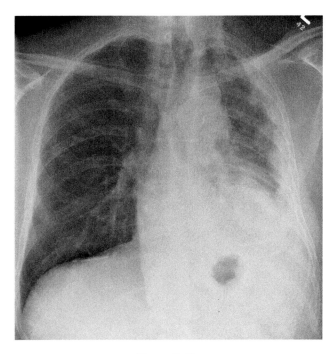

Figure 1.40a

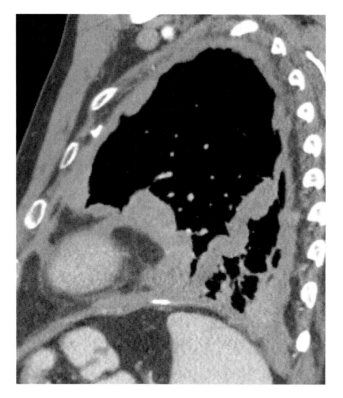

Figure 1.40b

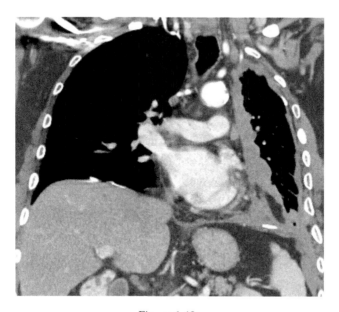

Figure 1.40c

Model answer

This is a PA radiograph of a skeletally mature individual (Figure 1.40a). The patient is rotated. The mediastinum is shifted to the left and the left hemithorax is smaller than the right. There is circumferential nodular pleural thickening extending from the apex to the base of the left hemithorax. Bilateral calcified pleural plaques are present. No bony abnormality is noted. The findings are strongly suspicious of mesothelioma due to previous asbestos exposure. A less likely differential diagnosis would be previous exposure to asbestos and concurrent pleural metastatic disease. Tumours that metastasize to the pleura include lung, breast, ovary and gastrointestinal neoplasms. A CT scan should be performed for further characterization of disease.

These are two images from a CT scan of the chest (Figures 1.40b, 1.40c). There is extensive left circumferential nodular pleural thickening which extends into the left major fissure. In some regions the pleural thickening is greater than 1 cm. There are bilateral calcified pleural plaques. There is probable invasion of the left hemidiaphragm.

The patient will need to be referred to a chest physician. The pleural disease is easily biopsied to obtain a definitive diagnosis but the patient (and clinician) should be aware of the possibility of tumour seeding into the biopsy tract, which is said to occur in up to 15% of cases.

Questions
1. **How do you differentiate benign from malignant pleural disease?**
   Malignant pleural thickening tends to be more than 1 cm thick, demonstrates nodularity, invades the chest wall, involves the mediastinal pleura and grows circumferentially around the lung.
2. **Can you diagnose mesothelioma without resorting to biopsy? What are the challenges with achieving a diagnosis? How would you suggest the biopsy be done?**
   The diagnostic yield is low with thoracentesis and cytology. Tissue diagnosis is usually required for diagnosis. However, it is difficult for the pathologist to separate some types of mesothelioma from adenocarcinoma, benign pleuritis and pleural plaque, and to distinguish reactive mesothelial hyperplasia from early mesothelioma. Immunohistochemistry stains are generally used, and a new special calretinin stain is most helpful. Electron microscopy is used as the gold standard in difficult cases. There is a move towards image-guided needle biopsy, which has a high diagnostic accuracy and lower incidence of seeding of tumour along the biopsy tract when compared to video-assisted thoracoscopic surgery.

Key points
- Mesothelioma is increasing in incidence.
- All forms of mesotheliomas are associated with asbestos exposure. Extrapleural sites of mesothelioma include the peritoneum, pericardium and scrotum.
- Infection (in particular, tuberculosis) can often be difficult to differentiate from pleural tumours on imaging.

Further reading
Müller NL, Silva CIS. *Imaging of the Chest*, Volume II. Philadelphia, PA: Saunders Elsevier, 2008; 1401–20.
Rubens MB, Padley SP. The pleura. In Sutton D, ed., *Textbook of Radiology and Imaging*, 7th edn. London: Elsevier, 2003; 87–107.

Images courtesy of Dr Nestor Müller, Vancouver General Hospital.

Cardiothoracic Case 41

JOHN CURTIS

Clinical history

17-year-old male with cough and wheeze.

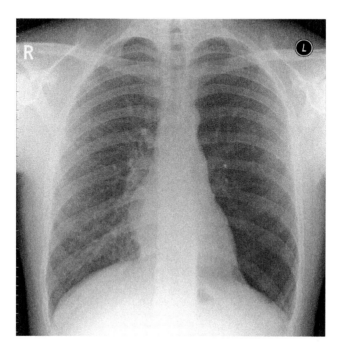

Figure 1.41a

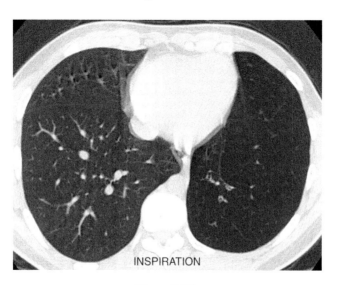

Figure 1.41b

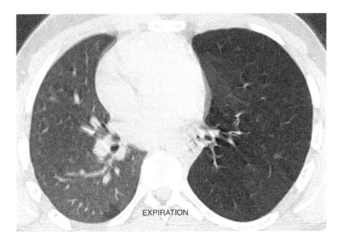

Figure 1.41c

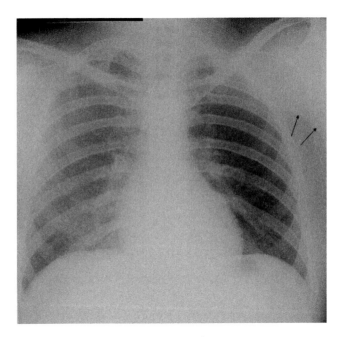

Figure 1.41d

Model answer

This PA chest radiograph of an adult male (Figure 1.41a) demonstrates unilateral hypertransradiancy of the left lung. There is global reduction in the pulmonary vasculature on the left side with a small left pulmonary artery. There is very mild volume loss in the left hemithorax. There are no obvious chest wall deformities and there is an impression of straightening of the left heart border. The heart is of normal size with otherwise normal mediastinal contours. I would like to obtain previous radiographs, and if this feature were long-standing this would point towards MacLeod's syndrome.

The reduced vascularity strongly points to left-sided pulmonary pathology rather than a soft tissue abnormality. The appearances may be due to MacLeod's syndrome (Swyer–James syndrome) or bronchial obstruction. An expiratory view demonstrating air trapping is very useful (Figures 1.41b, 1.41c). Ultimately an endobronchial lesion must be excluded.

Questions

1. What is MacLeod's syndrome?

This is also known as Swyer–James syndrome. It is a post-infective bronchiolitis in which submucosal fibrosis develops in the wall of medium-sized and small airways. This results in air trapping. The hypoxic environment results in chronic pulmonary artery vasoconstriction and subsequent underdevelopment of the pulmonary vasculature.

2. What are the other causes of unilateral hypertransradiancy?

Pulmonary causes (i.e. reduced vascular perfusion)

- Congenital
  - pulmonary artery aplasia
  - hypoplasia of lung
  - congenital lobar emphysema
  - proximal interruption of the pulmonary artery
- Acquired
  - pulmonary embolism
  - fibrosing mediastinitis
  - bronchial obstruction with hyperinflation ('ball-valve' effect) – e.g. endobronchial carcinoid
  - bronchial obstruction with compensatory hyperinflation of unaffected lobe – e.g. left lower lobe collapse due to endobronchial tumour and hyperinflation of the left upper lobe

Chest wall causes

- Absence of pectoralis major. This feature is characterized by asymmetry of the axillary folds (arrows on Figure 1.41d).
- Mastectomy
- Soft tissue excess on contralateral side – e.g. subcutaneous lipoma

Pleural thickening or effusion on supine radiographs

Technical factors

- Rotation: the side to which the patient is rotated appears hyperlucent
- 'Heel-toe' artefact of the x-ray beam

Key points

- Unilateral hypertransradiancy can be a challenging film in the viva and in practice.
- The first step is to look at the lung that is hypertransradiant and assess the vessels. If the number and size of vessels is reduced on the hypertransradiant side, the pathology is likely to be pulmonary. Conversely, if the vessels on this side are normal, there is either (a) a loss of soft tissue on the hypertransradiant side (e.g. Poland's syndrome, mastectomy) or (b) 'too much' soft tissue on the contralateral side (e.g. chest wall soft tissue mass or lipoma).
- MacLeod's syndrome is caused by a post-infective bronchiolitis in the developing lung (usually viral: measles, adenoviruses, occasionally mycoplasma). It usually affects one lung but may be segmental and bilateral.
  - The affected lung is aerated by collateral air drift through the pores of Kohn.
  - Reduced size of affected lung. Typically expiratory views demonstrate air trapping – hyperexpansion of the affected lung (Figures 1.41b, 1.41c). This is not seen with proximal interruption of the pulmonary artery.
  - Reduced number and size of pulmonary arteries. May be associated with bronchiectasis.
  - Clinical: often asymptomatic or wheeze with exertional dyspnoea.

• Identical radiographic features can be seen with slow-growing endobronchial tumours creating a 'ball-valve' effect, and it is essential to exclude such pathology with either bronchoscopy or multidetector CT. Conventional pulmonary angiography is not indicated.

Further reading

Davis SD. Case 28: proximal interruption of the right pulmonary artery. *Radiology* 2000; **217**: 437–40.

Pipavath SJ, Lynch DA, Cool C, Brown KK, Newell JD. Radiologic and pathologic features of bronchiolitis. *AJR Am J Roentgenol* 2005; **185**: 354–63.

Webb WR. Radiology of obstructive pulmonary disease. *AJR Am J Roentgenol* 1997; **169**: 637–47.

Cardiothoracic Case 42

JOHN CURTIS

Clinical history

Chest pain in a 40-year-old female who is otherwise well.

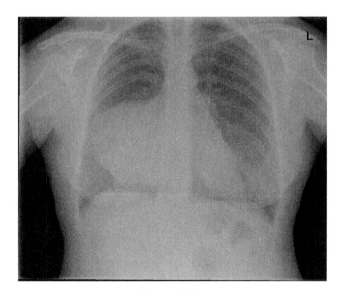

Figure 1.42a

Model answer

This frontal chest radiograph (Figure 1.42a) demonstrates a large mediastinal mass lesion that obscures the right heart border. It is sharp laterally and indistinct superomedially and inferomedially – typical of a non-pulmonary mediastinal lesion. It appears to be solitary. The heart appears normal in size. Lung fields are otherwise clear. No bony destruction.

The appearances suggest an anterior mediastinal mass lesion. The most likely diagnosis is a teratoma. The differential diagnosis is thymoma. Thyroid enlargement is very unlikely as the mass is not contiguous with the neck. Lymphoma is unlikely, as this appears to be a solitary lesion. I would like to carry out a CT of the thorax for further evaluation.

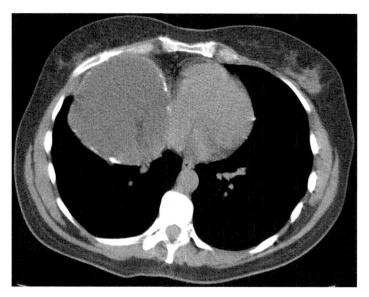

Figure 1.42b

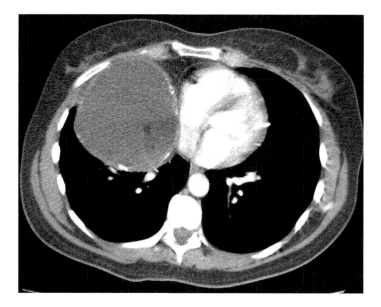

Figure 1.42c

Questions

1. **What does the CT show?**

Pre- and post-contrast-enhanced CT of the thorax (Figures 1.42b, 1.42c) demonstrates a large mass in the anterior mediastinum. There is rim calcification surrounding a predominantly fluid-containing cyst with a focal area of fat density. These appearances are diagnostic of teratoma and almost certainly the benign cystic variant – the so-called benign cystic dermoid.

- Look at the chest radiograph as if looking at the patient from the 'end of the bed' clinically. That way, you are less likely to overlook a mastectomy or mass lesions, e.g. in the neck or axillae.

Cardiothoracic Case 44

JOHN CURTIS

Clinical history

(a) A 13-year-old boy with acute shortness of breath.
(b) A 25-year-old man with cough and fever.

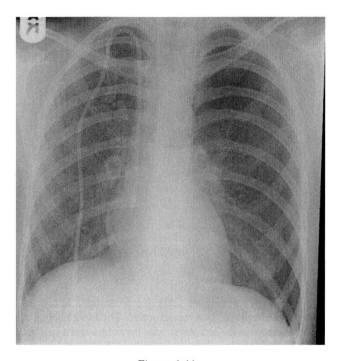

Figure 1.44a

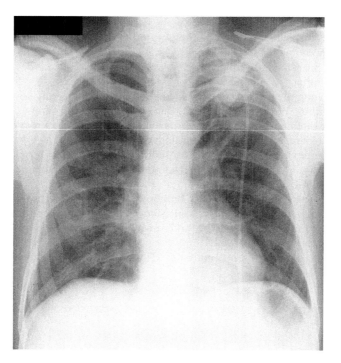

Figure 1.44b

Model answer

Figure 1.44a is a frontal chest radiograph demonstrating a left pneumothorax. There is a right-sided Hickman line with its tip in the right atrium, which is a suboptimal position as the tip of a Hickman line should ideally be at the cavoatrial junction. There is an ovoid mass lesion in the left lower lobe. The appearances suggest a metastasis in the left lower lobe in a patient receiving chemotherapy. The most likely diagnosis is an osteosarcoma metastasis in the lung, complicated by a pneumothorax. I would like to carry out a staging CT of the thorax for further evaluation with a view to discussion in the lung cancer or sarcoma multidisciplinary team meeting.

Figure 1.44b is a frontal chest radiograph demonstrating cavities in the left upper lobe and right mid zone both containing a soft tissue density mass and air-crescent signs. There are areas of consolidation adjacent to these cavitating lesions. The appearances are those of invasive aspergillosis. There is a left-sided Hickman line with its tip in the superior vena cava, which could suggest chemotherapy and an immunocompromised state. I would like to confirm this with an appropriate clinical history. The patient will require a CT scan of the chest to assess the degree of pulmonary involvement.

Questions

1. What other pathology should you look for in patients with a Hickman line?
- Bony pathology – destruction of bone may indicate metastatic disease.
- Barium swallow – may show oesophageal candidiasis and a Hickman line on the same image. These abnormalities should be linked and imply immunocompromised status.
- Mediastinal lymphadenopathy.
- Bilateral perihilar airspace shadowing without effusions or lymphadenopathy – think of *Pneumocystis jirovecii* pneumonia.

Key points

- Osteosarcoma metastases in the lung are often implicated in the development of pneumothorax. Necrosis of a metastatic lesion in the subpleural lung with a resulting bronchopleural fistula is the usual mechanism of the development of pneumothorax.
- Calcified lung metastases are very uncommon and more readily seen at CT than on plain films. When they do occur, think about metastases from osteosarcoma and other sarcomas and metastases from colon, ovarian and thyroid carcinoma.
- Invasive aspergillosis on the chest radiograph – 25% of cases may show no abnormality. Abnormalities include: nodular infiltrates, ground-glass opacification, consolidation and cavitation with air-crescent formation (which is more likely in the recovery phase of neutropenia).
- The air-crescent sign can be seen in both invasive aspergillosis and aspergilloma. Less typical causes of an air-crescent sign include lung abscess, necrotic lung tumour, pulmonary haematoma and tuberculous cavitation with Rasmussen aneurysm formation.
- Cavities may lead to pneumothorax (Figure 1.44c: arrows denote areas of aspergillosis).

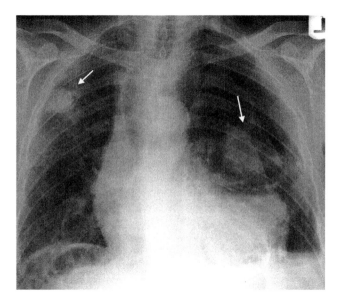

Figure 1.44c

Further reading

Buckingham SJ, Hansell DM. Aspergillus in the lung: diverse and coincident forms. *Eur Radiol* 2003; **13**: 1786–800.

Seo JB, Im JG, Goo JM, Chung MJ, Kim MY. Atypical pulmonary metastases: spectrum of radiologic findings. *Radiographics* 2001; **21**: 403–17.

Figure 1.44b courtesy of Dr Brian Eyes, University Hospital Aintree, Liverpool.

Vascular Case 45

KIAT T. TAN AND RICHARD J. T. OWEN

Clinical history

Young male track athlete presenting with exertional calf pain. Images were obtained using gadofosveset trisodium (Ablavar, formerly Vasovist).

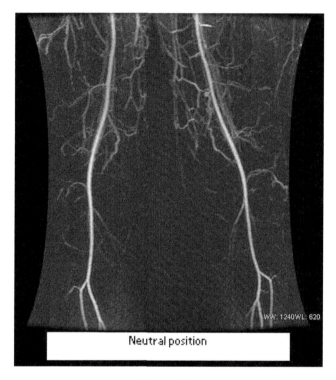

Figure 1.45a

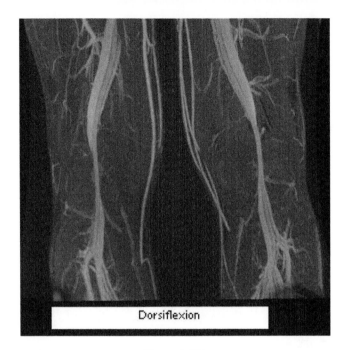

Figure 1.45b

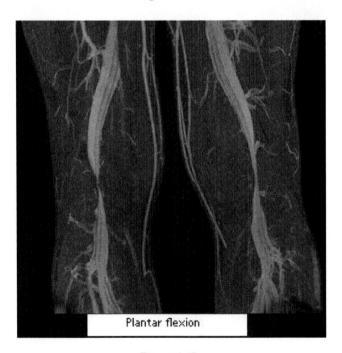

Figure 1.45c

Model answer

I am presented with three contrast-enhanced MR angiography images (Figures 1.45a–1.45c). The first is a sequence performed in the first-pass arterial phase, with the foot in a neutral position. The other two images are steady-state images with the foot in plantar and dorsiflexion. The MRAs with the foot in a neutral position and dorsi-flexion are normal. The image obtained in plantar flexion shows obliteration of the lumen of the right popliteal artery and some narrowing of the contralateral vessel. The findings are diagnostic of popliteal arterial entrapment syndrome. I would like to review the images on a workstation to confirm the diagnosis. In addition, I would like to obtain additional T1 imaging of the popliteal region to diagnose anatomical variants that could result in the syndrome. The result would need to be communicated to the referring clinician, as the patient will need to be referred for surgery.

Questions

1. **What are the causes of popliteal arterial entrapment?**
   The syndrome occurs due to compression of the artery by one (or more) of the following: (a) abnormal insertion of the lateral head of the gastrocnemius muscle; (b) a fibrous band; (c) anatomically normal muscle (also known as 'functional' popliteal arterial entrapment).
2. **Why did you suggest further T1-weighted imaging?**
   T1 imaging is excellent at delineating the anatomy around the knee joint. This enables the accurate detection of abnormal muscle insertion/fibrous bands. Axial T1 is the most useful view.
3. **Why do you recommend surgery?**
   Popliteal arterial entrapment (including the 'functional form') can lead to irreversible arteriosclerosis of the artery.

Key points

- Functional popliteal arterial entrapment tends to affect muscular young men and is believed to be due to calf muscle hypertrophy.
- A large proportion of 'normal' individuals demonstrate occlusion of the popliteal artery on plantar flexion. Therefore, MRI is used to exclude disease and delineate anatomy rather than for disease detection.
- Gadofosveset trisodium is a gadolinium-based blood-pool contrast agent that persists in the circulation rather than being excreted immediately. In contrast to conventional single-pass MRI contrast agents, blood-pool contrast agents enable repeated imaging of the circulation, thus enabling the stress views to be obtained.

Further reading

Macedo TA, Johnson CM, Hallett JW, Breen JF. Popliteal entrapment syndrome: role of imaging in the diagnosis. *AJR Am J Roentgenol* 2003; **181**: 1259–65.

Turnipseed WD. Functional popliteal artery entrapment syndrome: a poorly understood and often missed diagnosis that is frequently mistreated. *J Vasc Surg* 2009; **49**: 1189–95.

Vascular Case 46

KIAT T. TAN AND RICHARD J. T. OWEN

Clinical history
Severe abdominal pain.

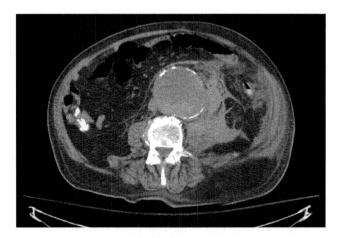

Figure 1.46a

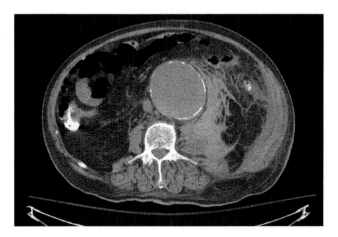

Figure 1.46b

Model answer
These are two non-contrast CT images of the abdomen (Figures 1.46a, 1.46b). The aorta is grossly enlarged. There is an apparent breach in the left lateral wall of the aorta, as evidenced by discontinuity of the calcified wall and loss of the adjacent fat plane. There is fluid of high attenuation in the left retroperitoneum. There is associated adjacent fat stranding and swelling of the left lateral abdominal wall muscles. The IVC is small, consistent with fluid depletion. The findings are consistent with a leaking abdominal aortic aneurysm. I would like to review the images on a

workstation to assess the extent of the aneurysm and leak. In addition, any coexisting morbidities should be reported. I will inform the on-call surgeon immediately, as the patient will require immediate intervention. Endovascular treatment may be an option, although this is limited to a few centres.

Questions

1. **Aortic size varies between individuals. How do you define an aneurysm?**

   An aneurysm is an abnormal dilatation of a blood vessel above 1.5 times its normal size. The upper limit of normal for the abdominal aorta is 2 cm. Therefore, an aortic aneurysm is an aortic segment that is larger than 3 cm.

2. **What do you know about the NHS abdominal aortic aneurysm screening programme? Who should be screened and at what age?**

   The programme is being introduced in England. Men are invited for a single ultrasound scan of the abdomen at the age of 65. Older men can self-refer for screening.

Key points

- Endovascular treatment of aortic aneurysm is increasingly being utilized. However, there is a lack of long-term data. Existing evidence suggests that the lower post-procedure complication rate of this procedure when compared to open repair is balanced out by a higher late complication rate.
- The choice between open and endovascular elective aneurysm repair should be based on patient preference. A reasonable approach is to recommend open repair to younger (and fitter) patients and endovascular treatment to older (less fit) patients.
- On plain radiography, a leaking aortic aneurysm may be present as a unilateral loss of a psoas outline. Always look for this sign (especially when given a history of renal colic in the FRCR exam!).

Further reading

EVAR trial participants. Endovascular aneurysm repair versus open repair in patients with abdominal aortic aneurysm (EVAR trial 1): randomised controlled trial. *Lancet* 2005; **365**: 2179–86.

Nicholson A, Patel J. The aorta, including intervention. In Adam A, Dixon AK, eds., *Grainger and Allison's Diagnostic Radiology*, 5th edn. London: Churchill Livingstone, 2008 (ebook).

UK Small Aneurysm Trial Participants. Mortality results for randomised controlled trial of early elective surgery or ultrasonographic surveillance for small abdominal aortic aneurysms. *Lancet* 1998; **352**: 1649–55.

Vascular Case 47

KIAT T. TAN AND RICHARD J. T. OWEN

Clinical history

16-year-old female. Symptoms of fever, arthralgia and transient ischaemic attack. Report the CT first.

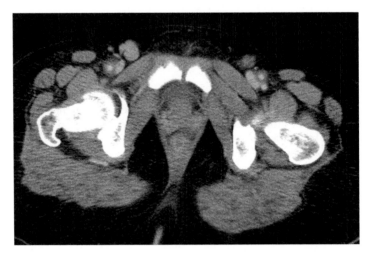

Figure 1.47a

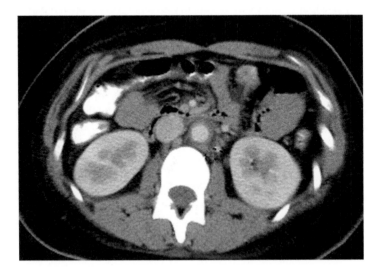

Figure 1.47b

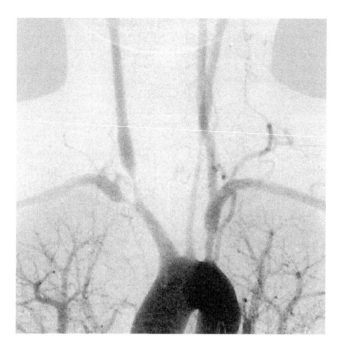

Figure 1.47c

Model answer

These are two images from a CT angiogram of the patient (Figures 1.47a, 1.47b). There is ill-defined circumferential thickening of the walls of the aorta and femoral arteries. The findings are suggestive of a large to medium-sized vessel vasculitic process, the most likely of which would be Takayasu's arteritis. I would like to review the rest of the imaging to look for involvement of other arteries.

The arch aortogram (Figure 1.47c) demonstrates smooth severe tapered stenoses at the origins of the right subclavian, right carotid and left carotid arteries. There is mild narrowing of the origin of the left subclavian artery. The right vertebral artery is not visualized and is likely to be occluded. There is hypertrophy of the left vertebral artery. The findings are consistent with Takayasu's arteritis and would fit the patient's clinical presentation.

I will communicate the results to the referring clinician. Treatment is by cortico-steroids and immunosuppressives to reduce vascular inflammation. A follow-up MRI is recommended.

Questions

1. **What are your differential diagnoses?**
   In an older patient, my differential diagnosis would include giant-cell arteritis. Infection should always be excluded in patients with vasculitis. Infections that cause aortitis include syphilis and tuberculosis.
2. **Why do you suggest MRI follow-up?**
   This young patient will require repeated imaging and radiation would be an issue long-term. In addition, there are some data to suggest that delayed contrast-enhanced MR imaging may be useful to detect active vascular inflammation.
3. **When should the patient be referred for angioplasty?**
   If the arterial narrowing persists despite resolution of active inflammation, the offending vessel could be angioplastied. Angioplasty of an actively inflamed vessel should be avoided if at all possible.

Key points

- Takayasu's arteritis is an inflammatory condition affecting the aorta, the pulmonary arteries and the major branches of the aorta.
- Early Takayasu's arteritis presents with fever, myalgia and arthralgia (the 'pre-pulseless stage'). The late stage of presentation ('pulseless stage') presents with ischaemic symptoms.
- Takayasu's arteritis is classified in four different types:
  type 1, where there is involvement of the branches of the arch
  type 2, a combination of types 1 and 3
  type 3, involvement of the aorta and its branches distal to the arch
  type 4, aneurysmal dilatation of the aorta

Further reading

Gotway MB, Araoz PA, Macedo TA, *et al*. Imaging findings in Takayasu's arteritis. *AJR Am J Roentgenol* 2005; **184**: 1945–50.

Nastri MV, Baptista LP, Baroni RH, *et al*. Gadolinium-enhanced three-dimensional MR angiography of Takayasu arteritis. *Radiographics* 2004; **24**: 773–86.

Vascular Case 48

KIAT T. TAN AND RICHARD J. T. OWEN

Clinical history

Young female. Hypertension.

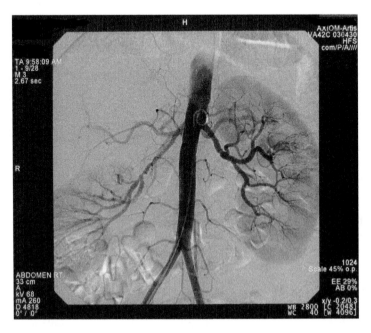

Figure 1.48

Model answer

This is a digitally subtracted flush aortogram performed with the pigtail catheter sited at the level of the renal arteries (Figure 1.48). The main renal arteries are abnormal bilaterally, with regions of stenoses in their mid-distal portions. These areas demonstrate beading, with alternating areas of stenosis and dilatation. The proximal renal arteries are normal. The aorta and other visualized arteries are normal. The findings are consistent with fibromuscular dysplasia (FMD). The patient will require angioplasty of the lesions. In addition, as FMD can cause carotid stenosis and is associated with intracerebral aneurysms, the patient should have a screening MR angiogram for the detection of these lesions.

Questions

1. **You mentioned renal and carotid arteries. Does FMD affect any other vessel?**
   Any other medium-sized vessel can be affected, including mesenteric, coeliac and iliac arteries.
2. **What is the major cause of renal artery stenosis?**
   Atherosclerosis.
3. **How do you differentiate atherosclerotic renal artery stenosis from fibromuscular dysplasia?**
   Atherosclerotic renal artery stenosis typically affects the origin of the renal artery. FMD usually affects the mid-distal renal artery and has a beaded appearance. In addition, FMD usually affects young patients while atherosclerotic disease affects older patients.
4. **Is the treatment for the hypertension associated with atherosclerotic renal artery stenosis different from that of FMD?**
   Yes. Angioplasty is the treatment of choice in FMD. There is no evidence to show that angioplasty is superior to optimal medical therapy to control hypertension in atherosclerotic renal artery stenosis.

Key points

- FMD is most commonly seen in young women.
- Atherosclerosis accounts for 90% of renal artery stenosis, with the remaining 10% due to FMD. Rare causes of renal artery stenosis include neurofibromatosis and congenital renal artery stenosis.
- Angioplasty alone is effective in the vast majority of patients with renal artery FMD. Stent placement is reserved for those who develop complications (e.g. rupture, dissection).

Further reading

Dubel GJ, Murphy TP. The role of percutaneous revascularization in renal artery stenosis. *Vasc Med* 2008; **13**: 141–56.

Olin JW, Pierce M. Contemporary management of fibromuscular dysplasia. *Curr Opin Cardiol* 2008; **23**: 527–36.

Vascular Case 49

KIAT T. TAN AND RICHARD J. T. OWEN

Clinical history
Abdominal pain and sepsis post-hepatic artery chemoembolization for hepatocellular carcinoma.

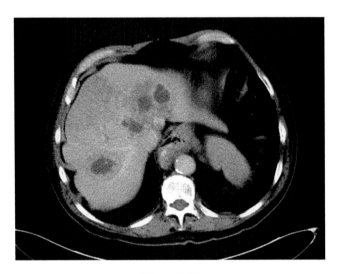

Figure 1.49

Model answer
This is a single axial image from an intravenous contrast-enhanced CT scan of the abdomen (Figure 1.49). There are four rounded hypoattenuating lesions with irregular thick enhancing rinds. There is a further wedge-shaped region of hypoattenuation in the periphery of the liver. The radiological differential diagnosis would be between disease recurrence in embolized regions and hepatic abscesses arising in necrotic tumour. In view of the history of sepsis, the latter is more likely. I will discuss the case with the referring clinician immediately, as the patient will need parenteral antibiotics, blood cultures and drainage of the abscesses. I would also like to review the rest of the imaging to look for other abscesses and complications of hepatic chemoembolization.

Questions
1. **Which conditions predispose to post-embolization hepatic abscesses?**
   Systemic sepsis, previous violation of the sphincter of Oddi with stenting or sphincterotomy, prior surgical treatments such as Roux-en-Y anastomoses and other hepatico-jejunostomies.
2. **What are the other complications of hepatic chemoembolization?**
   Liver failure, systemic effects of chemotherapy, embolization of adjacent structures (e.g. stomach, small intestine), complications of angiography, post-embolization syndrome.

Key points
- Chemoembolization is increasingly used in the treatment of hepatocellular carcinoma unsuitable for resection and as a bridge to transplantation. Some metastatic tumours (e.g. carcinoid) may also be suitable for chemoembolization.

- Chemoembolization involves the subselective catheterization of the artery (or as close as possible to the artery) supplying the tumour, with subsequent injection of chemotherapy into the catheter.
- Abscess can be difficult to differentiate from tumour necrosis and/or disease recurrence. Clinical history is key.

Further reading

Chung J, Yu JS, Chung JJ, Kim JH, Kim KW. Haemodynamic events and localised parenchymal changes following transcatheter arterial chemoembolisation for hepatic malignancy: interpretation of imaging findings. *Br J Radiol* 2010; **83**: 71–81.

Gates J, Hartnell GG, Stuart KE, Clouse ME. Chemoembolization of hepatic neoplasms: safety, complications and when to worry. *Radiographics* 1999; **19**: 399–414.

Vascular Case 50

KIAT T. TAN AND RICHARD J. T. OWEN

Clinical history

Young woman. Previous pregnancy-associated DVT. Now presenting with chest pain.

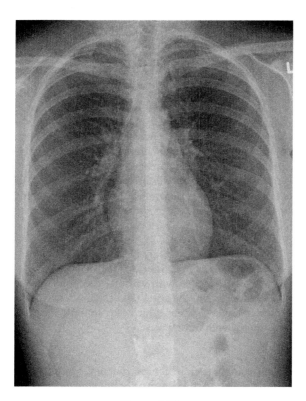

Figure 1.50a

Gastrointestinal Case 1

KIAT T. TAN AND RICHARD HOPKINS

Clinical history
Dysphagia and retrosternal pain. HIV-positive.

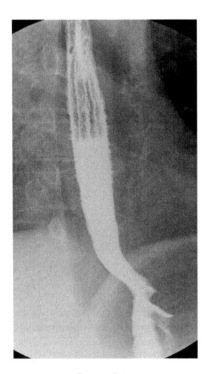

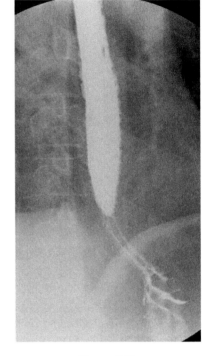

Figure 2.1a   Figure 2.1b

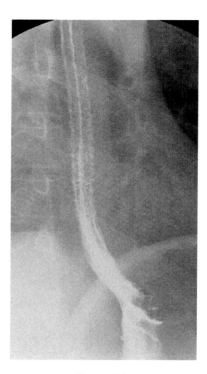

Figure 2.1c

Model answer

The barium swallow (Figures 2.1a–2.1c) shows a longitudinally arranged, shaggy serrated appearance of the middle and lower third of the oesophagus with innumerable small filling defects. Multiple tiny erosions and areas of ulceration are present. There is no evidence of obstruction or barium hold-up. No mass lesions identified. No stricture formation. Features are likely to represent candida oesophagitis, particularly given the history of HIV. This is an opportunistic infection of the oesophagus. I would like to examine the patient for evidence of oropharyngeal candidiasis, which is often manifested as white plaques in the mouth. As candida oesophagitis is an AIDS-defining illness in an HIV-positive patient, I would also like to discuss the case urgently with the referring clinician to ensure appropriate clinical management. Fungal cultures from the upper gastrointestinal tract can be obtained for definitive diagnosis.

Questions

1. **What are the symptoms associated with candida oesophagitis?**
   Symptoms include dysphagia, retrosternal chest pain and odynophagia. Oral thrush may be present. Weight loss is common. There may be associated nausea and vomiting. Fever is not typical of candida oesophagitis and may suggest another cause or fulminant systemic infection.

2. **Which patient groups are predisposed to candida oesophagitis?**
   Susceptible patient groups include individuals on inhaled steroid therapy or prolonged antibiotics, those who are HIV-positive, immunocompromised or elderly patients, or patients with delayed oesophageal emptying such as those with scleroderma, achalasia, strictures and post fundoplication.

Key points

- Candida oesophagitis is usually identified on barium studies as discrete, linear, or irregular plaque-like lesions separated by segments of normal intervening mucosa – mainly in the upper half of the oesophagus. In more advanced disease, coalescent plaques may produce a 'cobblestone' appearance or, in severe cases (usually in patients with AIDS), a grossly irregular or shaggy oesophagus caused by extensive plaque, pseudomembrane formation, intramural haemorrhage and ulcerations. In some cases, the disease can present with mycetoma formation, which may simulate an intramural neoplasm.

- Complications include dysphagia, progressive stricture formation, perforation, fistulas, and systemic candidiasis with dissemination into liver/spleen/kidneys and lungs.
- *Regarding aetiology of oesophagitis in patients with AIDS*: HIV, CMV and HSV can all cause oesophagitis. They typically cause large discrete ulcers, although severe disease can be difficult to distinguish radiologically from candida. *Mycobacterium tuberculosis* or atypical mycobacteria can also cause oesophageal ulceration.

Further reading

Federle M, Jeffrey RB, Anne VB. *Diagnostic Imaging of the Abdomen*. Salt Lake City, UT: Amirsys, 2004.

Roberts L, Gibbons R, Gibbons G, Rice RP, Thompson WM. Adult esophageal candidiasis: a radiographic spectrum. *Radiographics* 1987; **7**: 289–307.

Gastrointestinal Case 2

KIAT T. TAN AND RICHARD HOPKINS

Clinical history

Dysphagia. Report the chest radiograph first.

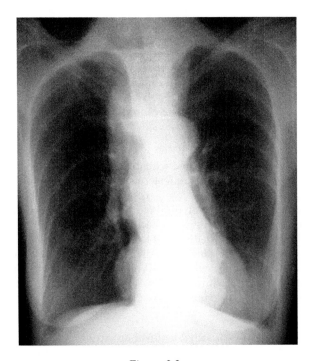

Figure 2.2a

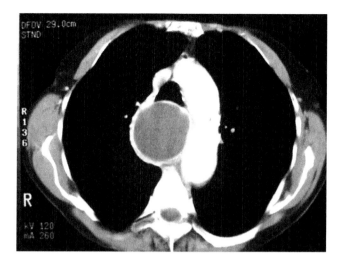

Figure 2.2b

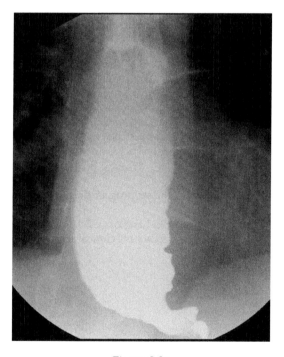

Figure 2.2c

Model answer

There is a gas-filled structure in the posterior mediastinum that extends from the upper mediastinum to the level of the gastro-oesophageal junction (Figures 2.2a, 2.2b). The features are of a dilated oesophagus.

The barium examination (Figure 2.2c) confirms the presence of a dilated oesophagus, together with a 'bird's-beak' lower oesophageal sphincter. Tertiary contractions are demonstrated in the distal oesophagus. The features are consistent with achalasia. The differential diagnoses include infiltrating carcinoma and Chagas' disease,

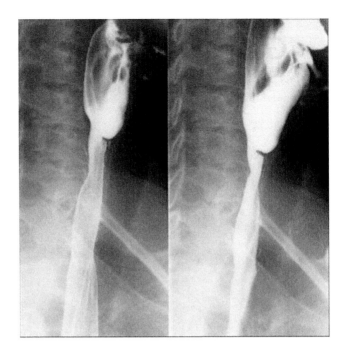

Figure 2.3b

Model answer

These are four images from a barium swallow study (Figures 2.3a, 2.3b). There are multiple, small, flask-shaped outpouchings that are of uniform depth. These findings are typical of oesophageal intramural pseudodiverticulosis. These are often associated with dysmotility and strictures, and there may be a link with oesophageal cancer. I would like to review the rest of the barium swallow study to look for these complications.

Questions

1. **What is oesophageal pseudodiverticulosis?**
   Anatomically, the pseudodiverticula are formed from dilatation of the oesophageal submucosal glands. They occur as a rare complication of oesophagitis.

Key points

- The pathogenesis of oesophageal pseudodiverticulosis is uncertain. However, stasis, blockage of the submucosal glands and inflammation are believed to be involved.
- The condition may cause dysphagia.

Further reading

Levine MS, Moolten DN, Herlinger H, Laufer I. Esophageal intramural pseudodiverticulosis: a reevaluation. *AJR Am J Roentgenol* 1986; **147**: 1165–70.

Mahajan SK, Warshauer DM, Bozymski EM. Esophageal intramural pseudo-diverticulosis: endoscopic and radiologic correlation. *Gastrointest Endosc* 1993; **39**: 565–7.

Gastrointestinal Case 4

KIAT T. TAN AND RICHARD HOPKINS

Clinical history

Repeated vomiting followed by severe chest pain. Report the chest radiograph first.

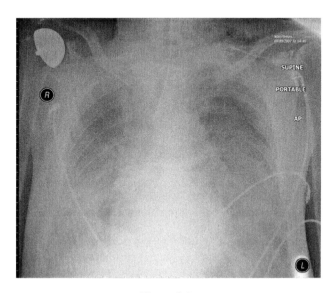

Figure 2.4a

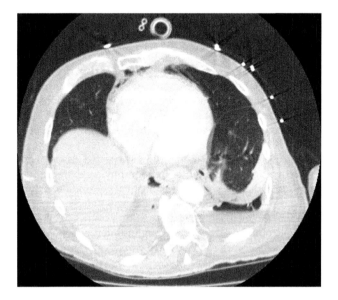

Figure 2.4b

Notes

The diagnosis is carcinoma of the left lower lobe bronchus with an associated mediastinal mass. There is extrinsic compression and invasion of the oesophagus where the mass is invading the mediastinum. The patient is not ventilating the left lung.

Further reading

Woodring JH. Unusual manifestations of lung cancer. *Radiol Clin North Am* 1990; **28**: 599–618.

Gastrointestinal Case 6

KIAT T. TAN AND RICHARD HOPKINS

Clinical history

History of haematemesis. Report the barium study first.

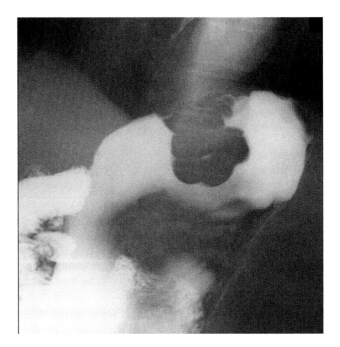

Figure 2.6a

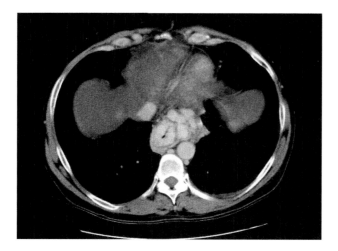

Figure 2.6b

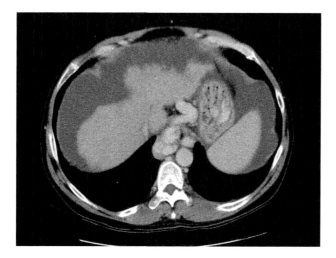

Figure 2.6c

Model answer

This is an image from an upper GI barium study (Figure 2.6a). The barium study shows a mass at the gastro-oesophageal junction. The mass is lobulated with a smooth edge, measuring several centimetres across and bulging into the lumen of the stomach. The differential diagnoses include gastro-oesophageal junction varices and neoplastic change. A clinical history would be useful. A CT scan is required for further characterization of the lesion.

The CT images are taken from the upper abdomen (Figures 2.6b, 2.6c). There are large enhancing vessels in the oesophagus and around the gastro-oesophageal junction consistent with the presence of varices. The liver has an irregular edge and there is ascites. The diagnosis is liver cirrhosis and gastro-oesophageal varices. I would like to review the rest of the imaging to look for other radiological evidence of cirrhosis as well its complications.

Questions
1. What are the common causes of cirrhosis?

Alcohol; viral hepatitis – hepatitis B and C; haemochromatosis; primary sclerosing cholangitis; primary biliary cirrhosis; cystic fibrosis; hepatic steatosis.

2. What are the CT features of cirrhosis?

- Irregular surface contour – this is due to regenerative nodules. It is often more conspicuous in the presence of ascitic fluid.
- Change in shape of the liver – enlargement of the caudate lobe, reduction in size of the right lobe.
- Widening of fissures between lobes.
- Fatty infiltration of the liver.
- Portal hypertension:
  - splenomegaly
  - recanalization of umbilical vein
  - portosystemic collaterals
  - increase in size of portal vein
  - ascites

3. What are the complications of liver cirrhosis that may be seen on a CT scan?

- Portal hypertension
- Hepatocellular carcinoma
- Portal vein thrombosis

Key points
- Cirrhosis is the end stage of a wide variety of chronic liver disease and is characterized by diffuse hepatic fibrosis and the presence of regenerating nodules.
- Radiologists are often asked to biopsy the cirrhotic liver. Check that coagulation and platelet count are acceptable before proceeding. Consider draining ascitic fluid prior to biopsy to reduce risk of bleeding. Transjugular liver biopsy should be considered in those at high risk of bleeding.

Further reading
Gupta AA, Kim DC, Krinsky GA, Lee VS. CT and MRI of cirrhosis and its mimics. *AJR Am J Roentgenol* 2004; **183**: 1595–601.

Kawamoto S, Soyer PA, Fishman EK, Bluemke DA. Nonneoplastic liver disease: evaluation with CT and MR imaging. *Radiographics* 1998; **18**: 827–48.

Gastrointestinal Case 7

KIAT T. TAN AND RICHARD HOPKINS

Clinical history
No history.

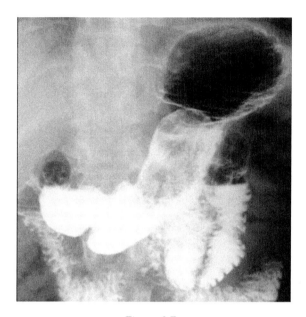

Figure 2.7a

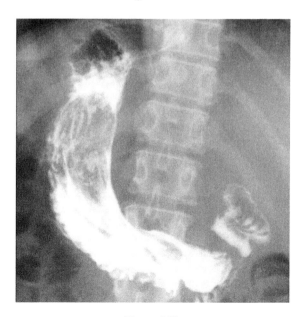

Figure 2.7b

Model answer

The two images (Figures 2.7a, 2.7b) are from a double-contrast barium meal examination and they show a large, ovoid mass in the body of the stomach. There is some speckled barium within the centre of the structure. The position of the mass is unchanged between the two images.

The features may be due to a bezoar, although a large mass such as a gastrointestinal stromal tumour (GIST) should also be considered. It would be possible to distinguish the two differentials if the mass could be confirmed as being freely mobile. Review of additional images from the study may help. I would like to obtain a clinical history of ingestion of hair or fibrous material from either the patient or the clinician in order to clinch the diagnosis. The patient will require further investigation by endoscopy or CT if a tumour is suspected.

Questions

1. **What are the radiological features of gastric bezoars?**
   On barium studies, bezoars are round or ovoid mottled or homogeneous masses. They can be mobile or immobile.

Key points

- A bezoar is a ball of hair or fibrous material trapped within the stomach, often caused by swallowing hair or fibrous materials.
- Prevalence of bezoars is greater among those with learning difficulties and in emotionally disturbed children, and they are most commonly seen in females aged 10–20 years.
- Other risk factors include gastroparesis, previous gastric surgery, including gastric bypass or vertical banded gastroplasty.

Further reading

Hewitt AN, Levine MS, Rubesin SE, Laufer I. Gastric bezoars: reassessment of clinical and radiographic findings in 19 patients. *Br J Radiol* 2009; **82**: 901–7.

Gastrointestinal Case 8

KIAT T. TAN AND RICHARD HOPKINS

Clinical history
No history.

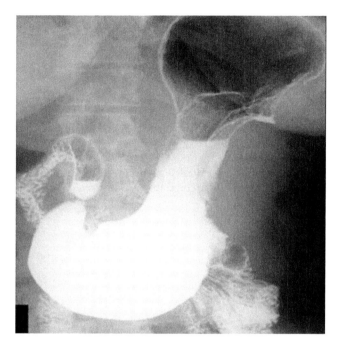

Figure 2.8

Model answer
This is a single image from a double-contrast barium meal examination (Figure 2.8). It shows a large mass arising from the greater curve of the stomach. The mass has a smooth surface. The fundus and antrum of the stomach and the duodenum are normal. Barium has passed freely into the proximal small bowel.

The differential diagnoses include adenocarcinoma, lymphoma, gastrointestinal stromal tumour and metastasis. I would like to review the rest of the imaging to look for other features of the tumour and also to find synchronous tumours. The patient will need an endoscopy with biopsy and a CT scan of the chest, abdomen and pelvis.

Questions
1. **What does an adenocarcinoma of a stomach look like on a barium study?**
   Gastric adenocarcinomas can present as an ulcerating mass, an intraluminal mass or a diffuse infiltrating lesion (i.e. linitis plastica).
2. **What are the risk factors for developing gastric adenocarcinoma?**
   Smoking, ingestion of nitrites (e.g. in preserved foods), *Helicobacter pylori* infection, atrophic gastritis, hereditary factors.

Key points

- There is a large amount of lymphoid tissue associated with mucosal surfaces (so-called mucosal-associated lymphoid tissue or MALT). Most gastric lymphomas are believed to arise from MALT. Indeed, low-grade gastric 'MALTomas' can occasionally resolve with treatment.
- Lymphomas of the stomach are indistinguishable from gastric adenocarcinomas. Gastric lymphomas tend to be more distensible than adenocarcinomas, and therefore 'distensible linitis plastica' (as opposed to the more usual non-distensible linitis plastica due to adenocarcinoma) is often due to lymphoma. Similarly, lymphomas are less likely to cause bowel obstruction than their carcinomatous counterpart.
- Staging of gastrointestinal lymphoma is the same as that of other non-Hodgkin's lymphoma.
- There is an association between gastrointestinal lymphoma and inflammatory diseases (e.g. *H. pylori* infection, Crohn's disease, coeliac disease, various auto-immune diseases). Immunosuppression, whether from drugs or HIV, is also a risk factor.

Notes

Biopsy of this mass showed it to be a lymphoma.

Further reading

Ghai S, Pattison J, Ghai S, *et al*. Primary gastrointestinal lymphoma: spectrum of imaging findings with pathologic correlation. *Radiographics* 2007; **27**: 1371–88.

Gastrointestinal Case 9

KIAT T. TAN AND RICHARD HOPKINS

Clinical history
No history.

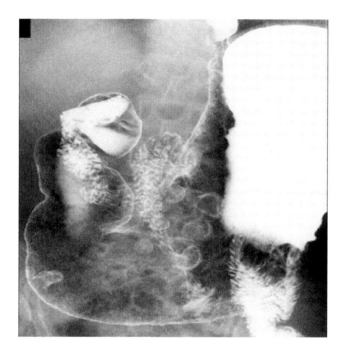

Figure 2.9a

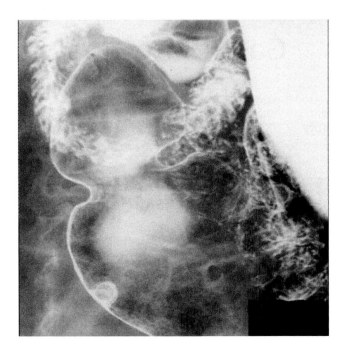

Figure 2.9b

Model answer

These are two images from a barium meal (Figures 2.9a, 2.9b). There are several ovoid polypoid lesions in the body and antrum of the stomach. These lesions are approximately 1 cm in diameter and are of similar size. The appearance is most likely to represent hyperplastic gastric polyps. A less likely differential diagnosis is multiple gastric adenomas. An endoscopy is recommended for direct visualization of the stomach. Endoscopic biopsies should be taken for histological study as well as for detection of *Helicobacter pylori*. If present, *H. pylori* should be eradicated to reduce the risk of malignancy.

Questions

1. **What is the usual location of gastric polyps?**
   Most gastric polyps are found in the antrum or body of the stomach.
2. **What is the underlying histology of most gastric polyps?**
   Approximately half of all polyps are solitary and half are multiple. Multiple polyps are usually hyperplastic. A minority of polyps are adenomas, and these are usually solitary. Multiple adenomas can occur in familial polyposis syndromes. A minority of miscellaneous conditions can mimic hyperplastic polyps and adenomas, including ectopic pancreas, small gastrointestinal stromal tumours (GISTs), submucosal metastases.
3. **How do you differentiate hyperplastic polyps from other polypoid lesions?**
   Hyperplastic polyps are smooth and less than 1 cm in diameter. The presence of ulceration, pedunculation or an irregular outline is an indication for urgent biopsy, although these features can sometimes be found in hyperplastic polyps. Adenomatous polyps tend to be larger than 1 cm and occur singly, although multiple lesions can sometimes be seen.

Key points

- Hyperplastic gastric polyps, although not premalignant, are associated with chronic atrophic gastritis, which is a risk factor for stomach malignancy.

- Chronic atrophic gastritis is most often due to either an autoimmune cause or *H. pylori* infection.

Further reading

Levine MS. Benign tumors. In: Gore RM, Levine MS, Laufer I, eds., *Textbook of Gastrointestinal Radiology*. Philadelphia, PA: Saunders, 1994; 628–58.

Wagner BJ, Brower AC. General case of the day: gastric hyperplastic polyps. *Radiographics* 1994; **14**: 682–5.

Gastrointestinal Case 10

KIAT T. TAN AND RICHARD HOPKINS

Clinical history

No history.

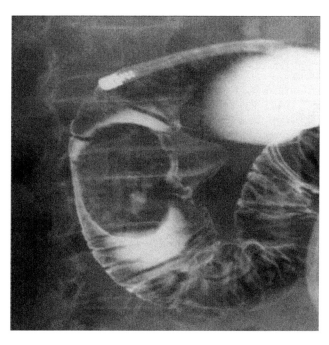

Figure 2.10a

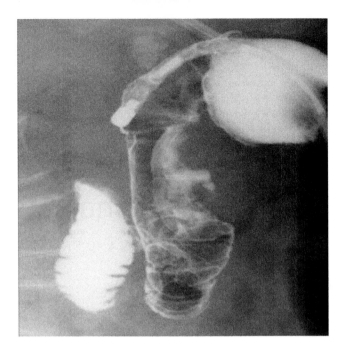

Figure 2.10b

Model answer

These are two images from a double-contrast barium study of the duodenum and proximal small bowel (Figures 2.10a, 2.10b). There is a naso-duodenal tube with its tip in the first part of the duodenum. There is a large, oval mass in the second part of the duodenum arising from its anterior wall. The mass is well defined and forms an obtuse angle to the bowel wall. There is some barium pooling in the centre of the mass, which would be consistent with ulceration. The remainder of the duodenum is normal and barium has passed freely through it.

The most likely diagnosis is a lesion that arises extraluminally, such as a gastro-intestinal stromal tumour. The differential diagnoses include lymphoma and ectopic pancreas. A carcinoma is less likely. The patient will require a CT scan and upper GI endoscopy with biopsy.

Questions

1. **In which locations within the GI tract do GISTs most commonly occur?**
   GISTs are most commonly found in the stomach (approximately two-thirds of cases) and small bowel (approximately one-third of cases), with a minority in the oesophagus and rectum.

Key points

- Gastrointestinal stromal tumours (GISTs) are the commonest mesenchymal tumour. They arise from the muscular layer of the bowel wall.
- GISTs often project exophytically out of the bowel and can be mistaken for a lesion that arises from an adjacent organ. They also often have an intraluminal component. However, presentation as an intraluminal polypoid mass (like adenocarcinoma) is uncommon.
- A CT scan often confirms the intramural origin of the tumour. Large tumours may cavitate or show central necrosis.

Notes
The histology showed GIST.

Further reading
Levy AD, Remotti HE, Thompson WM, Sobin LH, Miettinen M. Gastrointestinal stromal tumors: radiologic features with pathologic correlation. *Radiographics* 2003; **23**: 283–304.

Sandrasegaran K, Rajesh A, Rydberg J, *et al.* Gastrointestinal stromal tumors: clinical, radiologic, and pathologic features. *AJR Am J Roentgenol* 2005; **184**: 803–11.

Gastrointestinal Case 11

KIAT T. TAN AND RICHARD HOPKINS

Clinical history
No history.

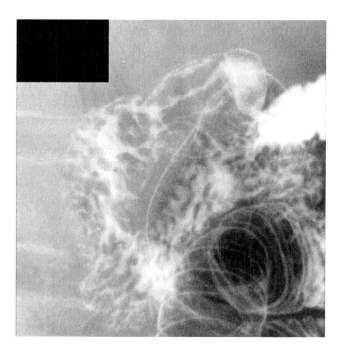

Figure 2.11a

Model answer

These are two axial images from an intravenous and oral contrast-enhanced CT scan of the abdomen (Figures 2.12a, 2.12b). There are multiple peri portal collateral vessels around the expected site of the portal vein. The main portal vein is not seen. Small collateral vessels are present around the gallbladder and body of the stomach. Splenomegaly is present. There is a small amount of pericholecystic fluid.

The appearance is of cavernous transformation of the portal vein. I would like to review the rest of the images on a workstation to look for conditions that would predispose to portal vein thrombosis, such as malignancy and infection. I would also like to document the presence of other features of portal hypertension, such as varices and recanalization of the umbilical veins. The clinical history would suggest an underlying prothrombotic state, and the patient should be investigated for this.

Questions

1. **What is cavernous transformation of the portal vein?**
   Cavernous transformation of the portal vein refers to the formation of collateral vessels in portal vein thrombosis. These collaterals could be either within or adjacent to the thrombosed vein and could occur within 6–20 days after the development of thrombosis.

2. **What are the causes of portal vein thrombosis?**
   Idiopathic, hepatobiliary/abdominal sepsis, cirrhosis, primary liver tumours, pancreatic malignancy, prothrombotic state (e.g. protein C deficiency, protein S deficiency, lupus anticoagulant syndrome).

Key points

- The liver has a dual blood supply. Therefore, acute portal vein thrombosis may not lead to liver infarction if the arterial blood supply is intact. Similarly, hepatic arterial occlusion alone does not lead to liver infarction.
- Symptoms from acute portal vein thrombosis may be minimal, with vague right upper quadrant pain or discomfort. Patients may be completely asymptomatic.
- Clinical presentation may not occur until the development of complications such as portal hypertension, liver dysfunction (usually in patients with cirrhosis or hepatic artery compromise) or thrombus progression (propagation of thrombus into the superior mesenteric vein (SMV) may occur, leading to small bowel mucosal oedema and venous ischaemia).

Further reading

Gallego C, Velasco M, Marcuello P, et al. Congenital and acquired anomalies of the portal venous system. *Radiographics* 2002; **22**: 141–59.

Ito K, Higuchi M, Kada T, et al. CT of acquired abnormalities of the portal venous system. *Radiographics* 1997; **17**: 897–917.

Gastrointestinal Case 13

KIAT T. TAN AND RICHARD HOPKINS

Clinical history

Patient with hepatitis C. Emergency admission with abdominal pain and shock.

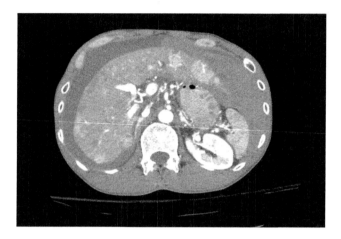

Figure 2.13a

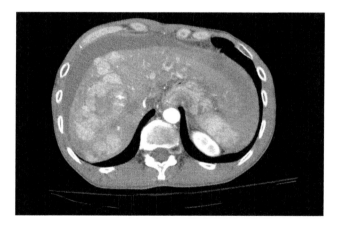

Figure 2.13b

Model answer

These are two images from an arterial-phase CT scan of the liver (Figures 2.13a, 2.13b). There are multiple hyperdense lesions of varying size within both lobes of the liver. Some of these appear to have areas of central necrosis. No lymphadenopathy is evident. Combined with the history of hepatitis C, the radiological features would be consistent with multicentric hepatocellular carcinoma (HCC). Multiple hypervascular liver metastases (such as from carcinoid, renal cell carcinoma, thyroid cancer and choriocarcinoma) is a differential diagnosis.

There is free fluid of varying high density around the liver and spleen, especially when compared to the cerebrospinal fluid in the spinal canal. This finding is suggestive of intraperitoneal haemorrhage. The density of the fluid is especially high around the left lobe of the liver, consistent with focal thrombus formation.

Taken together, the clinical and radiological features would be in keeping with bleeding from a ruptured HCC in the left lobe of the liver. I would like to review the rest of the imaging on a workstation to look for evidence of chronic liver disease as well as to assess for disease spread. In addition, review of pre-contrast and delayed imaging studies is essential, as it allows the determination of the contrast enhancement pattern of the tumour as well as assessment for active contrast extravasation. I will communicate the result to the clinician responsible for the patient. The patient will need fluid resuscitation. An urgent surgical referral is recommended. The patient may benefit from percutaneous endovascular treatment of the bleed by an interventional radiologist.

Questions

1. **How common is HCC rupture?**

   Approximately 10% of HCCs will be complicated by spontaneous rupture. Rupture-prone HCCs are usually located peripherally near the liver capsule. The patient often has an underlying coagulopathy from associated cirrhosis.

2. **What conditions are associated with HCC?**

   Most cases of HCC are seen in conjunction with cirrhosis from alcohol or hepatitis B, hepatitis C and haemochromatosis. Less common risk factors are alpha-1 -antitrypsin deficiency, anabolic steroid use, non-alcoholic steatohepatitis ('fatty infiltration of the liver'), exposure to thorotrast and oral contraceptive use.

Key points

- HCC is typically isodense to liver on unenhanced studies. The tumour enhances avidly with contrast on the arterial phase and is either hypodense or isodense to the liver on portal venous/delayed phases.
- The sentinel clot sign refers to the presence of hyperattenuating thrombus at the site of an intra-abdominal bleed. This sign is an especially specific indicator of the site of bleeding from a solid abdominal organ.
- Hepatic arteriography demonstrates hypervascular lesions throughout the liver (Figure 2.13c).

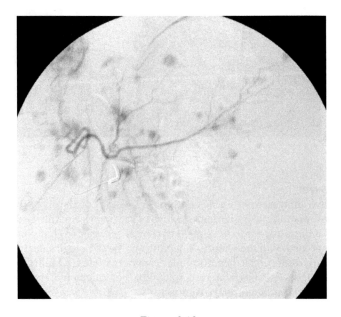

Figure 2.13c

Further reading

Choi BG, Park SH, Byun JY, *et al*. The findings of ruptured hepatocellular carcinoma on helical CT. *Br J Radiol* 2001; **74**: 142–6.

Orwig D, Federle MP. Localized clotted blood as evidence of visceral trauma on CT: the sentinel clot sign. *AJR Am J Roentgenol* 1989; **153**: 747–9.

Gastrointestinal Case 14

KIAT T. TAN AND RICHARD HOPKINS

Clinical history

No history.

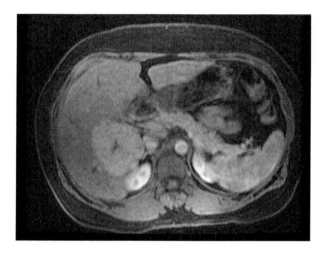

Figure 2.14a Arterial phase

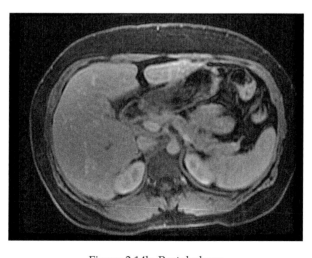

Figure 2.14b Portal phase

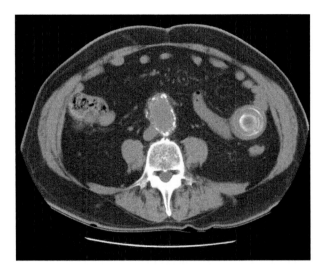

Figure 2.15b

Model answer

This is a frontal plain radiograph of the abdomen (Figure 2.15a). The nasogastric tube tip is just below the diaphragm while its side-hole is above the diaphragm. The tube should be advanced by at least 15 cm for optimal positioning and to prevent reflux of stomach contents into the oesophagus. A check radiograph is required post-NG tube manipulation. There is mild dilatation of the loops of small bowel in the left upper quadrant. Gas is outlined against the valvulae conniventes of the small bowel. There are subtle gas shadows projected over the right upper quadrant, suggestive of gas in a dilated biliary tree. No free gas. The large bowel gas pattern is normal, with no evidence of obstruction. A well-defined round calcified opacity, several centimetres in diameter, is seen overlying the left sacroiliac joint and iliac crest. An irregular calcified structure is seen within the right side of the pelvis, likely to be a calcified fibroid or mesenteric lymph node. The radiological findings are consistent with mechanical small bowel obstruction from gallstone ileus. The patient will need urgent surgical referral, and a CT scan should be obtained to confirm the diagnosis and delineate anatomy.

The single image from the CT scan (Figure 2.15b) shows a lamellar gallstone within the small bowel, consistent with gallstone ileus. No free gas. No small bowel dilatation. I would like to review the images on a workstation to look for the presence and location of the biliary-enteric fistula as well as the presence of other complications such as small bowel dilatation and free gas in the peritoneal cavity.

Questions

1. **What are the causes of small bowel obstruction?**

   Small bowel obstruction (SBO) occurs most commonly due to post-surgical adhesions or inguinal hernia. Other aetiologies (e.g. due to internal hernias and tumours) can have similar radiological appearances, and these often cannot be easily differentiated on the plain AXR. Gallstone ileus is a rare cause of SBO.

2. **What are the radiological features of gallstone ileus?**

   The classic features of gallstone ileus are signs of small bowel obstruction, gas in the biliary tree and a gallstone in an ectopic location. However, gallstones are calcified in less than a third of cases and are usually difficult to see on plain film. CT is therefore a useful tool in diagnosing gallstone ileus.

Key points
- Chronic gallbladder inflammation can allow the formation of a cholecystoduo-denal fistula and the subsequent passage of stone into the duodenum. This allows the movement of bowel gas into the biliary tree.

Further reading
Summerton SL, Hollander AC, Stassi J, Rosenberg HK, Carroll SF. US case of the day: gallstone ileus. *Radiographics* 1995; **15**: 493–5.

Gastrointestinal Case 16

KIAT T. TAN AND RICHARD HOPKINS

Clinical history
Right upper quadrant pain.

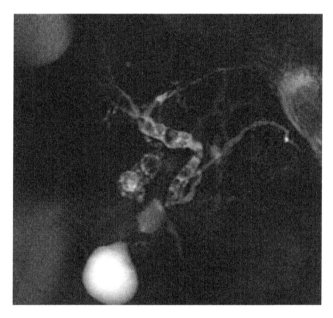

Figure 2.16a

to inform the referring clinician, as the condition may predispose to carcinoma of the gallbladder and the patient should be considered for cholecystectomy.

Questions
1. **Which other structures in the upper abdomen can calcify?**
   - Liver
     - granulomas
     - calcified metastases
   - Gallbladder
     - calcified gallstones
     - porcelain gallbladder
     - limey bile
   - Vascular
     - aorta
     - splenic artery
   - Renal
     - stones
     - cortical or medullary nephrocalcinosis
     - renal tumours
     - renal tuberculosis
     - xanthogranulomatous pyelonephritis
   - Adrenal
     - tuberculosis/infarction
   - Pancreas
     - chronic pancreatitis
   - Lymph nodes

Key points
- Porcelain gallbladder is so called because the gallbladder resembles fragile porcelain at surgery.
- The exact pathophysiology of porcelain gallbladder is uncertain, although it is believed to be related to gallstones and/or chronic inflammation.
- Porcelain gallbladder is often asymptomatic.
- Porcelain gallbladder is believed to be a risk factor for the development of carcinoma. Therefore, cholecystectomy is the recommended treatment of the condition. Open cholecystectomy is often the preferred option, to avoid seeding of tumour that may be present.

Further reading
Grand D, Horton KM, Fishman E. CT of the gallbladder: spectrum of disease. *AJR Am J Roentgenol* 2004; **183**: 163–70.
Stephen AE, Berger DL. Carcinoma in the porcelain gallbladder: a relationship revisited. *Surgery* 2001; **129**: 699–703.

Gastrointestinal Case 18

KIAT T. TAN AND RICHARD HOPKINS

Clinical history

No history

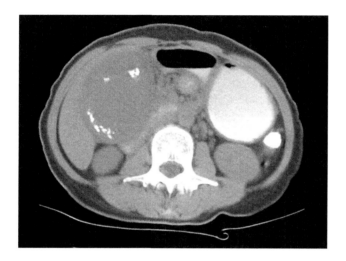

Figure 2.18a

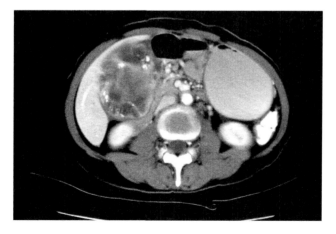

Figure 2.18b

Model answer

These are selected pre- and post-IV-contrast axial images from a CT scan of the abdomen (Figures 2.18a, 2.18b). There is a large, well-defined, rounded mass in the right upper quadrant abutting the liver and duodenum. There are foci of predominantly peripherally located calcification within this lesion. Following IV contrast the mass shows heterogeneous enhancement and intralesional septations. No intra- or extra-hepatic biliary dilatation is seen on the images provided. The gallbladder cannot be visualized separate to this lesion. No lymphadenopathy on the images provided. Findings are consistent with a gallbladder cancer in a pre-existing porcelain gallbladder. The patient will need to be referred to the gastroenterologist and will need to be discussed at the relevant multidisciplinary meeting. I would like to review the images on a workstation to look for evidence of disease spread, such as: (1) the presence of distant metastasis (especially to the liver); (2) peritoneal deposits; (3) invasion of adjacent structures; (4) enlarged lymph nodes; and (5) spread into the bile ducts.

Questions

1. **What are the predisposing causes of gallbladder cancer?**
   Risk factors include: porcelain gallbladder, gallbladder polyps larger than 2 cm, primary sclerosing cholangitis, inflammatory bowel disease, familial polyposis coli and congenital biliary anomalies.

2. **What are the radiological features of gallbladder cancer?**
   The disease presents as: (a) a mass replacing the gallbladder in the majority of cases; (b) gallbladder wall thickening; and (c) a polypoid lesion within an otherwise normal-looking gallbladder in a minority. Radiological findings of gallbladder cancer include pericholecystic infiltrations, dilatation of the biliary tree and lymphadenopathy in the porta hepatis. Necrosis, fistulas and abscess formation are common. The differential diagnoses include complicated cholecystitis, xanthogranulomatous cholecystitis and metastases to the gallbladder.

Key points

- Gallbladder cancer is most commonly found in the seventh decade of life.
- Gallbladder cancer has a poor prognosis, as it is often diagnosed at a late stage.
- The symptoms of gallbladder cancer are similar to those of gallstones.
- Gallbladder cancer can be difficult to differentiate from complicated cholecystitis. The presence of a low-attenuation intrahepatic rim around the gallbladder wall is a specific finding of cholecystitis.

Further reading

Grand D, Horton KM, Fishman E. CT of the gallbladder: spectrum of disease. *AJR Am J Roentgenol* 2004; **183**: 163–70.

Levy AD, Murakata LA, Rohrmann CA. Gallbladder carcinoma: radiologic–pathologic correlation. *Radiographics* 2001; **21**: 295–314.

Misra S, Chaturvedi A, Misra NC, Sharma ID. Carcinoma of the gallbladder. *Lancet Oncol* 2003; **4**: 167–76.

Gastrointestinal Case 19

KIAT T. TAN AND RICHARD HOPKINS

Clinical history
No history.

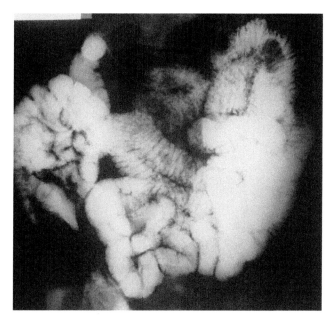

Figure 2.19

Model answer
This is a single image from a barium enteroclysis study (Figure 2.19). The naso-je-junal tube used for the barium infusion is seen in the proximal small bowel. The proximal and mid small bowel are filled with barium, which is of normal calibre, and the valvulae conniventes are of a normal appearance. There are three lobulated polypoid filling defects in the jejunum of varying sizes, the largest measuring up to approximately 2–3 cm diameter. There are also multiple small filling defects within the small bowel. The diagnosis is a polyposis syndrome, the most likely of which are Peutz–Jeghers syndrome and familial adenomatous polyposis. A clinical history and examination would be useful to differentiate between the two. Long-term cancer surveillance is required for both conditions.

Questions
1. **How can you differentiate between the Peutz–Jeghers syndrome and familial adenomatous polyposis (FAP) ?**
   Both conditions are inherited in an autosomal dominant fashion, and a family history would be useful in the diagnostic process. Peutz–Jeghers syndrome is characterized by mucocutaneous pigmentation along with the polyposis. Examination of the colon of an individual with FAP, whether by colonoscopy or barium enema, would reveal 'polyp carpeting' of the large intestine.

2. **What sort of polyps are associated with Peutz–Jeghers syndrome?**
   Intestinal hamartomatous polyps develop in the stomach, small intestine and colon (*as opposed to the adenomatous polyps of FAP*).

3. **What sorts of cancers are associated with Peutz–Jeghers syndrome?**
   Bowel, oesophagus, pancreas, testicle, cervix, lung, breast, uterus and ovary.

Key points

- Polyps may also cause intussusception and bowel obstruction.
- Other conditions that may give rise to hamartomatous polyps in the small bowel include Cowden's disease, juvenile polyposis and Cronkhite–Canada syndrome. The latter is typically associated with polyps that carpet the stomach.

Notes

This patient had Peutz–Jeghers syndrome.

Further reading

Cho GJ, Bergquist K, Schwartz AM. Peutz–Jeghers syndrome and hamartomatous polyposis syndrome: radiologic–pathologic correlation. *Radiographics* 1997; **17**: 785–91.

Half E, Bercovich D, Rozen P. Familial adenomatous polyposis. *Orphanet J Rare Dis* 2009; **4**: 22.

Gastrointestinal Case 20

KIAT T. TAN AND RICHARD HOPKINS

Clinical history

Abdominal pain. Report the barium study first.

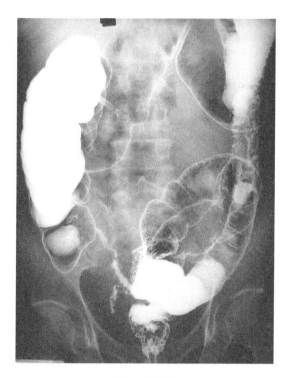

Figure 2.20a

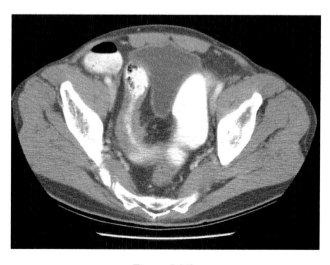

Figure 2.20b

Model answer

This is a single frontal projection from a barium enema series (Figure 2.20a). Barium has refluxed into the terminal ileum. The terminal ileum demonstrates luminal narrowing, rose-thorn ulcers (*or deep ulceration*), cobblestoning and possibly a linear ulcer in the mesenteric border. Part of the descending colon is also abnormal, with loss of the normal haustral pattern and rose-thorn ulcers. There is normal intervening bowel between the two abnormal areas. The diagnosis is Crohn's disease. No *evidence* of sacroiliitis demonstrated on the current examination.

The single image from the intravenous and oral contrast-enhanced CT scan (Figure 2.20b) shows a grossly thickened loop of small bowel, presumably the distal ileum seen on the barium study, associated with luminal narrowing. There is adjacent fat stranding, consistent with the transmural nature of the inflammation. The findings provide further evidence consistent with Crohn's disease. I would like to review the rest of the imaging to look for other features of the disease as well as its complications.

Questions

1. **What are the radiological features of Crohn's disease?**
   Early Crohn's disease is manifested by a granular appearance, due to villous oedema. This is typically followed by aphthous ulceration, which is seen on the barium study as a tiny collection of barium surrounded by a clear halo. More severe changes are longitudinal ulceration, deep ulcer cavities and transmural involvement. Cobblestoning is the result of normal or oedematous islands of mucosa between the linear ulcers. Crohn's disease typically affects discontinuous segments of bowel, thus giving rise to 'skip lesions'.
2. **What are the complications of Crohn's disease that can be detected radiologically?**
   Because of its transmural nature, Crohn's disease is often associated with strictures, fistulas and abscesses. Other complications include sacroiliitis, gallstones, sclerosing cholangitis, amyloidosis, autoimmune hepatitis, renal stones, thrombosis and gastrointestinal tumours.

Key points

- The radiologist is often asked to differentiate between Crohn's disease and ulcerative colitis. Crohn's disease typically: affects discontinuous segments of bowel; is transmural; is associated with discrete deep rose-thorn ulcers; and demonstrates cobblestoning. Longitudinal ulceration in the mesenteric border is pathognomonic of Crohn's disease. Ulcerative colitis affects the rectum and extends proximally in a continuous fashion. Ulcerative colitis can affect the terminal ileum as 'backwash ileitis', although this is almost always associated with caecal involvement.
- The predisposition to renal stones is the result of calcium malabsorption, resulting in increased oxalate excretion.
- Terminal ileum inflammation impairs the reabsorption of bile salts, thus increasing the risk of gallstones.
- Crohn's disease is associated with other inflammatory conditions, including inflammatory arthropathy (especially sacroiliitis), sclerosing cholangitis, autoimmune hepatitis, eye inflammation, skin lesions (e.g. pyoderma gangrenosum, erythema nodosum).

Further reading

Gore RM, Balthazar EJ, Ghahremani CG, Miller FH. CT features of ulcerative colitis and Crohn's disease. *AJR Am J Roentgenol* 1996; **167**: 3–15.

Halligan S. The small bowel and peritoneal cavity. In Sutton D, ed., *Textbook of Radiology and Imaging*, 7th edn. London: Elsevier, 2003; 615–34.

Gastrointestinal Case 21

KIAT T. TAN AND RICHARD HOPKINS

Clinical history

Colicky abdominal pain. Comment on the lesion in the right iliac fossa.

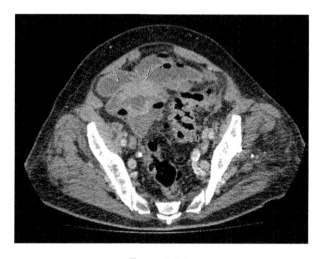

Figure 2.21a

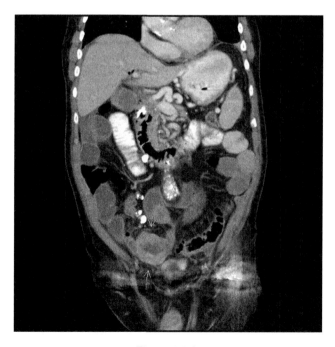

Figure 2.21b

Model answer

These are two images from an intravenous and oral contrast-enhanced scan of the abdomen (Figures 2.21a, 2.21b). There is gross irregular and eccentric ileal wall thickening. The bowel lumen appears well preserved. No evidence of hepato- or splenomegaly. No regional lymph nodes.

The features would be consistent with either small bowel lymphoma or carcinoma. I would like to review the rest of the CT scan to look for synchronous tumours as well as for evidence of metastatic disease. The patient will need to be discussed at the local cancer multidisciplinary meeting to plan management.

Questions

1. **Where are the typical locations for small bowel lymphoma?**
   Primary small bowel lymphoma may occur anywhere along the small bowel, but the distal ileum is more common than jejunum or duodenum.
2. **What are the risk factors for small bowel lymphoma?**
   Coeliac disease, AIDS, Crohn's disease, systemic lupus erythematosus.
3. **What are the CT signs of small bowel lymphoma?**
   A spectrum of CT signs are recognized in association with small bowel lymphoma:
   - polypoid mass arising from the bowel wall
   - intussusception
   - circumferential or eccentric bowel wall thickening (Figure 2.21c shows circumferential duodenal wall thickening)
   - thickening of the valvulae conniventes
   - soft tissue infiltrate around the bowel wall
   - aneurysmal/luminal dilatation or lack of functional stenosis
   - mesenteric lymph node enlargement
   - splenic enlargement

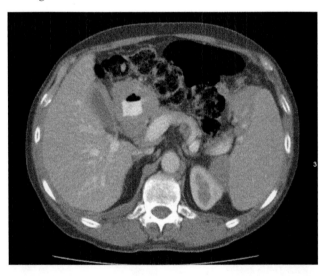

Figure 2.21c

Key points

- Primary small bowel lymphoma is usually of the B-cell-derived non-Hodgkin's type and usually affects the ileum.
- Small bowel lymphoma occurring in patients with coeliac disease is usually derived from T cells and most commonly affects the proximal small bowel.
- The bowel can also be secondarily involved by lymphoma arising elsewhere.

Further reading

Buckland JA, Fishman EK. CT evaluation of small bowel neoplasms: spectrum of disease. *Radiographics* 1999; **18**: 379–92.

Lee WK, Lau EW, Duddalwar VA, Stanley AJ, Ho YY. Abdominal manifestations of extranodal lymphoma: spectrum of imaging findings. *AJR Am J Roentgenol* 2008; **191**: 198–206.

Gastrointestinal Case 22

KIAT T. TAN AND RICHARD HOPKINS

Clinical history

Abdominal pain and distension.

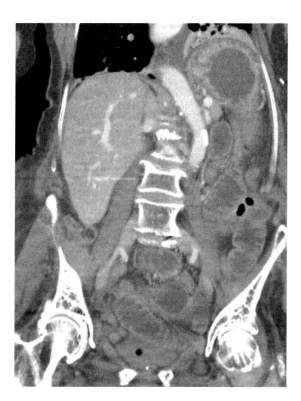

Figure 2.22a

Gastrointestinal Case 24

KIAT T. TAN AND RICHARD HOPKINS

Clinical history
Episodes of documented hypoglycaemia.

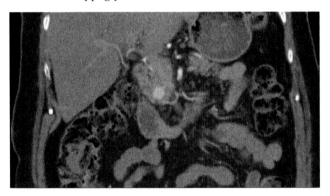

Figure 2.24

Model answer
This is a single coronal image from an arterial-phase CT scan of the upper abdomen (Figure 2.24). There is a small hypervascular lesion within the uncinate process of the pancreas, which measures approximately 1 cm in diameter. This is most likely to be an insulinoma, given the clinical history of hypoglycaemic episodes and the avid early enhancement in this arterial-phase study. Less likely diagnoses include other islet cell tumours of the pancreas or a hypervascular metastasis to the pancreas (renal cell carcinoma, melanoma). I would like to review the rest of the current CT study to look for synchronous tumours as well as for evidence of metastasis. I would like to discuss the result with the appropriate clinician and surgeon.

Questions
1. **How should you image islet cell tumours?**
   A dual- or triple-phase study is required. A dual-phase study is performed in the arterial and portal venous phases while a triple-phase study has an additional pancreatic phase.
2. **Which is the best phase for the detection of pancreatic tumour?**
   Some tumours are best detected on the arterial phase while others are better seen on the pancreatic or portal venous phases.
3. **Are all islet cell tumours functional?**
   Islet cell tumours can be either functional or non-functional. Functional tumours present with clinical features related to their hormone production, while non-functional tumours typically present later, with larger tumours and metastases.
4. **What syndromes are associated with islet cell tumours?**
   Islet cell tumours are associated with MEN-1 (parathyroid adenoma, pancreatic islet cell tumour, pituitary adenoma: the Ps) and von Hippel–Lindau (VHL) disease.

Key points

- Insulinoma is the most common type of functioning islet cell tumour, followed by gastrinoma.
- Ideally, biochemical confirmation of insulinoma should be performed prior to imaging. CT can detect up to 94% of tumours.
- Surgery results in a cure in over 90% of patients with insulinoma.
- Other islet cell tumours include gastrinomas, glucagonoma, VIPoma, somatostatinoma.

Further reading

Buetow PC, Miller DL, Parrino TV, Buck JL. Islet cell tumors of the pancreas: clinical, radiologic, and pathologic correlation in diagnosis and localization. *Radiographics* 1997; **17**: 453–72.

Fidler JL, Fletcher JG, Reading CC, *et al.* Preoperative detection of pancreatic insulinomas on multiphasic helical CT. *AJR Am J Roentgenol* 2003; **181**: 775–80.

Lewis RB, Lattin GE, Paal E. Pancreatic endocrine tumors: radiologic-clinicopathologic correlation. *Radiographics* 2010; **30**: 1445–64.

Gastrointestinal Case 25

KIAT T. TAN AND RICHARD HOPKINS

Clinical history

35-year-old female patient, previously fit and well, who presented with an upper GI bleed from oesophageal varices.

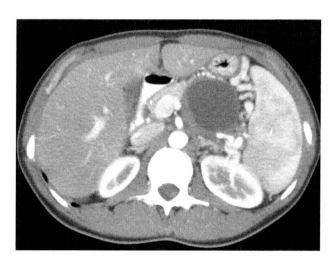

Figure 2.25

Model answer

This is a single axial image from a portal-venous-phase CT scan of the abdomen (Figure 2.25). There is a low-attenuation lesion of fluid attenuation in the body of the pancreas. The lesion is rounded and there is no lobulation. No internal septae or nodularity evident. The pancreas enhances normally elsewhere. The splenic vein is not visualized. There are multiple varices around the splenic hilum.

The features are most likely due to mucinous cystic neoplasm. Pseudocyst is a less likely diagnosis, as there is no history of pancreatitis and/or pancreatic calcification. The presence of varices would suggest splenic vein compromise due to the mass. I would like to review the rest of the CT study to define the size of the lesion, to look for evidence of metastasis and to further characterize the splenic and portal veins. If necessary, a Doppler ultrasound should be arranged to look at these vessels.

Surgical referral is advised. Ongoing management may include tumour markers, endoscopic ultrasound with guided fluid aspiration or surgical resection. If the splenic vein is thrombosed, selective embolization of the splenic artery should be considered to reduce blood flow to the spleen and thus the degree of variceal perfusion.

Questions

1. **What is the typical location for mucinous cystic tumours of the pancreas?**
   Typically they occur in the tail or body of the pancreas.
2. **Is this a benign lesion, and what is the treatment for this patient?**
   Although the histology of mucinous cystic tumours of the pancreas can range from benign to malignant, it is impossible to exclude malignancy on imaging and biopsy. In addition, all mucinous cystic tumours have malignant potential. Therefore, the treatment of choice for these lesions is complete surgical resection.
3. **What are the complications of splenic vein thrombosis?**
   Gastric varices may occur as blood is shunted through the small gastric veins. When large, these may rupture and lead to haematemesis.

Key points

- Pancreatic pseudocysts are rare without a history of pancreatitis. Conversely, mucinous cystic tumours can occur in a patient with a history of pancreatitis. It can be difficult to differentiate pancreatic pseudocysts from mucinous cystic tumours. Pseudocysts do not tend to have internal septation and intramural nodules.
- Mucinous cystic tumours typically have a smooth outline and can be unilocular or multilocated. The cysts are usually larger than 2 cm and are often found in the pancreatic body/tail. They typically have enhancing walls, intramural nodules and septae (although absence of these does not exclude mucinous cystic tumours). These tumours can demonstrate peripheral calcification.
- Serous cystadenomas usually have a *lobulated outline*, are composed of cysts ranging in size *0.2–2 cm* and are most often found in the *pancreatic head*. They may have *central calcification* and *do not demonstrate wall enhancement*.
- Single small (< 3 cm) unilocular thin-walled cystic pancreatic lesions in the absence of a history of pancreatitis present a diagnostic dilemma. A reasonable management approach is to arrange serial imaging of these lesions.
- Oligocystic (or macrocystic) serous cystadenoma can be difficult to differentiate from mucinous tumours.

Further reading

Acar M, Tatli S. Cystic tumors of the pancreas: a radiological perspective. *Diagn Interv Radiol* 2011; **17**: 143–9.

Kim YH, Saini S, Sahani D, *et al*. Imaging diagnosis of cystic pancreatic lesions: pseudocyst versus nonpseudocyst. *Radiographics* 2005; **25**: 671–85.

Sahani DV, Kadavigere R, Saokar A, *et al*. Cystic pancreatic lesions: a simple imaging-based classification system for guiding management. *Radiographics* 2005; **25**: 1471–84.

Gastrointestinal Case 26

KIAT T. TAN AND RICHARD HOPKINS

Clinical history

One-month history of epigastric pain radiating through to back.

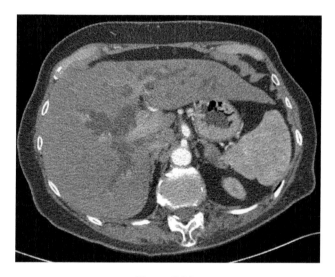

Figure 2.26a

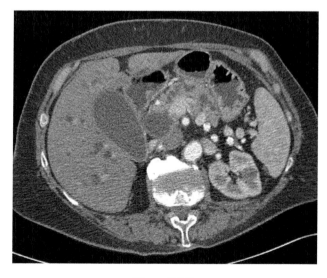

Figure 2.26b

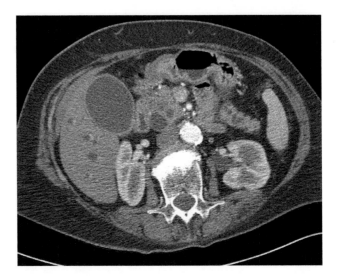

Figure 2.26c

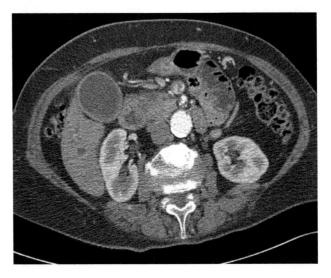

Figure 2.26d

Model answer

These are four axial images from an arterial-phase CT scan of the upper abdomen, and following a drink of water (Figures 2.26a–2.26d). There is biliary dilatation commencing at the level of the intrahepatic ducts and extending down to the level of the common bile duct. The common bile duct leads into an irregular low-density mass within the pancreatic head. The pancreatic duct is also dilated. The mass is abutting the superior mesenteric vein.

The radiological findings are consistent with biliary and pancreatic ductal obstruction due to carcinoma of the head of pancreas. I would like to review the rest of the images on a workstation to look for evidence of vascular compromise and metastasis. The patient should have endoscopic retrograde cholangiopancreatography so that a stent can be placed to relieve the biliary obstruction. If this is impossible, an interventional radiologist can place a drain or stent, via a percutaneous route, to relieve the obstruction. Biliary brushings should be obtained.

The case should be reviewed at an upper gastrointestinal multidisciplinary meeting, where full discussion with hepatobiliary surgeons and oncologists can be undertaken to plan treatment.

Questions

1. Is percutaneous biopsy appropriate prior to curative surgery?
No, full staging is required for such a patient but percutaneous biopsy may increase the risk of seeding and is not usually recommended. Preliminary surgical exploration may be performed prior to proceeding to a Whipple's procedure.

2. What do you understand by the 'double-duct' sign?
This is dilatation of both the common bile and pancreatic ducts. It indicates the presence of an obstructing lesion but is not a specific marker of pancreatic cancer.

3. What potential treatments are available if the patient is deemed inoperable?
Chemotherapy has been shown to improve survival in pancreatic cancer.

Key points

- The prognosis of pancreatic cancer is poor, with a one-year survival of 24% and five-year survival of less than 5%. Patients with disease in the pancreatic head tend to do better, as they are more likely to present early (due to biliary obstruction) and are more likely to have resectable tumours.
- The presence of tumour invasion of the portal and/or superior mesenteric veins is no longer considered a contraindication to surgical resection by many surgeons. Coeliac axis and/or superior mesenteric artery involvement is still considered to be a contraindication to surgery.
- Hepatic artery lymphadenopathy is indicative of poor prognosis.
- CT imaging of pancreatic cancer should be performed using a triple-phase protocol (pre-, arterial and portal venous). Pancreatic tumours are typically hypoattenuating relative to normal pancreas. 10% of tumours are isoattenuating to the pancreas.
- Biliary brushings performed during endoscopic retrograde cholangiopancreatography (ERCP) or percutaneous cholangiography has a sensitivity of up to 50% and a 100% specificity for malignancy.

Further reading

Baillie J, Paulson E, Vitellas K. Biliary imaging: a review. *Gastroenterology* 2003; **124**: 1686–99.

Brennan DD, Zamboni GA, Raptopoulos VD, Kruskal JB. Comprehensive preoperative assessment of pancreatic adenocarcinoma with 64-section volumetric CT. *Radiographics* 2007; **27**: 1653–66.

Kim JH, Kim MJ, Chung JJ, *et al.* Differential diagnosis of periampullary carcinomas at MR imaging. *Radiographics* 2002; **22**: 1335–52.

Tamm EP, Silverman PM, Charnsangavej C, Evans DB. Diagnosis, staging and surveillance of pancreatic cancer. *AJR Am J Roentgenol* 2003; **180**: 1311–23.

Case contributed by Dr Chris Cook, Weston General Hospital.

Gastrointestinal Case 27

KIAT T. TAN AND RICHARD HOPKINS

Clinical history

Hospital admission with severe upper abdominal pain. The three images are from different CT scans obtained at 3, 18 and 35 days after hospital admission. Please report these in sequence.

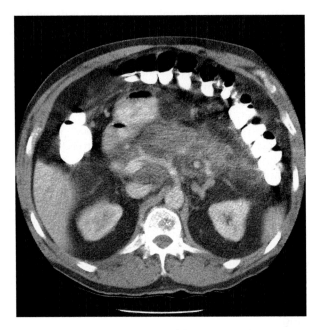

Figure 2.27a

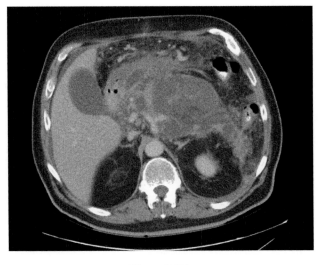

Figure 2.27b

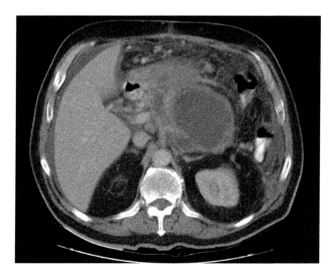

Figure 2.27c

Model answer

The axial image from the CT scan performed at three days (Figure 2.27a) shows a diffusely enlarged pancreas. There is some adjacent fat stranding. The findings are consistent with acute pancreatitis. I would like to review the rest of the images to look for the complications of pancreatitis.

By 18 days (Figure 2.27b) there is marked peripancreatic stranding and the development of septated loculated peripancreatic fluid collections. The findings are consistent with the development of an early pancreatic pseudocyst in the setting of severe pancreatitis.

At 35 days (Figure 2.27c) there is a thick-walled collection in the lesser sac anterior to the pancreas. There is a small amount of ascites. The findings are consistent with pseudocyst formation. I would like to review the rest of the imaging to assess the size and extent of the pseudocyst. I would like to discuss the radiological findings with the referring clinician in order to formulate an appropriate management plan.

Questions

1. **List the causes of acute pancreatitis**.
   Gallstones, alcohol, iatrogenic/trauma, autoimmune, infection, hyperlipidaemia, drugs, hypercalcaemia, pancreas divisum, idiopathic.

2. **What are the recognized complications of acute pancreatitis?**
   Pancreatic necrosis, pseudocyst formation, abscess, haemorrhage, fistula formation, portal vein thrombosis, pseudoaneurysm.

Key points

- A pancreatic pseudocyst is a collection of fluid which is walled off, usually in the upper abdomen, but does not have an epitheliased wall. Pseudocysts commonly form in the lesser sac, anterior to the pancreas, a few weeks after acute pancreatitis.
- Pancreatic pseudocysts can be thin- or thick-walled. Pseudocyst walls usually enhance with contrast and may calcify if chronic. They usually contain fluid of uniform low attenuation, although haemorrhagic cysts can be of high attenuation. The presence of septation and nodularity should raise the possibility of a mucinous tumour.

- Pancreatic pseudocysts should not be drained if small and asymptomatic. Large pseudocysts can become symptomatic due to gastric outlet obstruction or biliary obstruction. Pain is a common symptom. Conservative management is generally advised, but if drainage is necessary this can be performed, endoscopically, percutaneously or using a combined approach – cystogastrostomy.

Further reading

Demos TC, Posniak HV, Harmath C, Olson MC, Aranha G. Cystic lesions of the pancreas. *AJR Am J Roentgenol* 2002; **179**: 1375–88.

Sunnapwar A, Prasad SR, Menias CO, *et al*. Nonalcoholic, nonbiliary pancreatitis: cross-sectional imaging spectrum. *AJR Am J Roentgenol* 2010; **195**: 67–75.

Gastrointestinal Case 28

KIAT T. TAN AND RICHARD HOPKINS

Clinical history

Colicky abdominal pain and distension.

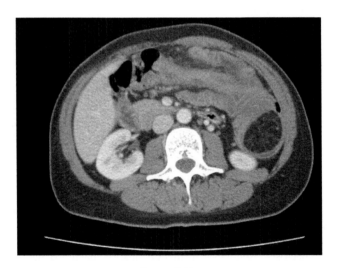

Figure 2.28a

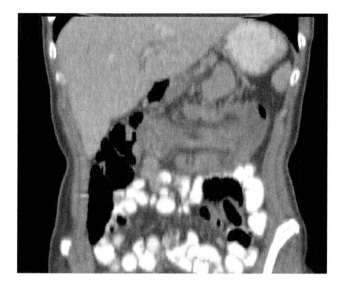

Figure 2.28b

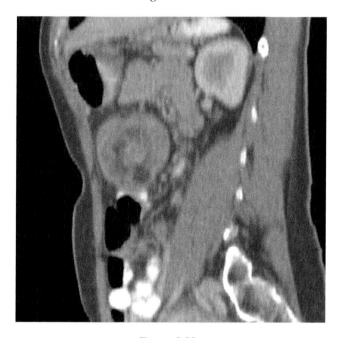

Figure 2.28c

Model answer

These are three images from an intravenous and oral contrast-enhanced CT scan of the abdomen (Figures 2.28a–2.28c).

The transverse colon is abnormal and a bowel-within-bowel appearance is demonstrated on the axial image. The lesion has an elongated appearance on coronal section. There is a mass that is of similar attenuation to fat in the centre of the lesion. The findings are due to colo-colic intussusception, with an intestinal lipoma acting as the lead point. No free gas to suggest perforation. I would like to review the rest of the imaging to assess the degree of bowel obstruction. The result will need to be communicated to the appropriate surgical team.

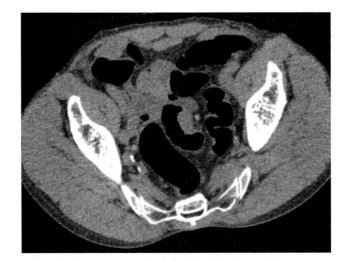

Figure 2.30b

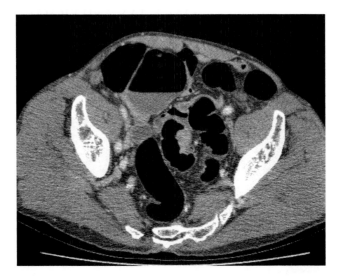

Figure 2.30c

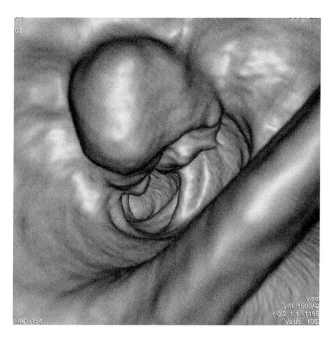

Figure 2.30d

Model answer

These are four images from a CT colonography study, with both supine and prone views (Figures 2.30a–2.30d). The supine study has been acquired with IV contrast. The colon is dilated due to insufflation of gas into the colon.

The axial images show an irregular polypoid lesion arising from the wall of the sigmoid colon, measuring approximately 2–3 cm in length, whose position remains constant on both the prone and supine images. There is evidence of contrast enhancement between the two series. The endoluminal view shows an irregular mass lesion arising from the bowel wall. There are at least three irregular hypodense lesions of varying sizes in the liver. The diagnosis is consistent with a primary sigmoid cancer that has metastasized to the liver. I would like to review the rest of the imaging to look for other sites of metastases. The patient will need to be discussed at the colorectal cancer multidisciplinary meeting for management planning.

Questions

1. **Why are images acquired in both supine and prone positions?**

   Faecal residue will change in position between the two series as the patient is rolled from prone to supine. Changing patient position makes it easier to differentiate between faecal residue and a polyp or mass lesion. Colonic loops will also change their position relative to adjacent anatomy. For this reason it is important to locate 'lesions' relative to easily identifiable structures such as a prominent haustral fold, a diverticulum or reference point which can be reviewed on both the supine and the prone study.

2. **How is the pneumocolon administered? What type of gas is used?**

   A rectal tube is inserted and gas is insufflated into the rectum, usually using an automated device which has pressure monitoring and volume measurements. CO_2 is commonly used as it is better absorbed following the study, which makes the procedure more pleasant for the patient. Buscopan is also given at the time of gas insufflation to reduce the abdominal discomfort.

3. **How do you differentiate faecal residue adherent to the bowel wall from a polyp?**

Position – polyps do not move between the prone and supine series.

Enhancement – polyps and colonic masses demonstrate contrast enhancement following IV contrast.

Gas bubbles – suspicious lesions need to be reviewed using a number of different CT windows including a 'lung window' setting which will better delineate tiny bubbles of gas. Any lesion containing tiny gas bubbles can be dismissed as faecal residue.

Configuration – polyps generally have a smooth, rolled edge, while faecal residue is often variable in configuration.

Key points

- Colon cancers can appear radiologically as: (a) annular strictures, (b) polypoid masses, (c) saddle lesions, which have features of both annular and polypoid lesions, (d) submucosal (rare, but may present with long smooth strictures with only subtle mucosal abnormality).
- Annular tumours are those that have penetrated to the circular layer of the smooth muscle wall of the colon, at the very least. The annular pattern is due to tumour infiltration of the lymphatics between muscle fibres.
- It is now clear that most adenocarcinomas are due to malignant transformation of adenomas. Therefore all polyps should be removed (if possible).

Further reading

Buetow PC, Buck JL, Carr NJ, Pantongrag-Brown L. From the archives of the AFIP. Colorectal adenocarcinoma: radiologic–pathologic correlation. *Radiographics* 1995; **15**: 127–46.

Pickhardt PJ, Kim DH. Colorectal cancer screening with CT colonography: key concepts regarding polyp prevalence, size, histology, morphology, and natural history. *AJR Am J Roentgenol* 2009; **193**: 40–6.

Silva AC, Hara AK, Leighton JA, Heppell JP. CT colonography with intravenous contrast material: varied appearances of colorectal carcinoma. *Radiographics* 2005; **25**: 1321–34.

Gastrointestinal Case 31

KIAT T. TAN AND RICHARD HOPKINS

Clinical history

Change in bowel habit. Report the barium enema first, followed by the CT and then the MRI. (In the exam, you might not be shown the MR images before you have presented the barium enema and the CT.)

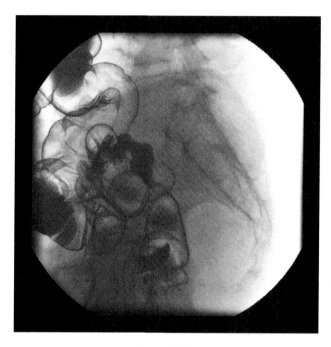

Figure 2.31a

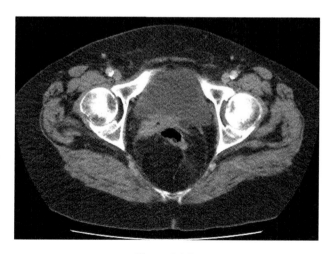

Figure 2.31b

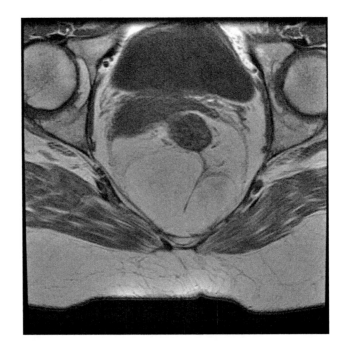

Figure 2.31c

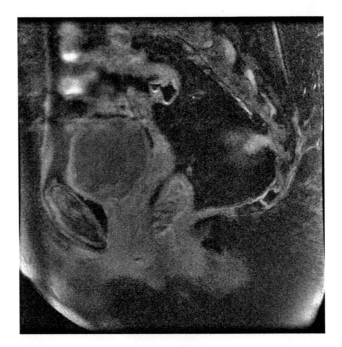

Figure 2.31d

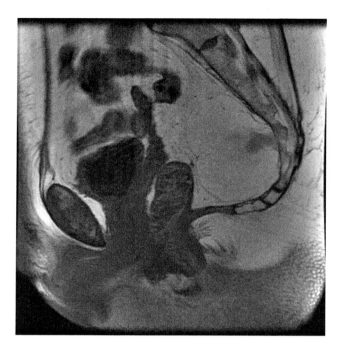

Figure 2.31e

Model answer

The image is a single lateral view of the rectum and sigmoid colon, taken from a double-contrast barium enema (Figure 2.31a). There is an area of underdistension in the rectosigmoid. Apart from this, the mucosal appearance is normal. No polyp or mass lesion is identified. The presacral space width is increased and the rectum is displaced anteriorly. No obvious bone destruction is present. No soft tissue calcification is present. Appearances are of a retrorectal mass. Further imaging by CT or MRI is required for further characterization of this finding.

I am presented with a single image from an intravenous contrast-enhanced CT scan of the pelvis (Figure 2.31b). There is a well-defined rounded soft tissue mass that is predominantly of fat attenuation, although higher-attenuating soft tissue is also present. There are no cystic areas. No calcification. The differential diagnoses would be between liposarcoma, presacral myelolipoma, teratoma and dermoid. I would like to review the rest of the images to look for features of each lesion. An MRI may provide additional information about the types of tissue present in the lesion.

These are three MRI images (Figures 2.31c–2.31e). The axial and sagittal T1 images show an encapsulated well-demarcated lesion that is generally of high signal, with a central area of intermediate signal. The intermediate signal area is in contact with the sacrum. The T1 high-signal region suppresses with fat saturation. The two major differential diagnoses would be between liposarcoma and presacral myelolipoma. Presacral dermoids and teratomas usually have a cystic component and are considered less likely. The lesion will need to be biopsied to exclude liposarcoma.

Questions
1. **What is a normal presacral width?**
   A presacral width of more than 15 mm is treated as suspicious, and anything above 20 mm should be regarded as abnormal.
2. **What are the main types of retrorectal mass lesions?**
   Classification of retrorectal masses includes:

- congenital
  - developmental cyst
  - teratoma
  - chordoma
- inflammatory lesions
  - abscess
- neurogenic
  - neuroblastoma
  - ganglioneuroma
- osseous
  - sarcoma
  - myeloma
- miscellaneous
  - lymphoma
  - myeloma
  - metastasis

Key points

- Myelolipomas are benign lesions made up of mature adipose cells and haemato-poietic cells. They are most commonly found in the adrenals, although they have been described in the presacral region. These lesions can calcify.
- Presacral liposarcomas usually do not have a capsule and have irregular contours. However, they cannot be reliably distinguished from myelolipomas on imaging alone.
- Dermoid cysts and teratomas may contain fat but usually have cystic components. Both of these lesions can calcify.

Notes

The lesion was found to be a presacral myelolipoma.

Further reading

Dann PH, Krinsky GA, Israel GM. Case 135: presacral myelolipoma. *Radiology* 2008; **248**: 314–16.

Kocaoglu M, Frush DP. Pediatric presacral masses. *Radiographics* 2006; **26**: 833–57.

Pereira JM, Sirlin CB, Pinto PS, Casola G. CT and MR imaging of extrahepatic fatty masses of the abdomen and pelvis: techniques, diagnosis, differential diagnosis, and pitfalls. *Radiographics* 2005; **25**: 69–85.

Gastrointestinal Case 32

KIAT T. TAN AND RICHARD HOPKINS

Clinical history
Abdominal pain, fever, unwell.

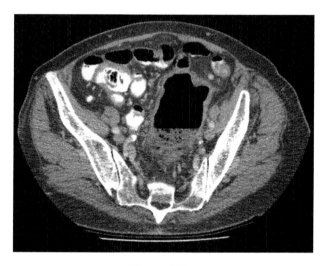

Figure 2.32a

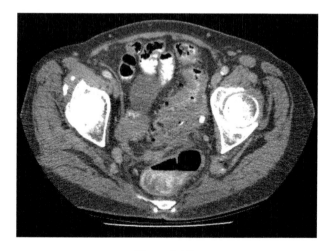

Figure 2.32b

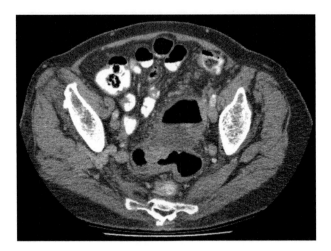

Figure 2.32c

Model answer

These are three images from an oral and intravenous contrast-enhanced CT scan of the abdomen and pelvis (Figures 2.32a–2.32c). There is a long segment of diverticulosis in the sigmoid colon. This segment is thick-walled and there is adjacent fat stranding. There is fluid tracking adjacent to the sigmoid colon. There is a large irregular thick-walled gas- and fluid-containing cavity in the pelvis. No pericolic lymph node evident. The appearance would be in keeping with a pelvic abscess complicating diverticular disease. A less likely differential diagnosis would be perforation of a colonic tumour with focal abscess formation. I would like to review the rest of the imaging to look for other pathology and for treatment planning. The clinician would need to be informed of the findings, as the collection will need to be drained.

Questions

1. **What are the complications of diverticular disease?**
   Rectal bleeding, stricture formation, large bowel obstruction, diverticulitis, perforation, abscess, peritonitis, fistula.

2. **What are the routes you would consider if you were to drain this abscess?**
   I would like to review the rest of the imaging for treatment planning. From the available images, an anterior transabdominal approach is not feasible because of the presence of overlying bowel. Either an ultrasound-guided transrectal or CT-guided transgluteal approach may be considered.

Key points

- Diverticulosis affects 5–10% of those over 45 years of age and 80% of those over 85.
- Diverticula are small outpouchings of mucosa and submucosa at the sites where blood vessels pierce the muscular layer of the wall.
- Complicated diverticulitis can be impossible to differentiate from colonic cancer. The presence of lymphadenopathy would favour cancer.
- Radiological drainage of pericolic abscesses could allow the inflammation to settle prior to surgery, which may allow for the definitive surgery to be carried out as a single-stage procedure.

Further reading

Harisinghani MG, Gervais DA, Hahn PF, *et al*. CT-guided transgluteal drainage of deep pelvic abscesses: indications, technique, procedure-related complications, and clinical outcome. *Radiographics* 2002; **22**: 1353–67.

Horton KM, Corl FM, Fishman EK. CT evaluation of the colon: inflammatory disease. *Radiographics* 2000; **20**: 399–418.

Gastrointestinal Case 33

KIAT T. TAN AND RICHARD HOPKINS

Clinical history

No history.

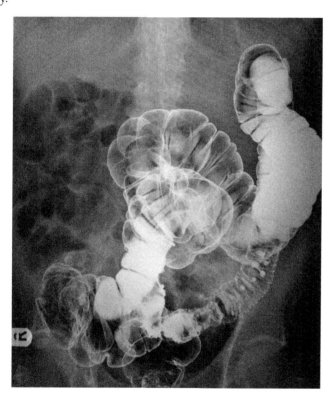

Figure 2.33

Model answer

The single image from a barium enema examination (Figure 2.33) shows features of diverticular disease in the sigmoid colon. The distribution of the bowel is abnormal, with the small bowel mainly situated in the right upper quadrant. The caecum is to the left of the midline and the ileum joins the caecum from the right. The findings are consistent with non-rotation of both small and large bowel. This is often an incidental finding, but there is an increased risk of volvulus.

Questions

1. **What do you understand by incomplete rotation, non-rotation and reversed rotation?**

   Non-rotation implies that the developing bowel has not rotated at all prior to assuming its final position in the abdomen. Non-rotation could affect either both small and large bowel or each in isolation. The non-rotated duodenum/jejunum lies to the right of the midline. The non-rotated caecum lies on the left.

   Incomplete rotation refers, as its name implies, to some but insufficient rotation. The radiological findings lie somewhere between non-rotation and complete rotation.

   Reverse rotation occurs when the transverse colon is situated posterior to the duodenum.

   NB: The exact embryological explanation for these observations is beyond the scope of this book, but the reader is directed to the excellent reviews listed below.

2. **What are the major radiological signs of malrotation?**

   The normal duodenojejunal junction (DJJ) is in the left upper quadrant, at or slightly lower than the level of the duodenal bulb. Malrotation should be suspected if the DJJ is situated to the right of the left vertebral pedicle. The position of the jejunum per se is not a reliable marker of rotation because of its mobility. A superior mesenteric vein that is either to the left or in front of the superior mesenteric artery is also a sign of malrotation. A corkscrew appearance of the small intestine is indicative of volvulus.

Key points

Review areas for 'normal-appearing barium enema' in viva situation:

- Skeletal abnormality. Check for bone metastases, sacroiliitis, hip abnormalities such as avascular necrosis.
- Bowel distribution. Malrotation of the bowel, bowel displaced by organomegaly (e.g. splenomegaly, liver enlargement from metastases).
- Serosal colonic pathology. The mucosa remains intact but extrinsic compression may cause stenosis or narrowing (e.g. serosal deposits from peritoneal malignancy, such as ovarian cancer).
- Endometriosis. Usually appears as a submucosal mid-rectal lesion in the anterior wall with a serrated appearance, best seen on the lateral projection.
- Abnormal calcification. Chronic pancreatitis, calcified gallstones, ovarian dermoid.

Further reading

Berrocal T, Lamas M, Gutierrez J, et al. Congenital anomalies of the small intestine, colon and rectum. *Radiographics* 1999; **19**: 1219–36.

Long FR, Kramer SS, Markowitz RI, Taylor GE. Radiographics patterns of intestinal malrotation in children. *Radiographics* 1996; **16**: 547–56.

Gastrointestinal Case 34

KIAT T. TAN AND RICHARD HOPKINS

Clinical history
Emergency department assessment. Abdominal pain. Very unwell systemically.

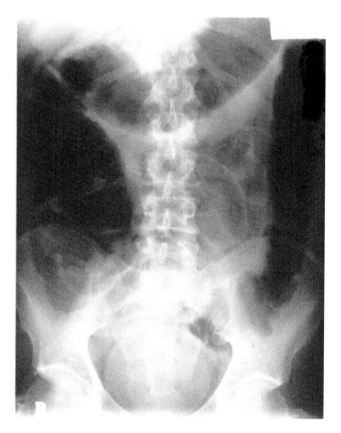

Figure 2.34

Model answer
This is a frontal plain abdominal radiograph of a skeletally mature patient (Figure 2.34). The caecum ascending, transverse, descending and the early part of the sigmoid colon are massively dilated, with associated loss of haustration. There is no gas within the rectum and more distal part of the sigmoid colon. Areas of thumbprinting and nodularity (also known as 'pseudopolyps') are evident in the large bowel. There is associated dilatation of the small bowel. Both the inner and outer walls of the small bowel loops are visible, consistent with a positive Rigler's sign, which is indicative of free gas in the peritoneal cavity. Sacroiliac joints are normal. The clinical and radiological findings are consistent with perforation of a hollow viscus due to toxic megacolon, which is most often due to ulcerative colitis. I will discuss the case with the referring team, as additional history would be helpful to elucidate the exact cause of the problem. The surgical team will need to be informed, as the patient will need an urgent laparotomy.

Questions

1. **What are the causes of toxic megacolon?**

   Toxic megacolon can result from any cause of colitis, including ulcerative colitis, Crohn's disease, *Clostridium difficile* colitis, other infective colitis and ischaemic colitis.

2. **The surgical registrar wishes to have a water-soluble contrast study or another imaging study to delineate anatomy prior to laparotomy. What is your advice?**

   Toxic megacolon is an absolute contraindication to contrast enema studies. Most surgeons would operate without further imaging. A CT may be performed if it does not delay laparotomy.

3. **How do you differentiate megacolon due to colitis from other causes of large bowel dilatation?**

   This can be difficult in a small number of cases. A clinical history of colitis is helpful. Thumbprinting, bowel wall nodularity and loss of haustral pattern all point toward a diagnosis of toxic megacolon.

4. **In the absence of perforation, how could you differentiate between those patients who could be managed medically and those who need urgent surgery?**

   The treatment should be guided by the clinical picture. Patients who present with a severe flare of ulcerative colitis should have daily abdominal radiographs to detect increasing large bowel dilatation and/or perforation. Surgical treatment should be considered if there is no reduction in colonic dilatation after 48 hours of optimal medical treatment. The presence of small bowel distension is a marker of poor response to medical treatment.

Key points

- Megacolon refers to gross dilatation of the large bowel not due to mechanical obstruction. Toxic megacolon occurs when the colonic diameter is larger than 5.5 cm in association with evidence of systemic toxicity.
- Toxic megacolon has a mortality of around 5%. Toxic megacolon complicated by perforation has a mortality rate of around 20%.
- The classic signs of peritonitis may be absent in patients with perforation due to corticosteroid use. The radiologist may be the first person to diagnose peritonitis in toxic megacolon.

Further reading

Ambrosini R, Barchiesi A, Di Mizio V, *et al*. Inflammatory chronic disease of the colon: how to image. *Eur J Radiol* 2007; **61**: 442–8.

Bartram CI, Taylor S. The large bowel. In Adam A, Dixon AK, eds., *Grainger and Allison's Diagnostic Radiology*, 5th edn. London: Churchill Livingstone, 2008 (ebook).

Gastrointestinal Case 35

KIAT T. TAN AND RICHARD HOPKINS

Clinical history
Abdominal pain. Loose stools with blood and mucus.

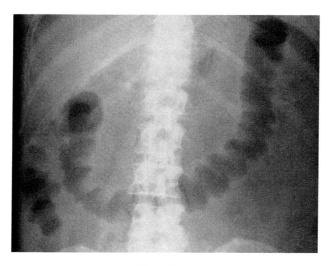

Figure 2.35

Model answer
This is a limited upper abdominal radiograph of a skeletally mature patient (Figure 2.35). There are multiple smooth scalloped defects in the transverse colon and the hepatic flexure, which are often referred to as 'thumbprinting'. This finding is non-specific and could be due to either oedema or submucosal haemorrhage. Colitis (of whatever cause) is the most common cause of this finding. A clinical history from either the patient or the referring clinician is essential to guide further investigation and management.

Questions
1. What are the common causes of thumbprinting on a plain film?
   Inflammatory bowel disease (IBD, e.g. Crohn's disease and ulcerative colitis), ischaemia, infective colitis (e.g. pseudomembranous colitis), malignancy (e.g. lymphoma, metastases).

Further reading
Kawamoto S, Horton KM, Fishman EK. Pseudomembranous colitis: spectrum of imaging findings with clinical and pathologic correlation. *Radiographics* 1999; **19**: 887–97.

Gastrointestinal Case 36

KIAT T. TAN AND RICHARD HOPKINS

Clinical history
80-year-old female patient. Past history of carcinoma of cervix.

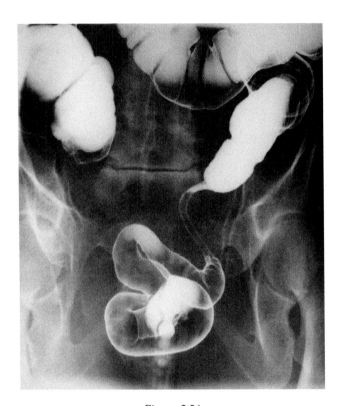

Figure 2.36

Model answer
This single image from a barium enema series (Figure 2.36) shows a long smooth narrowing at the level of the rectosigmoid junction. No evidence of proximal dilatation of the bowel is present. There is no evidence of mucosal destruction and there is no sign of the 'shouldering' typically found with a malignant tumour. The mucosal detail in the superior part of the stricture and the adjacent colon are obscured by barium. There is a ring shadow in the inferior part of the stricture. Minor bony sclerosis is present at the L5/S1 level.

The radiological features suggest a benign pathology. Given the history of carcinoma cervix the most likely diagnosis is a stricture secondary to radiotherapy. Radiotherapy is a common treatment for carcinoma of the cervix. The appearances are not typical for the other causes of benign strictures such as diverticular disease, ischaemia and inflammatory bowel disease.

Questions

1. **What are the causes of colorectal strictures?**
   - Malignant:
     - carcinoma
     - extrinsic compression from peritoneal malignancy
   - Benign:
     - diverticular stricture
     - ischaemia
     - inflammatory bowel disease
     - radiotherapy
     - postoperative
     - infection – lymphogranuloma venereum

Key points

- The radiological diagnosis of colonic scirrhous carcinoma can be problematic. However, there are often subtle mucosal abnormalities which could point towards the underlying diagnosis.
- The differentiation between polyp, faecal residue and diverticulum is usually straightforward, although they appear similar when viewed on face. Diverticula can be shown to be outpouchings of the bowel wall, while residue is usually freely mobile.

Further reading

Balthazar EJ, Siegel SE, Megibow AJ, Scholes J, Gordon R. CT in patients with scirrhous carcinoma of the GI tract: imaging findings and value for tumor detection and staging. *AJR Am J Roentgenol* 1995; **165**: 839–45.

Halligan S. The large bowel. In Sutton D, ed., *Textbook of Radiology and Imaging*, 7th edn. London: Elsevier, 2003; 635–63.

Gastrointestinal Case 37

KIAT T. TAN AND RICHARD HOPKINS

Clinical history
No history.

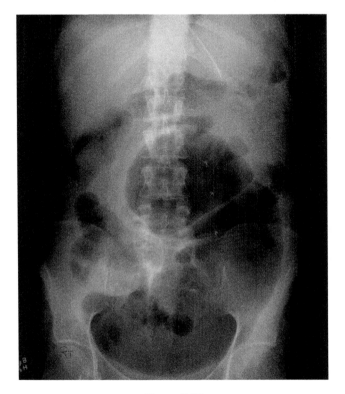

Figure 2.37

Model answer
This is a frontal abdominal radiograph of an adult patient (Figure 2.37). The naso-gastric tube tip is projected below the diaphragm. However, the side-hole of the NG tube is just at the level of the diaphragm and could be intraoesophageal. For optimal positioning, the tube should be advanced by another 10–15 cm and a repeat check radiograph obtained. A markedly distended loop of large bowel is seen to extend from the right lower quadrant to the mid abdomen, with a smooth superior aspect and a tapering inferior end. Gas is seen in the transverse colon but not in the rectum, and no free gas is demonstrated, suggesting that there is no perforation. The bowel gas pattern elsewhere is normal, with no evidence of small bowel dilatation. The bones are normal.

Features are of caecal volvulus. The findings should be communicated to the surgical team, as surgical treatment is usually required.

Questions

1. Why is no small bowel distension demonstrated?

This is usually a feature of early cases and is due to ileocaecal valve competence. In this case it may also have been decompressed by the gastric tube.

2. When would you perform a contrast enema study?

If there are no contraindications and the diagnosis is unclear from plain radiography, a contrast enema may be useful. The characteristic feature of caecal volvulus is a beak-like termination of normal colon at the site of obstruction. A barium enema can occasionally reduce the volvulus.

Key points

- Caecal volvulus can be caused by rotation of the ascending colon around its longitudinal axis in the axial plane, or by the caecum folding anteromedially to the ascending colon – the caecal bascule. Axial torsion is demonstrated here, as the distended caecum is seen low in the abdomen. The caecal bascule usually occupies a higher position.

Further reading

Consorti ET, Liu TH. Diagnosis and treatment of caecal volvulus. *Postgrad Med J* 2005; **81**: 772–6.

Perret RS, Kunberger LE. Case 44: cecal volvulus. *AJR Am J Roentgenol* 1998; **171**: 855, 859, 860.

Peterson CM, Anderson JS, Hara AK, Carenza JW, Menias CO. Volvulus of the gastrointestinal tract: appearances at multimodality imaging. *Radiographics* 2009; **29**: 1281–93.

Gastrointestinal Case 38

KIAT T. TAN AND RICHARD HOPKINS

Clinical history

Abdominal pain and distension in a 68-year-old male arteriopath.

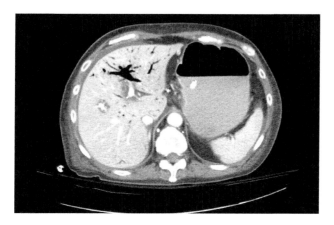

Figure 2.38a

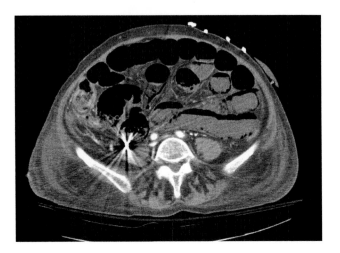

Figure 2.38b

Model answer

These are two images from an intravenous contrast-enhanced CT scan (Figures 2.38a, 2.38b). The stomach and small bowel are distended. There is gas in the bowel wall. Gas is also seen in the branches of the superior mesenteric vein. These extend into the intrahepatic portal vein branches. There is no free gas. Subcutaneous oedema is noted.

The clinical and radiological findings would be consistent with acute mesenteric ischaemia. I would like to review the rest of the images to assess the coeliac axis, superior mesenteric artery and inferior mesenteric artery. In addition, thrombus in the portal venous system should also be sought. The case will need to be discussed with the surgeon. If the patient is for further active management, he should have an echocardiogram to look for a source of emboli.

Questions

1. **How is gas in the portal vein distinguished from pneumobilia?**
   Gas in the biliary tree is observed centrally and does not extend to the liver capsule.
2. **Does portomesenteric gas always indicate mesenteric ischaemia?**
   No. Gas crosses from the bowel lumen into the mesenteric vessels when there is increased bowel wall permeability due to conditions such as inflammatory bowel disease, intestinal distension, blunt trauma, diverticulitis and abscess, but the most common cause is intestinal ischaemia with bowel necrosis.
3. **What is this patients's prognosis?**
   The prognosis of acute mesenteric ischaemia is poor in the presence of portal venous gas, with a mortality rate of up to 90%.

Key points

- Mesenteric ischaemia can be either acute or chronic.
- Acute mesenteric ischaemia can be due to arterial thrombosis, arterial embolism, venous thrombosis or a diverse group of diseases collectively known as non-occlusive mesenteric ischaemia. The latter group includes vasospasm (e.g. from cocaine) and low-output states (e.g. toxic shock, cardiac failure).
- Radiological features of acute mesenteric ischaemia include bowel wall thickening, evidence of vascular occlusion, increased bowel wall enhancement *as well as*

lack of bowel wall enhancement, bowel wall gas and portal vein gas. Absence of vascular obstruction per se *does not exclude* acute mesenteric ischaemia.

- It is important to search for a source of emboli in acute arterial occlusion. Pay particular attention to the left atrial appendage and left ventricle on CT.
- The presence of portal vein gas does not necessarily indicate a poor prognosis in the absence of bowel ischaemia.

Further reading

Rha SE, Ha HK, Lee SH, *et al.* CT and MR imaging findings of bowel ischemia from various primary causes. *Radiographics* 2000; **20**: 29–42.

Sebastia C, Quiroga S, Espin E, *et al.* Portomesenteric vein gas: pathologic mechanisms, CT findings, and prognosis. *Radiographics* 2000; **20**: 1213–24.

Gastrointestinal Case 39

KIAT T. TAN AND RICHARD HOPKINS

Clinical history
Abdominal pain. Outpatient scan.

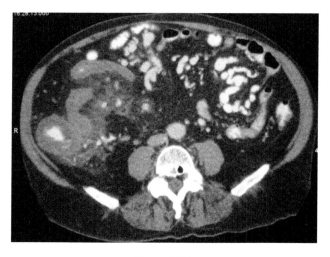

Figure 2.39a

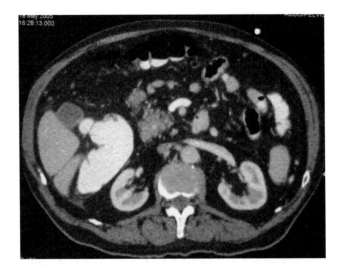

Figure 2.39b

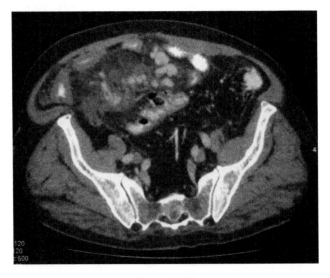

Figure 2.39c

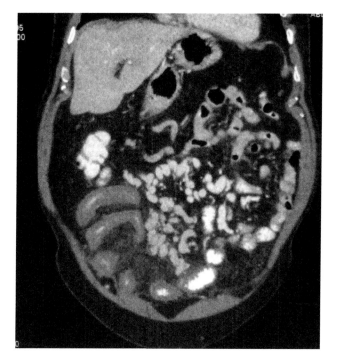

Figure 2.39d

Model answer

These are three axial images and one coronal image from an intravenous and oral enhanced CT scan of the abdomen (Figures 2.39a–2.39d). The distal small bowel, caecum and ascending colon are oedematous. Multiple collateral vessels are seen in the mid abdomen and right iliac fossa. There is 'misting' and infiltration of the small bowel mesentery, surrounding and tracking along the superior mesenteric vessels. A 'halo' of low attenuation can be seen around the branches of the superior mesenteric artery (Figure 2.39a). Multiple serpentine collateral vessels are present.

The diagnosis is sclerosing mesenteritis, with secondary midgut congestion due to compromise of the superior mesenteric vein branches. I would like to review the rest of the imaging to assess the extent of venous obstruction, as well as the size of the affected area. In addition, as sclerosing mesenteritis is associated with other inflammatory diseases as well as malignancy, the imaging features of these should be sought on the CT scan. I would like to discuss the case with the referring surgeon to plan management.

Questions

1. What are the differential diagnoses for sclerosing mesenteritis?

The imaging features of this case are of classic sclerosing mesenteritis, and there is no differential diagnosis. A 'halo' around the mesenteric vessels is not found in any of the major differential diagnoses of this condition. If the imaging features are not as typical, the differential diagnoses include:

- Carcinoid – mesenteric masses, calcification and retraction can occur in both carcinoid and sclerosing mesenteritis. Mesenteric calcification is a recognized feature of both entities (although not present in the case above). Clinical presentation, biochemical investigations (5-HIAA) and octreotide imaging can help to distinguish the two pathologies.

- Superior mesenteric vein (SMV) thrombosis – this would give a similar pattern of oedema to the case example above. After the acute episode, collateral vessels, as demonstrated above, may develop, but mesenteric infiltration is not a feature.
- Mesenteric tumours – desmoid tumour, peritoneal carcinomatosis and lymphoma may demonstrate infiltrate and mass lesions in the mesentery. Lymphoma does not usually cause vascular obstruction.

2. **What conditions are associated with sclerosing mesenteritis?**

Autoimmune conditions (such as sclerosing cholangitis, retroperitoneal fibrosis, Riedel's thyroiditis, orbital pseudotumour) and malignancy (lymphoma, breast, lung, melanoma).

Key points
- Sclerosing mesenteritis is an inflammatory condition of uncertain aetiology.
- The condition can be classified into three overlapping subgroups: panniculitis, where there is fat inflammation; lipodystrophy, caused by fat necrosis; and retractile mesenteritis, which is due to fibrosis.
- Treatment is by steroids, colchicine, progesterone, immunosuppression. Resection could be attempted in selected cases.

Further reading
Horton KM, Lawler LP, Fishman EK. CT findings in sclerosing mesenteritis (panniculitis): spectrum of disease. *Radiographcis* 2003; **23**: 1561–7.

Gastrointestinal Case 40

KIAT T. TAN AND RICHARD HOPKINS

Clinical history
Outpatient CT scan performed for right-sided abdominal fullness and abdominal discomfort.

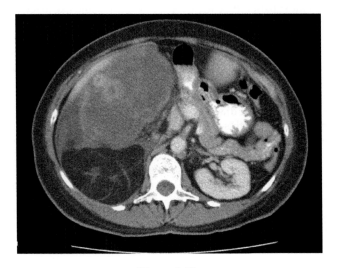

Figure 2.40a

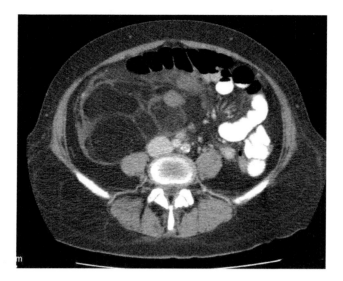

Figure 2.40b

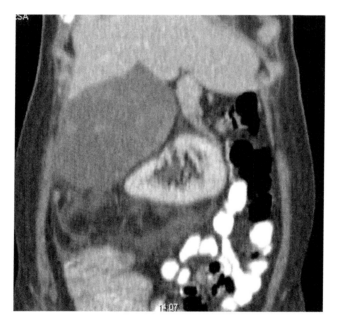

Figure 2.40c

Model answer

These CT images (Figures 2.40a–2.40c) show a large retroperitoneal mass that is posterolateral to the right kidney and lateral to the right psoas muscle. The mass is closely related to the inferior vena cava and displaces the kidney, ascending colon and duodenum anteriorly. The lesion is composed of tissue that is of fat density as well as mixed soft tissue attenuation. There are coarse septations within the mass and areas of heterogeneous enhancement.

The location of the mass and the density of the tumour is typical of liposarcoma. Referral to the regional sarcoma multidisciplinary team is required.

Questions

1. What are the clues to indicate a tumour is retroperitoneal?

Anterior displacement of retroperitoneal organs is an indication that a tumour is retroperitoneal in origin: kidneys; adrenal glands; ureters; ascending and descending colon; pancreas; duodenum; major vessels, aorta, IVC.

2. Name some tumours that occur in the retroperitoneum.

- Liposarcoma
- Neurogenic tumours
- Schwannomas (the most common tumour of peripheral nerves)
- Ganglioneuromas (typically located along the sympathetic chain, larger, rounded, and more commonly calcified than nerve sheath tumours)
- Paragangliomas and haemangiopericytomas (very vascular)
- Desmoid tumours
- Leiomyomas
- Leiomyosarcomas (tend to develop massive cystic degeneration)
- Rhabdomyosarcomas
- Lymphoma

Key points

- Liposarcoma can affect adults of all ages and is the most common sarcoma in adults.
- Liposarcoma is believed to arise from mesenchymal cells rather than pre-existing fat cells.
- Common sites of liposarcoma include the limbs (especially the lower limb), retroperitoneum and mesenteric region.
- Intra-abdominal liposarcomas can grow to massive proportions.

Further reading

Nishino M, Hayakawa K, Minami M, *et al*. Primary retroperitoneal neoplasms: CT and MR imaging findings with anatomic and pathologic diagnostic clues. *Radiographics* 2003; **23**: 45–57.

Pereira JM, Sirlin CB, Pinto PS, Casola G. CT and MR imaging of extrahepatic fatty masses of the abdomen and pelvis: techniques, diagnosis, differential diagnosis, and pitfalls. *Radiographics* 2005; **25**: 69–85.

Gastrointestinal Case 41

KIAT T. TAN AND RICHARD HOPKINS

Clinical history

Dull back pain for several months. Medially displaced ureters on intravenous urography.

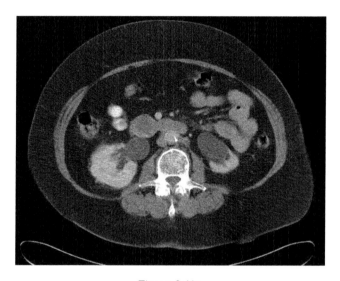

Figure 2.41a

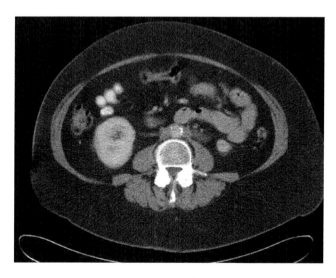

Figure 2.41b

Model answer

These are two selected images from an intravenous and oral contrast-enhanced CT scan of the abdomen (Figures 2.41a, 2.41b). There is dilatation of both renal collecting systems. The left kidney is small. A cuff of soft tissue is seen surrounding the aorta and IVC.

Retroperitoneal fibrosis or lymphoma are both possible causes for this appearance. The presence of a small left kidney would be consistent with chronic obstructive uropathy due to obstruction by the retroperitoneal soft tissue.

The patient will require hydration to reduce the risk of contrast nephropathy. In addition, careful monitoring of renal function is required. A review of the medical history, including a drug history, would help to narrow the differential diagnoses. I would like to review the rest of the imaging to assess the extent of the disease. In addition, I would like to discuss the case with the clinician, as a retrograde ureteric stent – or, if this is impossible or unsuccessful, a nephrostomy – may be required to prevent further loss of renal function.

Questions

1. **What are the causes of retroperitoneal fibrosis (RPF)?**

   More than half of cases of retroperitoneal fibrosis are believed to be due to an autoimmune disease. Other causes include drugs such as methysergide and tumours (e.g. lymphoma). The retroperitoneum following treatment of lymphoma can have an appearance on CT very similar to primary RPF.

Key points

- Classically, the ureters are displaced medially in retroperitoneal fibrosis. However, the position of the ureter may be normal.
- The middle third of the ureter is commonly affected, and approximately three-quarters of ureteric obstruction occurs bilaterally. Treatment is by ureteric stenting.
- Other causes of medially deviated ureters include normal variant and pelvic lipomatosis.

Further reading

Cronin CG, Lohan DG, Blake MA, *et al.* Retroperitoneal fibrosis: a review of clinical features and imaging findings. *AJR Am J Roentgenol* 2008; **191**: 423–31

Case contributed by Dr Chris Cook, Weston General Hospital.

Gastrointestinal Case 42

KIAT T. TAN AND RICHARD HOPKINS

Clinical history
Middle-aged patient with a long-term condition and current symptoms of diarrhoea, malabsorption and abdominal pain.

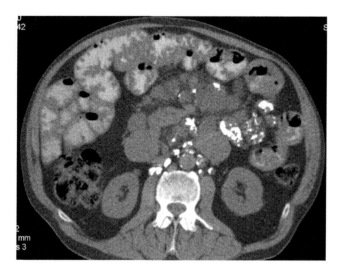

Figure 2.42

Model answer
The CT image with oral contrast (Figure 2.42) shows diffuse, symmetric thickening of the valvulae conniventes. Multiple calcified lymph nodes are present in the retroperitoneum and also in the small bowel mesentery. The affected small bowel loops are mildly dilated. The differential diagnoses include intestinal tuberculosis (e.g. tabes mesenterica), amyloidosis, previously treated lymphoma or two separate pathologies.

I would like to review the rest of the imaging to look for evidence that would favour one or the other diagnosis. A clinical history would be invaluable. Comparison with previous imaging to look for progression is required.

Questions
1. **What are the causes of small bowel fold thickening?**
   Crohn's disease, infection, oedematous states (e.g. cirrhosis, heart failure), infiltrative conditions (e.g. amyloid, lymphoma), haemorrhage into bowel wall.
2. **What are the causes of intra-abdominal lymph node calcification?**
   Previous exposure to tuberculosis (also histoplasmosis); previously treated lymphoma; amyloid; sclerosing mesenteritis.

Key points
- Amyloidosis refers to a diverse group of diseases that are due to deposition of insoluble protein fibres in various organs.

- Bowel wall thickening, hepatosplenomegaly, macroglossia and gallbladder wall thickening are gastrointestinal features of amyloidosis.
- Amyloid protein can also be deposited in the mesentery and lymph nodes. These deposits may calcify.

Notes

The diagnosis is amyloidosis.

Further reading

Georgiades CS, Neyman EG, Barish MA, Fishman EK. Amyloidosis: review and CT manifestations. *Radiographics* 2004; **24**: 405–16.

Kim SH, Han JK, Lee KH, *et al*. Abdominal amyloidosis: spectrum of radiologic findings. *Clin Radiol* 2003; **58**: 610–20.

Gastrointestinal Case 43

KIAT T. TAN AND RICHARD HOPKINS

Clinical history

No history.

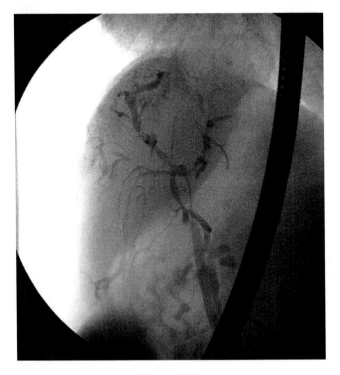

Figure 2.43

Model answer

The single image from an ERCP (endoscopic retrograde cholangiopancreatography) examination (Figure 2.43) shows multiple strictures in the intra- and extrahepatic biliary tree. There are also areas of focal dilatation in the biliary tree, which gives rise to a beaded appearance. A stent is seen in the common bile duct. The findings are consistent with sclerosing cholangitis, which could either be primary or secondary. A medical history would be invaluable, and monitoring of liver function is mandatory. The patient will need radiological follow-up to detect the development of cholangiocarcinoma.

Questions

1. **What are the causes of sclerosing cholangitis?**
   Sclerosing cholangitis can be primary or secondary. Primary sclerosing cholangitis is believed to be an autoimmune condition, and there is a strong association with other inflammatory conditions such as inflammatory bowel disease, retroperitoneal fibrosis and Sjögren's syndrome. Secondary sclerosing cholangitis could be due to chronic biliary infection (e.g. bacterial or parasitic), AIDS, eosinophilic cholangitis, intraductal stones, malignancy, trauma, ischaemia post liver transplantation and hepatic transarterial chemoembolization.
2. **What are the complications of primary sclerosing cholangitis (PSC)?**
   Biliary cirrhosis (and all the complications of cirrhosis), infection, biliary stone, development of cholangiocarcinoma (up to 15% of those with PSC).

Key points

- Secondary sclerosing cholangitis needs to be excluded before a diagnosis of PSC is made.
- Up to 75% of patients with PSC have inflammatory bowel disease.
- Symptoms include pruritus, jaundice, fatigue and right upper quadrant pain. Some patients present with secondary bacterial infection. Up to 40% of patients are asymptomatic.
- Cholangiocarcinoma in patients with PSC can be difficult to diagnose. Clinical features include rapid deterioration in symptoms and biliary obstruction. Imaging features are often non-specific. Radiological findings that could suggest cholangiocarcinoma include rapidly progressive stricturing, a polypoid lesion within the bile duct and the presence of shouldering in a stricture. Biliary brushing (whether performed endoscopically or percutaneously) is specific but not sensitive for cholangiocarcinoma.

Further reading

Abdalian R, Heathcote EJ. Sclerosing cholangitis: a focus on secondary causes. *Hepatology* 2006; **44**: 1063–74.

Vitellas KM, Keogan MT, Freed KS, *et al*. Radiologic manifestations of sclerosing cholangitis with emphasis on MR cholangiopancreatography 1. *Radiographics* 2000; **20**: 959–75.

Gastrointestinal Case 44

KIAT T. TAN AND RICHARD HOPKINS

Clinical history

Admitted via emergency department following road traffic accident. Report the CT first.

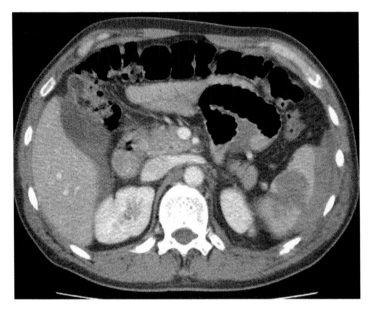

Figure 2.44a

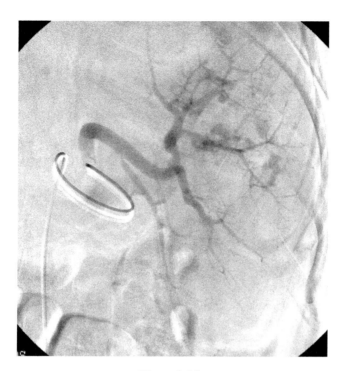

Figure 2.44b

Model answer

This is a single image from an intravenous and oral contrast-enhanced CT scan of the abdomen (Figure 2.44a). There is a large splenic laceration which extends from the hilum of the spleen to the lateral side of the capsule. A subcapsular haematoma is seen, along with free intra-abdominal bleeding. An associated left-sided rib fracture is evident. A focus of high attenuation is evident at the hilum of the spleen. It is uncertain if this represents active contrast extravasation or part of a splenic artery. The findings would be consistent with a traumatic splenic injury that is of at least grade III severity.

I would like to review the rest of the imaging to further assess the degree of splenic injury, the degree of intraperitoneal bleeding, the presence of active contrast extravasation and the presence of coexisting injury. The result will need to be communicated to the referring clinician and the on-call interventional radiologist for further management.

This is an image from a selective angiogram of the splenic artery (Figure 2.44b). Multiple abnormal contrast blushes are seen in the superior and middle branches of the splenic artery. These are consistent with contrast extravasation and/or pseudoaneurysms. There is a stenosis in the inferior branch of the splenic artery, which may represent focal spasm. The patient will require splenic arterial embolization with coils. Post-embolization CT follow-up is required within a few days. Even though splenic function is likely to be preserved in patients who have undergone successful splenic artery embolization, these patients should nonetheless receive the same precautions as those who have undergone splenectomy.

Questions

1. **How is splenic trauma managed?**
   Stable patients with grade I–II splenic injury and no evidence of other abdominal injury can usually be safely observed. The presence of active contrast extravasation

and/or pseudoaneurysm is an indication for angiography. Haemodynamically stable grade III–IV splenic injury patients (with no other indication for surgery) should have angiography + embolization. Grade V injuries with complete splenic devascularization can be treated either surgically or endovascularly (*although at least one of the authors prefers the former*). Unstable patients (and those with other significant organ injury) usually proceed directly to surgery. However, some centres do perform splenic embolization on appropriately resuscitated unstable patients with isolated splenic injury.

2. **What are the possible complications of splenic injury?**
Delayed rupture of the spleen is a known complication, usually occurring within 1–2 weeks of the acute injury. This is often due to rupture of a contained subcapsular haematoma. Other complications include pseudoaneurysm formation (and risk of rupture), splenic necrosis, splenic pseudocyst formation, recurrent bleeding, infection of haematoma/necrotic splenic tissue and hyposplenism.

Key points

- The spleen is the most commonly injured abdominal organ.
- An inferior left-sided rib fracture on a chest radiograph may be the only indication of a splenic injury on initial assessment. Other chest radiographic features include an elevated left hemidiaphragm and a left pleural effusion.
- The American Association of Trauma Surgery classification of splenic injury is as follows:
    Grade I – subcapsular haematoma of less than 10% surface area OR a capsular tear that is less than 1 cm in maximal depth.
    Grade II – subcapsular haematoma of 10–50% of surface area OR intraparenchymal haematoma of less than 5 cm in diameter OR laceration 1–3 cm in maximal depth that does not involve a parenchymal vessel.
    Grade III – subcapsular haematoma of more than 50% of surface area OR intraparenchymal haematoma of more than 5 cm in diameter OR expanding haematoma OR laceration more than 3 cm in depth OR laceration involving parenchymal vessel.
    Grade IV – laceration of segmental/hilar vessel with devascularization of more than 25% of the spleen.
    Grade V – shattered spleen and/or hilar vascular injury.
- It is currently uncertain if central splenic embolization or subselective embolization of the splenic artery branches should be the preferred endovascular treatment. There is some evidence to favour the former, although this is still being debated.

Further reading

Lubner M, Menias C, Rucker C, *et al*. Blood in the belly: CT findings of hemoperitoneum. *Radiographics* 2007; **27**: 109–25.

Raikhlin A, Baerlocher MO, Asch MR, Myers A. Imaging and transcatheter arterial embolization for traumatic splenic injuries: review of the literature. *Can J Surg* 2008; **51**: 464–72.

Acknowledgements

Richard Hopkins would like to acknowledge the help of the following people in the preparation of this chapter: Dr Matt Shaw, Dr Chris Cook, Dr S. Gandhi, Dr G. Clague, Dr R. Singh, Dr J. Rowlands, Dr A. Isaac.

MSK Case 1

HAN WEI AW-YEANG

Clinical history

Painful foot on activity.

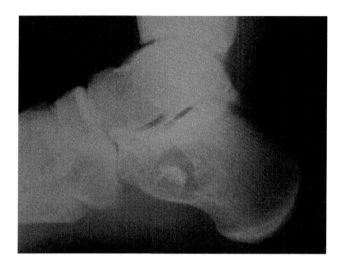

Figure 3.1a

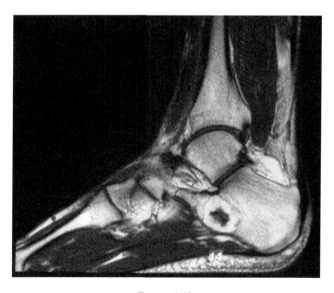

Figure 3.1b

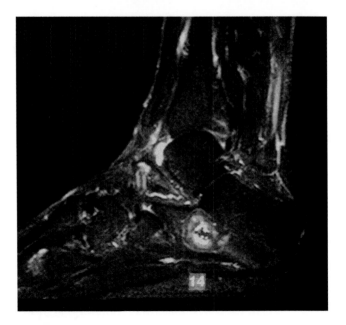

Figure 3.1c

Model answer

This is a single lateral view of a skeletally mature foot (Figure 3.1a) showing a well-defined lucency at the base of the calcaneal neck. There is an irregular focus of sclerosis centrally in this lucency. No fracture.

Sagittal T1 and STIR sequences of the foot (Figures 3.1b, 3.1c) show that the periphery of the lucent lesion contains fat (high signal on T1 which has saturated out on the STIR). The centre has remained low signal, consistent with calcification. There are some cystic areas around the calcification. The lesion is an intraosseous lipoma of the calcaneus.

Questions

1. **What might be demonstrated on bone scintigraphy?**
   Mild increased tracer activity.
2. **Is there a risk of malignancy?**
   No.

Key points

- Intraosseous lipomas are most frequently detected in the fourth and fifth decades of life.
- Sites of occurrence include intertrochanteric region of the proximal femur (34%), tibia (13%), fibula (10%), calcaneus (8%) and ilium (8%). Long bone involvement is usually metaphyseal.
- Central calcification is thought to be either due to fat necrosis or mesenchymal in nature. Absence of calcification raises the possibility of a unicameral bone cyst on plain films. CT and MR are diagnostic.
- Symptomatic intraosseous lipomas may be treated by curettage.

Further reading

Bertram C, Popken F, Rütt J. Intraosseous lipoma of the calcaneus. *Langenbecks Arch Surg* 2001; **386**: 313–17.

Kwak HS, Lee KB, Lee SY, Han YM. MR findings of calcaneal intraosseous lipoma with hemorrhage. *AJR Am J Roentgenol* 2005; **185**: 1378–9.

Murphey MD, Carroll JF, Flemming DJ, *et al*. From the archives of the AFIP. Benign musculoskeletal lipomatous lesions. *Radiographics* 2004; **24**: 1433–66.

MSK Case 2

HAN WEI AW-YEANG

Clinical history

Painful foot.

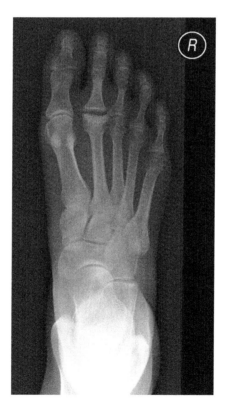

Figure 3.2a

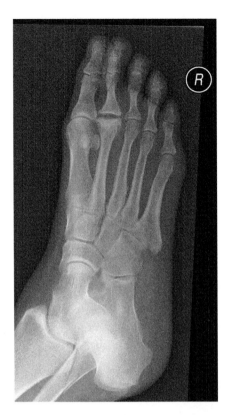

Figure 3.2b

Model answer

Two views of the right foot (Figures 3.2a, 3.2b) show widening of the second metatarsophalangeal joint space with associated flattening, sclerosis and concavity of the subchondral bone in the second metatarsal head. There are also degenerative changes in the base of the proximal phalanx. The appearances are consistent with Freiberg's disease, or avascular necrosis of the second metatarsal head. There is a spiral fracture of the distal fibula.

Questions

1. **What is the aetiology of Freiberg's infraction?**
   It is thought to be trauma. Unlike other causes of avascular necrosis, it is not associated with the usual causes such as steroids or alcohol.
2. **Can any other metatarsals be affected?**
   Yes, the third and fourth metatarsal heads. The second and third metatarsals are the least mobile, possibly making them more susceptible to repeated microtrauma.
3. **Who is typically affected?**
   Adolescent girls. Females are affected five times more frequently than males, in contrast to other osteochondroses, where there is a male preponderance.

Key points

- Initial radiographs show flattening of the head of the second metatarsal with mild sclerosis. Later there is widening of the joint space.
- Freiberg's infraction may be associated with loose bodies of fragmented bone within the joint.

Further reading

Tachdjian MO. Freiberg's infraction. In *Pediatric Orthopedics*, 2nd edn. Philadelphia, PA: Saunders, 1990; 1006–10.

Thompson FM, Hamilton WG. Problems of the second metatarsophalangeal joint. *Orthopedics* 1987; **10**: 83–9.

MSK Case 3

HAN WEI AW-YEANG AND JOHN CURTIS

Clinical history

Painful knee.

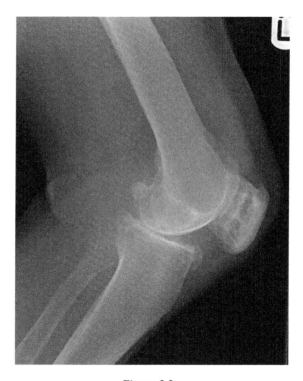

Figure 3.3a

Model answer

This is a single lateral view of a skeletally mature knee (Figure 3.3a). There is generalized tibiofemoral and patellofemoral degenerative change with loss of joint space and osteophyte formation. The patella is abnormal, with coarse trabeculation, cortical thickening and bony expansion.

The appearances are consistent with Paget's disease of the patella. There is no evidence of fracture or malignant transformation.

Questions
1. What are the complications of Paget's disease?

Secondary osteoarthritis, pathological fracture, spinal stenosis, conductive deafness and sarcomas. Paget's disease of the skull base can lead to sensorineural deafness, optic atrophy and hydrocephalus secondary to platybasia.

Key points

- Paget's disease can involve any bone in the skeleton but commonly affects long bones such as the femur and tibia (approx 35%) and the bony pelvis (up to 75%).
- Involvement of the ribs, fibula and bones of the hand and foot is uncommon. It is not uncommon, however, for these sites to prevail in the FRCR examination (Figure 3.3b)!
- In long bones osteolysis almost always starts in a subchondral position and spreads into the metadiaphysis, and this has been likened to a 'blade of grass' (Figure 3.3c).

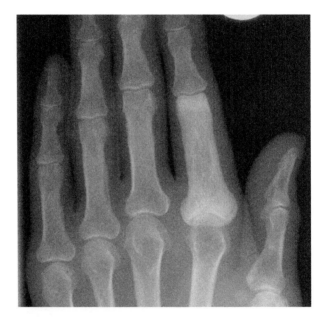

Figure 3.3b

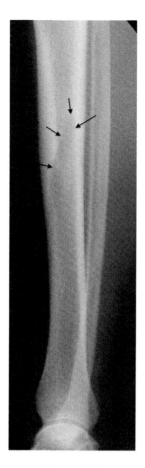

Figure 3.3c

Further reading

Gordon L. Paget's disease of the patella. *J Bone Joint Surg Am* 1958; **40**: 1423–5.

Smith SE, Murphey MD, Motamedi K, *et al*. From the archives of the AFIP. Radiologic spectrum of Paget disease of bone and its complications with pathologic correlation. *Radiographics* 2002; **22**: 1191–216.

Stull MA, Moser RP, Vinh TN, Kransdorf MJ, Callaghan JJ. Paget's disease of the patella. *Skeletal Radiol* 1990; **19**: 407–10.

MSK Case 4

HAN WEI AW-YEANG

Clinical history
Painful knee.

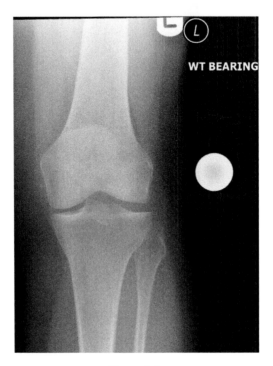

Figure 3.4a

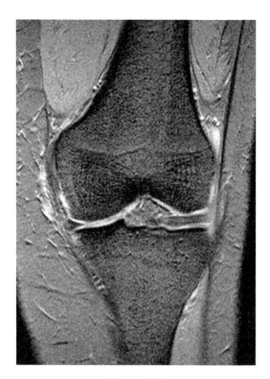

Figure 3.4b

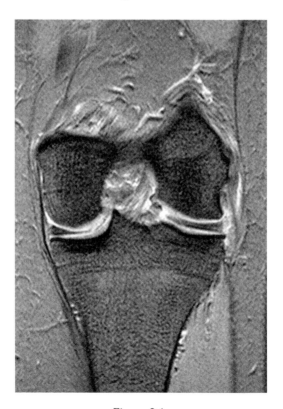

Figure 3.4c

Model answer

On the weight-bearing frontal x-ray of the left knee (Figure 3.4a) there is no bony abnormality. Increased joint space is noted in the lateral tibiofemoral compartment, with hypoplasia of the lateral tibial eminence.

On the two coronal fat-saturated proton-density MRI images of the knee (Figures 3.4b, 3.4c), the lateral meniscus is larger than expected and extends towards the intercondylar notch. The appearances are consistent with a discoid lateral meniscus. No visible tears are demonstrated on these limited views.

Further assessment of the sagittal images would be useful to see if this is a Wrisberg variant of discoid meniscus, which is hypermobile and therefore unstable because there is no connection of meniscus to the meniscofemoral ligament of Wrisberg.

Questions

1. **Which is more common – a discoid medial or lateral meniscus?**
   Discoid lateral menisci are much more common.
2. **What is the frequency of bilateral discoid meniscus?**
   20%.

Key points

- A discoid meniscus has a broad shape, which gives rise to a thickened 'bow-tie' appearance of the lateral meniscus.
- A discoid meniscus can cause a snap as the femoral condyle articulates with a thickened lateral meniscus posteriorly. This causes repeated microtrauma and may predispose to meniscal tearing by minimal trauma.

Further reading

Helms CA. The meniscus: recent advances in MR imaging of the knee. *AJR Am J Roentgenol* 2002; **179**: 1115–22.

Ryu KN, Kim IS, Kim EJ. MR imaging of tears of discoid lateral menisci. *AJR Am J Roentgenol* 1998; **171**: 963–7.

MSK Case 5

HAN WEI AW-YEANG

Clinical history
Post-ictal patient with shoulder pain.

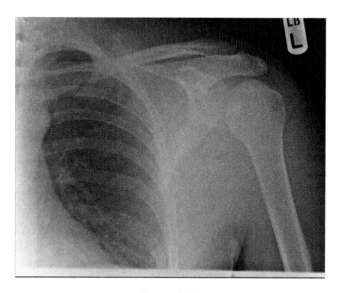

Figure 3.5a

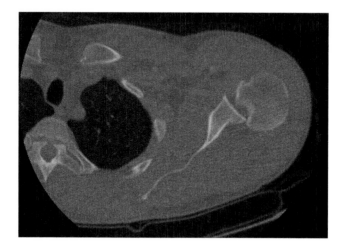

Figure 3.5b

Model answer
The single AP radiograph of the left shoulder (Figure 3.5a) shows loss of congruity of the glenohumeral articulation. The humeral head is also symmetrically round, consistent with the 'lightbulb' sign. This is suggestive of a posterior dislocation of the shoulder,

The axial CT of the left shoulder (Figure 3.5b) confirms that the humeral head is dislocated posteriorly relative to the glenoid. There is also a defect in the anteromedial aspect of the humeral head, which is known as the reverse Hill–Sachs deformity.

Questions
1. What are the associated injuries?
A tear in the posterior aspect of the glenoid labrum (reverse Bankart lesion) and fracture/injury to the anterior humeral head.

Key points
- Posterior dislocations are rare, comprising only 4% of shoulder dislocations, and are a consequence of severe adduction and internal rotation caused by muscular contraction. They are often associated with a seizure or electrical injury. They can very rarely be bilateral, when seizure is by far the likeliest cause.
- Posterior dislocations are less likely than anterior dislocations to cause neurovascular injury but are frequently associated with posterior glenoid fractures and an anterior compression injury to the head of the humerus (reverse Hill–Sachs injury)
- Radiographic findings are subtle and include the 'trough line sign' or reverse Hill–Sachs deformity (Figure 3.5c, arrows) and loss of congruity of the humeral head and glenoid fossa. A scapular 'Y' or axillary projection will readily make this diagnosis.

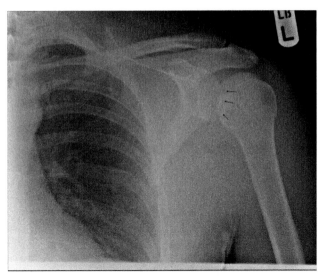

Figure 3.5c

Further reading
Gor DM. Signs in imaging: the trough line sign. *Radiology* 2002; **224**: 485–6.

Griffith JF, Antonio GE, Yung PS, *et al.* Prevalence, pattern, and spectrum of glenoid bone loss in anterior shoulder dislocation: CT analysis of 218 patients. *AJR Am J Roentgenol* 2008; **190**: 1247–54.

Saupe N, White LM, Bleakney R, *et al.* Acute traumatic posterior shoulder dislocation: MR findings. *Radiology* 2008; **248**: 185–93.

MSK Case 6

HAN WEI AW-YEANG

Clinical history

Painful knee.

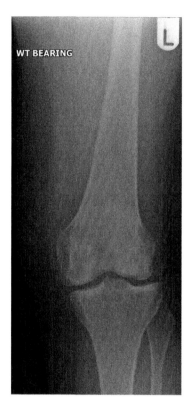

Figure 3.6a

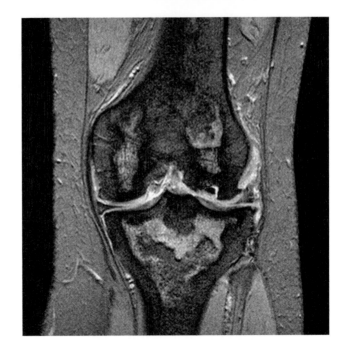

Figure 3.6b

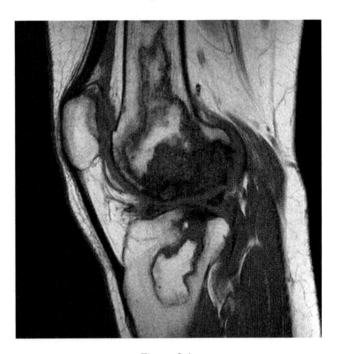

Figure 3.6c

Model answer

On the weight-bearing frontal x-ray of the left knee (Figure 3.6a) there are patchy areas of sclerosis and lucency in the subchondral regions of the femoral condyles and tibial plateaux. A small bony defect is demonstrated in the lateral femoral condyle, which is affecting the articular surface.

These are a coronal proton-density (PD) fat-saturated MRI image and a sagittal T1 MRI image (Figures 3.6b, 3.6c). They show curvilinear areas of abnormal marrow signal affecting the metaphyseal regions of the distal femur and proximal tibia. The double-line sign is apparent on the coronal PD fat-sat image, showing high-signal areas outlined by low-signal lines. On T1 the decreased signal indicates granulation tissue and sclerotic bone. The appearances are consistent with bone infarct or osteonecrosis.

On correlating with the radiographic abnormality, there is an osteochondral fragment still attached to the femur.

Questions
1. **What are the common causes of bone infarcts?**
   Trauma, radiotherapy, steroid use, diabetes, infection, sickle cell disease and autoimmune conditions such as systemic lupus erythematosus.
2. **What are the complications of bone infarcts?**
   Secondary osteoarthritis, osteochondral lesions and malignancy (fibrosarcoma and malignant fibrous histiocytoma).

Key points
- Bone infarction is caused by a reduced blood supply to bone and is associated with many causes. It is always worth looking at the whole radiograph to search for clues that reveal the overall diagnosis – e.g. 'H-shaped' vertebrae in sickle cell disease.
- MR imaging classically demonstrates the 'double-line sign', which is the interface between normal and ischaemic bone. On T2-weighted imaging this interface comprises a narrow low-signal line (bone sclerosis) and inner high-signal zone (granulation tissue). On T1-weighted imaging this interface is a line of low signal (granulation tissue and sclerotic bone).
- Bone scintigraphy will demonstrate a 'cold' lesion in early ischaemic change and a 'hot' lesion some weeks to months after this when there is reparative bone healing and revascularization. Note that bone scans may be normal if imaging occurs between these two stages of the ischaemic process.

Further reading
Blacksin MF, Finzel KC, Benevenia J. Osteomyelitis originating in and around bone infarcts: giant sequestrum phenomena. *AJR Am J Roentgenol* 2001; **176**: 387–91.
Hara H, Akisue T, Fujimoto T, *et al.* Magnetic resonance imaging of medullary bone infarction in the early stage. *Clin Imaging* 2008; **32**: 147–51.
Zurlo JV. The double-line sign. *Radiology* 1999; **212**: 541–2.

MSK Case 7

HAN WEI AW-YEANG

Clinical history
Backache, generally unwell.

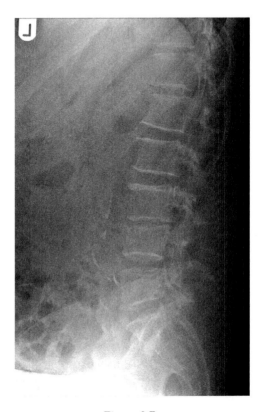

Figure 3.7a

Model answer
This is a sagittal x-ray of the lumbar spine (Figure 3.7a) showing destruction of the anterior aspect of the superior end plate of L4 vertebra, with associated loss of disc height between L3 and L4.

Questions
1. **What would you do next to confirm it?**
   An MRI scan would confirm the diagnosis.
2. **Describe the features on MRI?**
   On the sagittal T2-weighted image (Figure 3.7b), abnormal changes are seen at the L3/L4 disc. There is loss of disc height and high-signal change within the disc, with abnormal high-signal change in the marrow of the adjacent vertebrae. On the axial T2-weighted image (Figure 3.7c), high-signal abnormalities are noted in the psoas muscles bilaterally, consistent with abscesses. The diagnosis is L3/L4 discitis with associated psoas abscess collections.

3. **What are the common organisms responsible for this condition?**
   Staphylococcus aureus, *Escherichia coli* and *Proteus* spp.

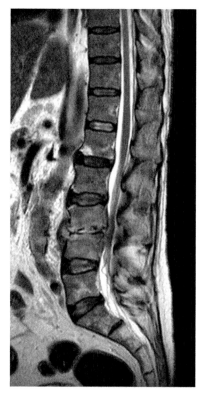

Figure 3.7b

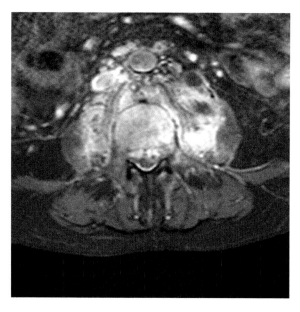

Figure 3.7c

Key points

- When dealing with patients with infective discitis, remember the rule of 50s:
  - 50% of patients are older than 50.
  - Fever is only present in 50%.
  - The urinary tract is the source of the pathogen in 50%.
  - *Staphylococcus aureus* is the causative organism in 50%.
  - The lumbar spine is affected in 50% of cases.
  - 50% of cases have more than three months of symptoms at presentation.
- In adults infective discitis is most commonly caused by haematogenous spread of pathogens into the bone marrow of vertebral bodies and then to the disc.
- The anterior portion of the vertebral body is richly vascularized and is the first site of involvement.
- Children will develop disc infection by direct haematogenous spread before vertebral involvement, since the disc has a rich blood supply. In adult infective discitis without initial vertebral involvement, iatrogenic causes are implicated, e.g. lumbar puncture.
- Only 25% of patients will have radiographic abnormalities at the onset of symptoms. These include blurring of the end plate. Later there is disc space narrowing.
- MR is the most sensitive modality to detect early change. It is also useful to detect associated epidural collections.

Further reading

Balériaux DL, Neugroschl C. Spinal and spinal cord infection. *Eur Radiol* 2004; **14**: E72–83

Conaughty JM, Chen J, Martinez OV, *et al*. Efficacy of linezolid versus vancomycin in the treatment of methicillin-resistant Staphylococcus aureus discitis: a controlled animal model. *Spine* 2006; **31**: E830–2.

Cottle L, Riordan T. Infectious spondylodiscitis. *J Infect* 2008; **56**: 401–12.

Ehara S. Spondylodiskitis. *AJR Am J Roentgenol* 1999; **172**: 1450–1.

Images courtesy of Dr Ravi Adapala, Arrowe Park Hospital, Wirral.

MSK Case 8

JOHN CURTIS

Clinical history
18-year-old male with muscle weakness.

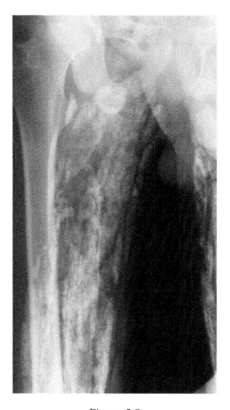

Figure 3.8

Model answer
The radiograph (Figure 3.8) demonstrates sheet-like calcification, which follows the fascial planes, together with amorphous rounded calcific densities in both thighs. No bone or joint abnormalities are present. The diagnosis is calcinosis universalis. As it is commonly associated with connective tissue disease it would be important to exclude dermatomyositis as the underlying cause.

Questions
1. **What may be demonstrated on MRI?**
   Inflammatory myositis.

Key points
- Calcinosis universalis usually affects children and young adults and may be idiopathic or associated with dermatomyositis. It is more common in females.

- Unlike tumoral calcinosis and scleroderma (calcinosis circumscripta), the calcification in calcinosis universalis is confined to muscles and fascial planes.
- Clinically there may be a violaceous facial rash and a high incidence of internal malignancies, although this is less likely in children.
- It is associated with muscle weakness and acro-osteolyis.
- It is characterized by calcium deposition but no bone formation.

Further reading
Olsen KM, Chew FS. Tumoral calcinosis: pearls, polemics, and alternative possibilities. *Radiographics* 2006; **26**: 871–85.

MSK Case 9

JOHN CURTIS

Clinical history
Twisting injury to the ankle in a 30-year-old male.

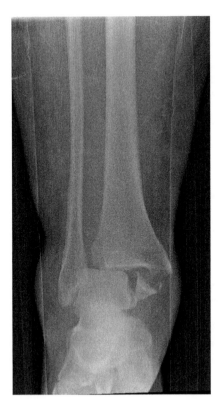

Figure 3.9a

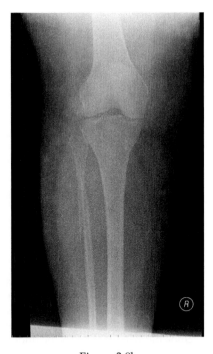

Figure 3.9b

Model answer

These AP radiographs (Figures 3.9a, 3.9b) demonstrate a spiral fracture through the proximal third of the fibula. There is widening of the tibiofibular syndesmosis and a fracture of the medial malleolus. There is probable rupture of the deep deltoid ligament. The appearances are those of a Maisonneuve fracture. Incidentally, there are varicose veins present.

Questions

1. **What is the mechanism of injury?**
   Pronation–extension forces lead to this unstable injury.
2. **Is this stable or unstable?**
   These fractures are laterally unstable.

Key points

- This injury is the lower limb equivalent of the Monteggia and Galeazzi fractures. It is more serious than initial radiographs may suggest.
- The fibrous/bony ring which is formed by the talus, both malleoli, distal tibiofibular syndesmosis and collateral ligaments is disrupted following the pronation–external rotation force. Subsequently the interosseous membrane is torn, leading to a fracture of the proximal fibula.
- The injury is often unstable and usually requires internal fixation.
- A Maisonneuve fracture should be considered in any apparently isolated posterior malleolar fracture and when there is lateral talar displacement. A view of the entire tibia and fibula is then required to exclude this injury.

Further reading

Barron D, Branfoot T. Imaging trauma of the appendicular skeleton. *Imaging* 2003; **15**: 324–40.

MSK Case 10

JOHN CURTIS

Clinical history
55-year-old male diabetic with painful hands.

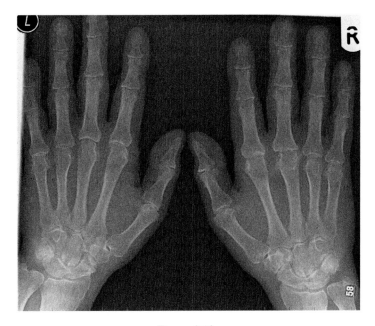

Figure 3.10a

Model answer
This radiograph (Figure 3.10a) demonstrates moderate degenerative change in the second to fifth metacarpophalangeal (MCP) joints of the left hand and severe degenerative change in the second and third MCP joints of the right hand. In addition, there are beak-like osteophytes involving the radial aspects of the second and third MCP joints of both hands and the fifth MCP joint on the left hand. There is no evidence of chondrocalcinosis in the triangular fibrocartilage (TFC). The appearances are essentially symmetrical and most likely those of haemochromatosis. This diagnosis would explain diabetes.

Questions
1. **What are the other manifestations of haemochromatosis?**
   Skin pigmentation, pancreatic iron deposition (diabetes mellitus), pituitary iron deposition with consequent hormone deficiency, cirrhosis, cardiomyopathy.

Key points
- Idiopathic calcium pyrophosphate dihydrate (CPPD) deposition disease and haemochromatosis have a propensity to cause a symmetrical arthropathy involving the second and third MCP joints. In the case of haemochromatosis the fourth and fifth MCP joints tend to be involved, unlike in idiopathic CPPD. The beak-like

osteophytes (Figure 3.10b, black arrows) are characteristic and may also occur in the hip and shoulder.

- It is worth telling the examiner that you are searching for chondrocalcinosis in the TFC (Figure 3.10b, white arrow). Chondrocalcinosis occurs in 30% of patients with haemochromatosis.
- Most patients with haemochromatosis are male and become symptomatic in the fifth decade of life. Both CPPD crystals and iron may deposit within the same joint.

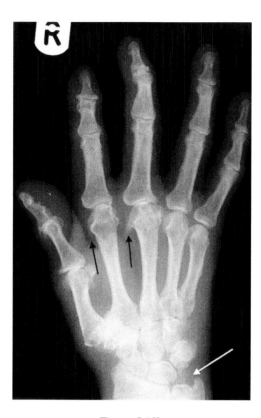

Figure 3.10b

Further reading

Jacobson JA, Girish G, Jiang Y, Sabb BJ. Radiographic evaluation of arthritis: degenerative joint disease and variations. *Radiology* 2008; **248**; 737–47.

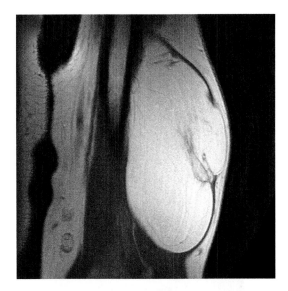

Figure 3.11d

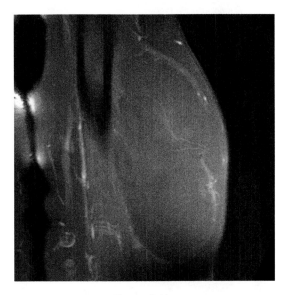

Figure 3.11e

Model answer

XR (Figures 3.11a, 3.11b). These are orthogonal views of the upper arm, showing a well-defined lucent mass in the soft tissues of the arm with a well-defined rim of soft tissue density. No bone changes.

MRI (Figures 3.11c–3.11e). Axial and sagittal T1 and sagittal STIR sequences of the upper arm demonstrate a well-defined homogeneous fat-signal mass within the soft tissues of the arm, bordered by a rim of soft tissue signal, likely to be muscle. The signal of the mass is isointense to subcutaneous fat. There are a few linear strands within the lesion in keeping with fibrous septa but no evidence of nodules. There is complete suppression of the fat signal on the STIR images. The appearances are those of a benign intramuscular lipoma of the upper arm.

Questions
1. **How frequent are lipomas compared to liposarcomas?**
   100 : 1.
2. **Is there a risk of malignancy?**
   No.

Key points
- Lipomas are most frequently detected in the fifth and sixth decades of life.
- Lipomas are multiple in up to 15% of cases.
- Lipomas in the retroperitoneum are very rare and should be considered liposarcomas until proven otherwise.
- Thin septa (< 2 mm) are seen in up to 50% of lipomas. The presence of thick septa, enhancement, nodules and incomplete suppression on STIR sequences strongly suggest liposarcoma.
- Fat that interdigitates with muscle is a feature of benignity and is not seen in liposarcomas.

Further reading
Murphey MD, Carroll JF, Flemming DJ, *et al.* From the archives of the AFIP: benign musculoskeletal lipomatous lesions. *Radiographics* 2004; **24**: 1433–66.

MSK Case 12

JOHN CURTIS

Clinical history
Painful swollen thigh in a 30-year-old male.

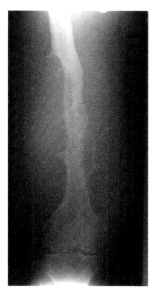

Figure 3.12a

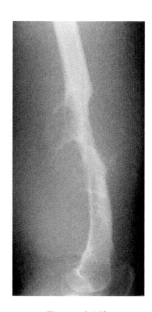

Figure 3.12b

Questions
1. What are the causes of unilateral muscle wasting?
Stroke, old polio and one-sided neglect.

Key points
- Duchenne muscular dystrophy is an X-linked recessive inherited disorder and is characterized by profound and progressive muscle weakness in boys and young men. Spontaneous mutations account for a third of cases.
- Muscular weakness is inexorable, leading to death in the early 20s from respiratory failure and infection. Contractures are common.
- All muscles are affected and become atrophic, eventually being replaced by fat.
- Pseudohypertrophy of the soleus muscles is a characteristic clinical feature, a result of fatty infiltration of muscle.

Further reading
Schreiber A, Smith WL, Ionasescu V, *et al.* Magnetic resonance imaging of children with Duchenne muscular dystrophy. *Pediatric Radiology* 1987; **17**: 495–7.

MSK Case 14

JOHN CURTIS

Clinical history
50-year-old male with bone pain.

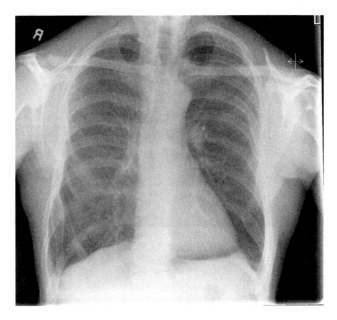

Figure 3.14a

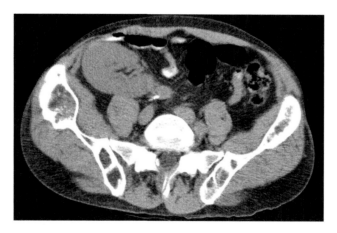

Figure 3.14b

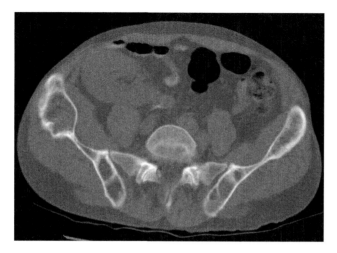

Figure 3.14c

Model answer

The frontal chest radiograph (Figure 3.14a) demonstrates focal expansion of the anterolateral portions of the right ribs and posterior aspects of the left ribs. There is soft tissue calcification overlying the left shoulder. There are surgical clips in the right side of the neck. The heart is normal size. Lungs clear.

CT of the lower abdomen without IV contrast (Figures 3.14b, 3.14c) reveals expansile, lucent bone lesions without extraosseous soft tissue extension. There is a transplant kidney in the right iliac fossa.

The appearances are those of multiple brown tumours and metastatic calcification in a patient with hyperparathyroidism secondary to renal failure. The patient has undergone a parathyroidectomy for tertiary hyperparathyroidism and a renal transplant.

Questions

1. **In which bones are brown tumours usually found?**
   Mandible, pelvis, ribs and femur.

Key points

- Brown tumours appear radiographically as single or multiple focal lytic areas that are generally well demarcated and often cause expansion of bone. They most commonly involve the facial bones, pelvis, ribs, and femur and are the result of osteoclastic resorption.
- Brown tumours are localized collections of giant cells and fibrous tissue and are often expansile well-defined lucent lesions. They are often associated with other features of hyperparathyroidism. Large expansile lesions may mimic neoplasms. They may undergo necrosis and form true cysts (osteitis fibrosa cystica).
- Brown tumours are frequently multiple, and may be cortical or medullary in location.

Further reading

Chew FS, Huang-Hellinger F. Brown tumor. *AJR Am J Roentgenol* 1993; **160**: 752.

Eisenberg RL. Bubbly lesions of bone. *AJR Am J Roentgenol* 2009; **193**: W79–94.

Miller TT. Bone tumors and tumorlike conditions: analysis with conventional radiography. *Radiology* 2008: **246**; 662–74.

MSK Case 15

JOHN CURTIS

Clinical history

Painful swollen joints in both feet in a 50-year-old male.

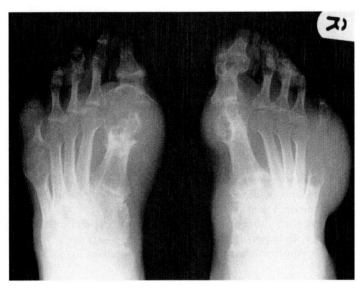

Figure 3.15

Model answer

This DP view of both feet (Figure 3.15) demonstrates extensive soft tissue swelling, notably at the metatarsophalangeal (MTP) joints of the left big toe and both little toes. There is associated bone destruction on both sides of all involved joints. There are well-defined juxta-articular erosions (intraosseous tophi) involving the right big toe interphalangeal joint. There is periarticular osteopenia. In the left big toe MTP joint there are 'clasps' of mineralization at the periphery of the soft tissue tophi formed by the margin of the expanded bone ends. The appearances are those of chronic tophaceous gout.

Questions

1. **Name three causes of hyperuricaemia.**
   Hypothyroidism, glomerulonephritis, glycogen storage diseases.
2. **What is the difference in appearances of the crystals in pseudogout and gout?**
   Gout is characterized by urate crystals, which are needle-shaped and exhibit negative birefringence to polarized light. Pseudogout is characterized by calcium pyrophosphate dihydrate (CPPD) crystals, which are rhomboid-shaped and positively birefringent.

Key points

- Gout is due to hyperuricaemia and may be idiopathic or related to other disorders – primary gout is due to an inborn metabolic error, secondary gout is due to other pathology such as myeloproliferative disorders, renal disease and endocrine abnormalities.
- Idiopathic gout is more common in men (20 : 1) and typically occurs in the fifth decade.
- Acute gout is characterized by the presence of monosodium urate crystals within the joint and periarticular soft tissues followed by an intense inflammatory response. Usually only one joint is affected in the early stages and there is usually a lag of about five years from the onset of symptoms to the appearance of radiological signs.
- Gout typically produces well-defined erosions, often 'punched out' with sclerotic margins and overhanging edges. Soft tissue swelling due to urate deposition is common. The big toe MTP joint, tarsal joints and interphalangeal joints of the hands are the most frequently affected areas.
- Joint spaces and bone density around the joints are preserved until late on in the disease, unlike rheumatoid arthritis, which is characterized by early periarticular osteopenia.
- Tophaceous gout results in urate deposition within the articular cartilage, synovium and subchondral bone in addition to periarticular tissues. Subsequent loss of articular cartilage allows urates to enter the subchondral bone, causing intraosseous tophi.

Further reading

Grainger AJ, McGonagle D. Imaging in rheumatology. *Imaging* 2003; **15**: 286–97.
Jacobson JA, Girish G, Jiang Y, Sabb BJ. Radiographic evaluation of arthritis: degenerative joint disease and variations. *Radiology* 2008; **248**: 737–47.
Sheldon PJ, Forrester DM, Learch TJ. Imaging of intraarticular masses. *Radiographics* 2005; **25**: 105–19.

Image courtesy of Dr Brian Eyes, University Hospital Aintree, Liverpool.

MSK Case 16

JOHN CURTIS

Clinical history
Ankle pain and reduced joint movement in a 40-year-old male.

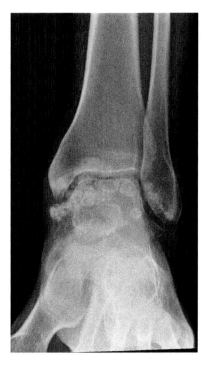

Figure 3.16a

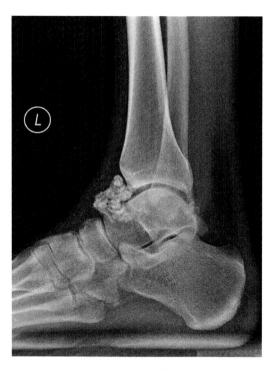

Figure 3.16b

Model answer

These AP and lateral radiographic views of the ankle (Figures 3.16a, 3.16b) demonstrate multiple ossific loose bodies in the anterior ankle joint. There is no joint space narrowing or osteophytic lipping. The ossific loose bodies have a uniform shape and are of approximately the same size, evenly distributed in the anterior joint. No periarticular osteopenia. The lack of degenerative joint changes and the uniformity and multiplicity of loose bodies suggests that this is primary synovial osteochondromatosis.

Questions

1. **Is this likely to affect other joints?**
   No, this condition is typically monoarticular.
2. **Is there a risk of malignancy?**
   Yes. Although the risk is low, chondrosarcomatous transformation has been described.

Key points

- Primary synovial osteochondromatosis (PSO) is an uncommon condition caused by metaplasia or benign neoplasia of connective tissue beneath the synovium. In stage I cartilaginous nodules (usually more than five) are formed (chondromas), which subsequently calcify in approximately 30% of cases (osteochondromas). When these lesions break free from the synovium (stage II) they become intra-articular loose bodies. Stage III is inactive disease but with the presence of persistent intra-articular nodules.
- PSO usually affects the young and middle-aged but may occur at any age from childhood to the eighth decade. Men are more frequently affected than women (2 : 1). Symptoms include pain, swelling and restricted movement.

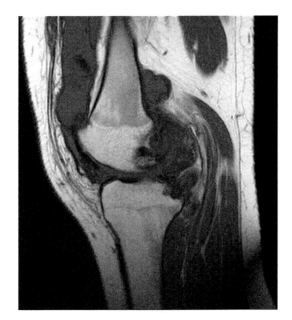

Figure 3.17d

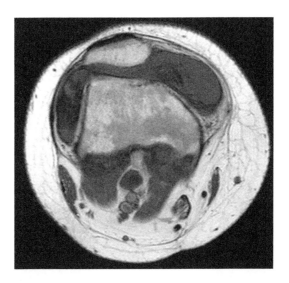

Figure 3.17e

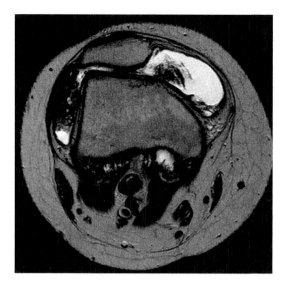

Figure 3.17f

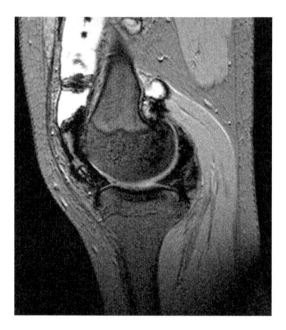

Figure 3.17g

Model answer

The MRI images of the knee (Figures 3.17a–3.17g) demonstrate a large suprapatellar joint effusion with a diffuse distribution of multiple nodules of low signal on all sequences. The appearances are most likely to be due to intra-articular pigmented villonodular synovitis (PVNS).

Questions

1. What are the differential diagnoses?

Synovial haemangioma. The absence of multiple vessels makes this unlikely.

Haemophiliac haemarthrosis can be considered only if the patient is male and there is a positive history of haemophilia.

2. **Which is more likely to calcify – PVNS or synovial sarcoma?**
   Synovial sarcoma. Calcification in PVNS is very rare, while calcification in synovial sarcomas occurs commonly.

Key points

- Pigmented villonodular synovitis (PVNS) is a rare benign neoplasm of synovium characterized by synovial proliferation and haemosiderin deposition. It may be intra- or extra-articular. When intra-articular it may be diffuse or localized, but extra-articular PVNS is always focal. Extra-articular disease is confined to the tendon sheath or bursa. PVNS tends to be monoarticular.
- Localized disease accounts for 77% cases and is associated with an intra-articular mass. Diffuse intra-articular disease accounts for 23% of cases and is associated with effusions and erosion of bone both sides of the joint. Diffuse intra-articular PVNS has an incidence of about 2 per million population. There is equal sex incidence. Diffuse PVNS involves the knee in up to 80% of cases, followed by the hip and ankle. In 'tight' joints such as the hip and ankle, there is frequently erosion of bone (occurring in 90% of cases involving the hip).
- Patients are in their third to fifth decade at presentation and typically complain of long-standing symptoms of pain and swelling. Bloody effusions may be elicited in the history.
- Radiographs of affected joints may be normal or demonstrate effusions (may be radiodense), soft tissue swelling and bony erosion. There is no periarticular osteopenia. Calcification is very rare and the joint space is preserved.
- MRI demonstrates low signal intensity within the haemosiderin-stained synovial tissue on all sequences – it is intermediate to low signal on T1-weighted images and low signal on T2-weighted images because haemosiderin reduces T2 relaxation times. MRI is more sensitive than radiography in the detection of erosions.
- PVNS tissue may enhance after gadolinium.
- A characteristic 'blooming' artefact occurs on gradient echo images. This is a magnetic-susceptibility low-signal artefact caused by haemosiderin, making the low-signal tissue appear even bigger.

Further reading

Garner HW, Ortiguera CJ, Nakhleh RE. Pigmented villonodular synovitis. *Radiographics* 2008; **28**: 1519–23.

Murphey MD, Rhee JH, Lewis RB, et al. Pigmented villonodular synovitis: radiologic–pathologic correlation. *Radiographics* 2008; **28**: 1493–518.

Sheldon PJ, Forrester DM, Learch TJ. Imaging of intraarticular masses. *Radiographics* 2005; **25**: 105–19.

MSK Case 18

JOHN CURTIS

Clinical history
Middle-aged male with bilateral hip and back pain.

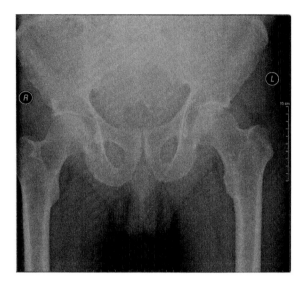

Figure 3.18a

Model answer
There is a destructive lesion of the sacrum with evident loss of the sacral ala (Figure 3.18a). There is an area of lucency in the right femoral neck, raising the possibility of an aggressive lytic lesion here. The appearances suggest disseminated malignancy. The differential diagnosis lies between a lytic metastasis or primary bone neoplasm such as chordoma and giant-cell tumour. Another possibility could be direct invasion by a rectal carcinoma. Lytic metastatic disease is much more likely.

Questions
1. **What are the causes of lytic bone metastases?**
   Carcinoma of the breast, bronchus, kidney and thyroid. Myeloma may also give similar appearances and is always worth remembering.
2. **What investigation would you advise next?**
   Chest radiograph and bone scan followed by CT of the pelvis to include the right hip.

Key points
- This is a common viva film in the FRCR examination. Absence of the sacrum may be difficult to detect, since it is a midline abnormality and is less readily identified than a lateral abnormality. *However, to avoid mistakes, it is worth looking at the sacrum as your first action when assessing a pelvic radiograph.*
- A bone scan is useful in identifying other lesions for radiotherapy purposes, and to establish whether the bone destruction is solitary or multiple.

- Note that myeloma is likely to be 'cold' on bone scans.
- A chest radiograph is a simple effective first-line investigation, searching for a bronchial carcinoma. Do not forget to look at the breast shadows in females.
- Chordoma (Figures 3.18b, 3.18c) is a rare tumour, accounting for up to 4% of all primary bone tumours. Radiographically it is very similar in appearance to a sacral metastasis. After myeloma it is the commonest adult malignant primary spinal tumour. 50% of chordomas are located in the sacrum, with the remainder distributed in the clivus and rest of the spine.

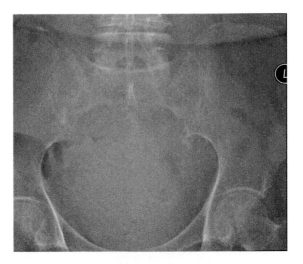

Figure 3.18b

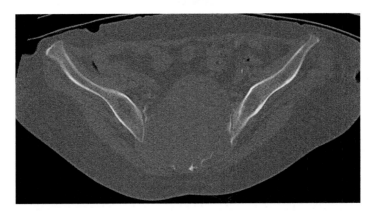

Figure 3.18c

Further reading

Erlemann R. Imaging and differential diagnosis of primary bone tumors and tumor-like lesions of the spine. *Eur J Radiol* 2006; **58**: 48–67.

JOHN CURTIS

Clinical history
65-year-old male with bone pain.

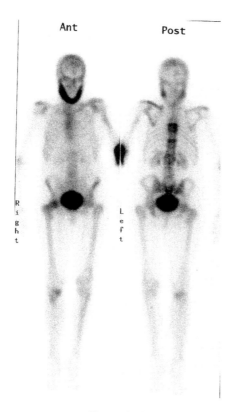

Figure 3.19

Model answer
This is an isotope bone scan (Figure 3.19) demonstrating intense homogeneous uptake of tracer in the mandible (Abraham Lincoln sign). There is increased uptake in two contiguous mid-thoracic vertebrae, a lower thoracic and an upper lumbar vertebra and the proximal right femur. There is mild increased uptake of tracer in the left scapula.

These findings need plain film correlation. The appearances are most likely those of Paget's disease. Serum alkaline phosphatase estimations are required.

Questions
1. **What is the reason for encouraging frequent micturition following injection of ^{99m}Tc-MDP?**

It encourages bladder emptying, thereby reducing radiation dose to the gonads.

Key points

- Paget's disease of the mandible produces a characteristic appearance on bone scintigraphy resembling Abraham Lincoln, the 16th President of the United States.
- Paget's disease, when affecting a long bone such as the femur, produces a continuous area of increased tracer activity that starts in a subarticular position.
- It is important to obtain plain film correlation of the mandible to (1) confirm the diagnosis and (2) exclude osteosarcoma, which may be a concern if the patient has mandibular pain.

Further reading

Patel MB, Bhalla A. Paget's disease of the mandible. *N Engl J Med* 2008; **358**: 625.

MSK Case 20

JOHN CURTIS

Clinical history

An elderly female with bone pain.

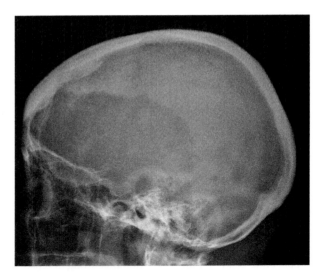

Figure 3.20a

Model answer

AP pelvis x-ray (Figure 3.21a). This demonstrates sclerosis of the femoral heads. There is some flattening of the lateral aspect of the right femoral head. The inferior end plate of the L5 vertebral body is depressed and it resembles an H-shape.

AP lumbar spine (Figure 3.21b). This demonstrates H-shaped vertebrae at all levels. At the bottom corner of the film there is a suggestion of a metallic right hip prosthesis.

AP chest radiograph (Figure 3.21c). This demonstrates bilateral pleural effusions and right mid-zone consolidation suggestive of heart failure with coexisting infection, infarction or pulmonary oedema. The tip of the right internal jugular line lies in the right atrium. There is the 'snow cap' sign of patchy subchondral sclerosis in the right humeral head. There is a left humeral prosthesis.

The combined signs are those of sickle cell disease with avascular necrosis in the femoral heads, leading to a femoral prosthesis on the right side. The H-shaped vertebrae are virtually pathognomonic of sickle cell disease.

Questions

1. **What are the causes of consolidation in a patient with sickle cell disease who presents with chest pain?**
   This can be very non-specific, and three conditions – oedema, infection and infarction – are all implicated. Clinical correlation is necessary to determine the cause of consolidation, and when this is not possible empirical therapy for all three conditions is instituted.

2. **What are the causes of H-shaped vertebrae?**
   - Sickle cell disease.
   - Gaucher's disease.
   In both conditions there is occlusion of end-arteries that supply the central end plate. This results in infarction and bone softening, which over time leads to end-plate depression. This eventually leads to the so-called H-shaped configuration of vertebrae (Figure 3.21d). The periphery of the end plate is unaffected because of its blood supply from a rich capillary network. In sickle cell disease the spleen is usually small or absent due to auto-infarction, whereas in Gaucher's disease the spleen is often moderately enlarged.

3. **What complications may occur in sickle cell disease?**
   - Infection – salmonellae are implicated in 50% of cases of osteomyelitis and septic arthritis.
   - Avascular necrosis (AVN) – subchondral ends of long bones, and in extreme cases generalized avascular necrosis.
   - AVN of a metacarpal or metatarsal will lead to shortening.
   - Renal papillary necrosis.
   - Cholelithiasis secondary to haemolytic anaemia.
   - Splenic atrophy and infarction – increased susceptibility to infection with encapsulated organisms.
   - Pulmonary infarction and infection.
   - Heart failure secondary to anaemia.

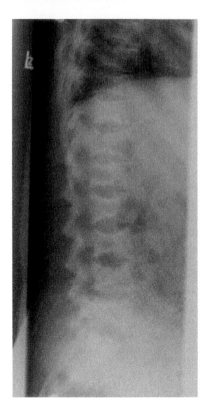

Figure 3.21d

Key points

- Avascular necrosis of one or both of the femoral heads on a pelvic radiograph has a number of causes. This film is a common scenario in the viva part of the FRCR examination. It is worth thinking of the associated features that may help determine the underlying cause of AVN:
  - Ileostomy bag (Figure 3.21e). This indicates steroid use in ulcerative colitis prior to surgery.
  - Ankylosing spondylitis (Figure 3.21f). Non-steroidal anti-inflammatory drugs used in this condition can lead to AVN (note the right hip prosthesis) and also renal papillary necrosis. So look for it (in the form of calcified papillae) on abdominal radiographs.
  - Renal transplant clips in the iliac fossa or a calcified rejected renal transplant indicate current or previous treatment with steroids.
  - In sickle cell disease always look for H-shaped vertebrae in the lumbar spine on the film.
  - Splenomegaly – myelofibrosis and Gaucher's disease. Both conditions lead to AVN of the femoral heads, and in the case of Gaucher's disease the development of H-shaped vertebrae in addition.
  - Pancreatic calcification on an abdominal radiograph suggests chronic pancreatitis and a possible aetiology for AVN.
  - An abdominal radiograph that demonstrates AVN of the femoral head, H-shaped vertebrae, a small spleen (high splenic flexure) and gallstones or cholecystectomy is indicative of sickle cell disease.

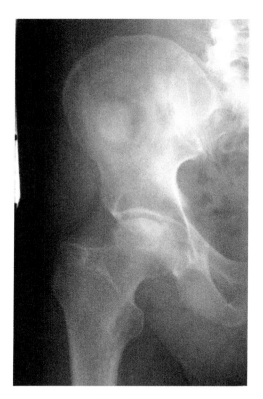

Figure 3.21e

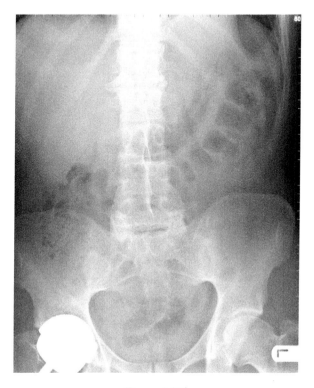

Figure 3.21f

Further reading

Ejindu VC, Hine AL, Mashayekhi M, Shorvon PJ, Misra RR. Musculoskeletal mani-festations of sickle cell disease. *Radiographics* 2007; **27**: 1005–21.

Lonergan GJ, Cline DB, Abbondanzo SL. Sickle cell anemia. *Radiographics* 2001; **21**: 971–94.

Madani G, Papadopoulou A, Holloway B, et al. The radiological manifestations of sickle cell disease. *Clin Radiol* 2007; **62**: 528–38.

McCann C, Mondal D, Curtis J. 2_148 The Musculoskeletal Manifestations of the Haemoglobinopathies. *Radiology Integrated Training Initiative*. Royal College of Radiologists, 2010.

Resnick D. Hemoglobinopathies and other anemias. In Resnick D, ed., *Diagnosis of Bone and Joint Disorders*, 4th edn. Philadelphia, PA: Saunders, 2002; 2146–87.

Images courtesy of Dr Priya Healey, Royal Liverpool University Hospital, Liverpool (Figures 3.21a–3.21c), and Dr Otto Chan, London (Figure 3.21d).

MSK Case 22

JOHN CURTIS

Clinical history
Non-specific pelvic pain of short duration in a 50-year-old male. No other history.

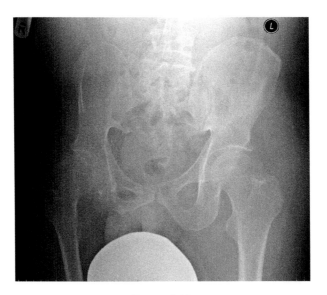

Figure 3.22

Model answer
The AP radiograph of the pelvis (Figure 3.22) demonstrates poor development of the right iliac bone, femoral head and proximal femur with associated osteopenia and marked soft tissue atrophy. No additional features.

The diagnosis is that of old poliomyelitis affecting the right pelvic girdle and thigh.

Questions
1. **What are the causes of underdevelopment of bone?**
   - Poliomyelitis.
   - Previous radiotherapy during growth.

Key points
- This is a viva 'Aunt Minnie'. These appearances – osteoporosis, growth retardation and muscle wasting – are virtually pathognomonic of old polio.

MSK Case 23

JOHN CURTIS

Clinical history
Elderly male who is constitutionally unwell with chest pain.

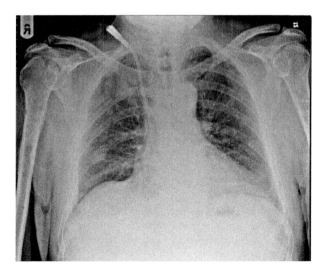

Figure 3.23a

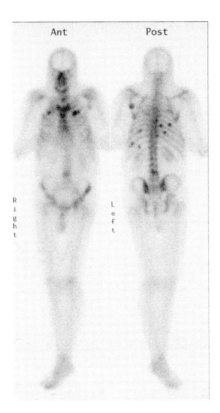

Figure 3.23b

Model answer

The chest radiograph (Figure 3.23a) demonstrates a destructive lesion occupying the posterior right fourth rib, with associated soft tissue mass that appears as an area of increased density. There is a healing fracture of the posterior right seventh rib. Pleural-based shadowing is present in the right costophrenic angle. There is a right internal jugular line in situ with its tip in the right atrium. There are multiple 'punched-out' well-defined lytic lesions in the right humerus and small lytic foci in the clavicles.

The bone scan (Figure 3.23b) demonstrates multiple discrete foci of increased tracer activity involving the posterior ribs and left scapula. There is increased tracer activity in the lower lumbar spine. There is no abnormal tracer activity in the humeri.

The appearances are likely to be due to multiple myeloma. The foci of increased tracer activity in the ribs can be explained by fractures, which may be apparent or non-apparent on the chest radiograph. The differential diagnosis for the combined appearances is lytic metastases, but this is much less likely.

Questions

1. **What are the common causes of multiple lytic bone lesions?**
   Multiple myeloma. Metastases from carcinoma of the breast, bronchus, kidney and thyroid. The latter two produce expansile lesions.
2. **What investigations would be required?**
   Bone marrow biopsy, serum electrophoresis and Bence–Jones protein estimation.

3. What would rib metastases look like on a bone scan?

As rib involvement is infiltrative it causes linear tracer uptake, unlike fractures, which produce focal uptake.

Key points

- Increased uptake of tracer on a ^{99m}Tc-MDP bone scan occurs with osteoblastic activity and so will not occur with multiple myeloma unless there is a healing process following fracture. In fact the plasma cells in myeloma produce an osteoclastic stimulating factor, which causes the characteristic osteolytic lesions and inhibits osteoblasts.
- Classically myeloma produces well-defined lytic lesions of uniform size and shape.
- Solitary lesions are plasmacytomas, and they tend to involve the spine, ribs, iliac bone and femur.
- Common sites of involvement in myeloma include:
  - skull
  - spine
  - ribs
- Metastases and myeloma may appear similar. However, sites of involvement more suggestive of myeloma include:
  - mandible
  - clavicle (especially distal end)
  - sternum
  - vertebral bodies without involvement of posterior elements (unlike metastases)

Further reading

Angtuaco EJ, Fassas AB, Walker R, Sethi R, Barlogie B. Multiple myeloma: clinical review and diagnostic imaging. *Radiology* 2004; **231**: 11–23.

MSK Case 24

JOHN CURTIS

Clinical history
18-year-old male with backache.

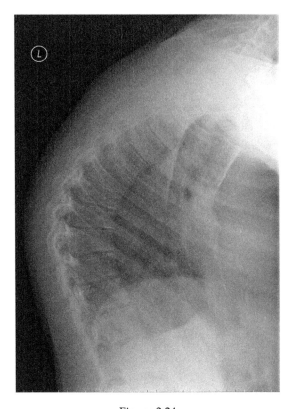

Figure 3.24

Model answer
This is a lateral thoracic spine radiograph (Figure 3.24) that demonstrates marked kyphosis. In the kyphotic section there is lucent irregularity of the end plates, reactive sclerosis and loss of disc height at multiple levels. There is anterior wedging of several contiguous vertebrae. The appearances are those of Scheuermann's disease.

Questions
1. **What is the pathology in Scheuermann's disease?**
   Intraosseous displacement of disc through the end plate. This is thought to be stress-related and leads to reactive sclerosis and disc space narrowing.

Key points
- Scheuermann's disease, or kyphosis dorsalis juvenalis, was thought to be due to osteochondritis, but it is now thought to be stress-related intraosseous extension of disc through the end plate. This leads to anterior wedging and kyphosis.

- The defect in the bone is lucent and associated with a reactive sclerosis. This lesion is synonymous with the term Schmorl's node.
- Patients, who are typically aged between 13 and 17, complain of backache and kyphosis.

Further reading
Afshani E, Kuhn JP. Common causes of low back pain in children. *Radiographics* 1991; **11**: 269–91.

MSK Case 25

JOHN CURTIS

Clinical history
Spot diagnosis.

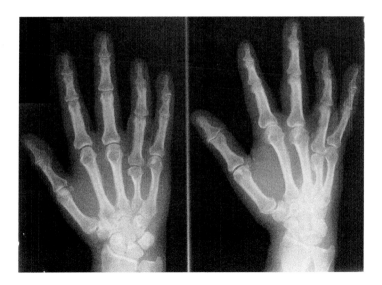

Figure 3.25

Model answer
DP and oblique views of the hand (Figure 3.25) demonstrate a short fourth metacarpal. The differential diagnosis is wide, as this can be seen in many conditions:
- idiopathic
- secondary to trauma or infection
- Turner's syndrome (often with associated Madelung's deformity)
- pseudohypoparathyroidism and pseudopseudohypoparathyroidism
- Gorlin's syndrome (basal cell naevus syndrome)
- sickle cell disease with metacarpal infarction
- familial type 1 diabetes mellitus (solitary short fifth metacarpal)

Key points
- Do not make a diagnosis of Turner's syndrome unless the patient is female!
- Pseudohypoparathyroidism (PHP) and pseudopseudohypoparathyroidism (PPHP) share identical phenotypic features of short stature and shortening of the first and fourth metacarpals. The biochemistry in PPHP is normal. The biochemistry in PHP is low/normal serum calcium with normal/increased parathyroid hormone levels.

MSK Case 26

JOHN CURTIS

Clinical history

Hand radiograph in a 43-year-old woman.

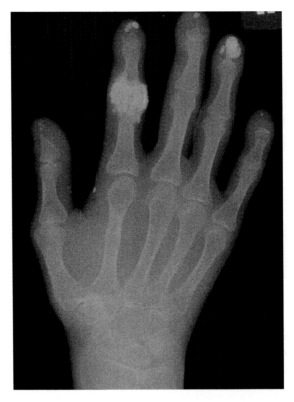

Figure 3.26a

Model answer

This radiograph (Figure 3.26a) demonstrates acro-osteolysis and sclerodactyly affecting all terminal phalanges. The bone destruction affects the distal phalangeal tufts and appears disproportionate compared with the degree of soft tissue atrophy. There is subcutaneous calcification adjacent to the resorbed phalanges and in the periarticular region around the proximal interphalangeal joint of the index finger. No articular erosions. The appearances are those of scleroderma (progressive systemic sclerosis).

Questions
1. **What are the causes of acro-osteolysis?**
- Tuft resorption:
  - scleroderma
  - thermal injury (heat or cold)
  - hyperparathyroidism
  - psoriasis
  - epidermolysis bullosa
- Mid-phalangeal resorption:
  - familial
  - chemical – polyvinyl chloride
  - connective tissue disease
  - hyperparathyroidism (see Figure 3.40b)
  - (rarely in scleroderma)
- Periarticular erosions (DIP joint):
  - psoriasis
  - gout
  - thermal injury
  - scleroderma
  - hyperparathyroidism

2. **What are the other hand and wrist manifestations of scleroderma?**
- Flexion deformity of fingers.
- Soft tissue atrophy, especially over finger tips.
- Arthropathy – joint erosions may be seen especially in the metacarpophalangeal, proximal interphalangeal and radiocarpal joints. The first carpometacarpal joint is a classical site of involvement in scleroderma with erosion and subluxation.
- Acro-osteosclerosis – sclerosis in the distal tip of the terminal phalanges.
- Soft tissue calcification in the hand is amorphous in composition, occurring in up to 30% of cases, and may be:
  - subcutaneous
  - tendinous
  - capsular
  - intra-articular

Key points
- Scleroderma may be associated with other manifestations of the so-called CREST syndrome: Calcinosis of subcutaneous tissue, Raynaud's phenomenon, oEsophageal dysmotility, Sclerodactyly and Telangiectasia.
- Some patients have additional features, which are in keeping with systemic lupus erythematosus or dermatomyositis, and are said to have mixed connective tissue disease.
- Calcification occurs in 'pressure' areas where the underlying bone is close to the skin surface, e.g. the prepatellar region (Figure 3.26b), finger tips and ischial tuberosities.
- Erosions may occur in the distal ulna and radius away from the joint, in the ribs and at the mandibular angles.
- Changes in the hands invariably exceed those present in the feet.

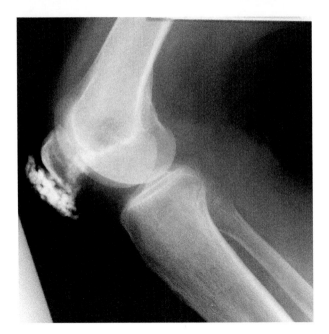

Figure 3.26b

Further reading

Bassett LW, Blocka KLN, Furst DE, Clements PJ, Gold RH. Skeletal findings in progressive systemic sclerosis (scleroderma). *AJR Am J Roentgenol* 1981; **136**: 1121–6.

Jones SN, Stoker DJ. Radiology at your fingertips: lesions of the terminal phalanx. *Clin Radiol* 1988; **39**: 478–85.

MSK Case 27

JOHN CURTIS

Clinical history
Sterile pyuria in a young adult male.

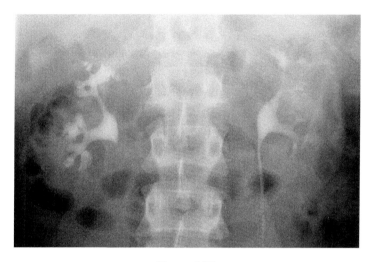

Figure 3.27

Model answer
This is a close-up of a full-length AP radiograph from an IVU series (Figure 3.27), which demonstrates bilateral renal papillary necrosis. This manifests as contrast material filling central excavations in the papillae of both kidneys, giving the 'golf-ball-on-tee' appearance. There are 'H-shaped' lumbar vertebrae. The appearances are most likely due to sickle cell disease. No evidence of radio-opaque gallstones or cholecystectomy clips.

Questions
1. **What are the causes of renal papillary necrosis (RPN)?**
   A – analgesic use/abuse
   D – diabetes mellitus, dehydration
   I – infants in shock
   P – pyelonephritis
   O – obstructive uropathy
   S – sickle cell disease, shock
   E – ethanol
2. **What are the causes of sterile pyuria?**
   - partially treated urinary tract infections
   - stone disease
   - renal papillary necrosis
   - urethritis
   - tuberculosis

Key points

- This is a viva 'Aunt Minnie' film – the combined appearances of RPN and H-shaped vertebrae are virtually pathognomonic of sickle cell disease. RPN is caused by a number of conditions that ultimately lead to ischaemia of the renal papillae (see mnemonic ADIPOSE above). In sickle cell disease, sickling of erythrocytes is more likely to occur in the hypertonic and relatively hypoxic environment of the renal medulla, which leads to RPN.
- RPN is characterized radiologically by the swelling of the papilla, which gives rise to calyceal excavation of contrast, which sits within the calyx – the so-called golf-ball-on-tee sign.
- Eventually progression of the process leads to forniceal excavation, which in turn gives rise to the 'lobster claw' appearance, the 'signet ring' appearance and eventually the 'clubbed calyx' appearance.
- Once a diagnosis of sickle cell disease has been suggested, look around the rest of the film for associated signs – e.g. avascular necrosis of the hip, cholelithiasis, cholecystectomy clips, renal stones, splenic atrophy (splenic flexure high up in the left upper quadrant), and mention these signs to the examiner.

Further reading

Dyer RB, Chen MYM, Zagoria RJ. Classic signs in uroradiology. *Radiographics* 2004; **24**: S247–80.

Dyer RB, Chen MYM, Zagoria RJ. Intravenous urography: technique and interpretation. *Radiographics* 2001; **21**: 799–824.

Hartman MS. The golf ball-on-tee sign. *Radiology* 2006; **239**: 297–8.

Jung DC, Kim SH, Jung SI, Hwang SI, Kim SH. Renal papillary necrosis: review and comparison of findings at multi-detector row CT and intravenous urography. *Radiographics* 2006; **26**: 1827–36.

Lonergan GJ, Cline DB, Abbondanzo SL. Sickle cell anemia. *Radiographics* 2001; **21**: 971–94.

Image courtesy of Dr Otto Chan, London.

MSK Case 28

JOHN CURTIS

Clinical history
Generalized bone pains and general fatigue.

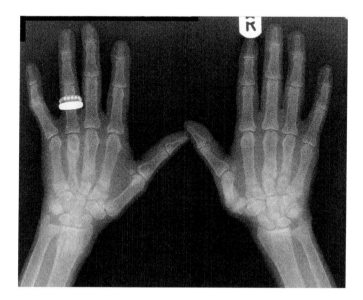

Figure 3.28a

Model answer
This is a radiograph of both hands of a skeletally mature female (Figure 3.28a). There is generalized osteopenia. There are wide band-like areas of reduced density traversing the base of all metacarpals of the right hand and the second and third metacarpals of the left hand. The lucent bands are perpendicular to the long axis of the bone, and have sclerotic margins with localized periosteal new bone on the cortical margin. The appearances are those of multiple Looser's zones associated with osteomalacia. The hands are an atypical site for Looser's zones, suggesting severe disease.

Questions
1. **What percentage of daily vitamin D requirements is obtained in the diet? What foods are rich in vitamin D?**
   Approximately 10% of vitamin D is provided by diet. Foods rich in vitamin D include oily fish, liver, eggs and fortified breakfast cereals. Approximately 90% of vitamin D is produced by ultraviolet light in combination with a sterol precursor (cholecalciferol), present in the deep layers of the skin.
2. **What are the causes/risk factors for the development of vitamin D deficiency?**
   Vitamin D is a fat-soluble vitamin and is produced by 25-hydroxylation in the liver and 1-hydroxylation in the kidneys to produce 1,25-dihydrocholecalciferol (vitamin D).
   - Poor intake of vitamin D – poor nutrition.

- Poor absorption of vitamin D – gastric surgery, biliary disease, diseases of the terminal ileum, coeliac disease, chronic pancreatic disease (rarely). Poor absorption is the commonest cause of vitamin D deficiency in the United States.
- Renal disease – failure to 1-hydroxylate.
- Liver disease – failure to 25-hydroxylate.
- Drugs – e.g. anticonvulsants, rifampicin.
- Dark skin – dark skin is less efficient than light skin at manufacturing vitamin D.
- The very young and very old.
- House-bound individuals.
- Pregnancy.
- Alcoholism.
- X-linked hypophosphataemic rickets.
- Fanconi's anaemia.
- Tumour-associated osteomalacia – e.g. giant-cell tumour, non-ossifying fibroma.

Key points

- Osteomalacia is the manifestation of systemic disease in the *mature* skeleton and is due to defective mineralization (calcification) of osteoid. It is caused by a deficiency of vitamin D. The biochemistry is identical to rickets except that rickets affects the *immature* skeleton. Unlike rickets, osteomalacia has no effect on the growth plate.
- The key biochemical effect of vitamin D deficiency is a reduced availability of calcium and/or phosphate for effective osteoid mineralization. This manifests as undermineralization of both cortical and trabecular bone, leading to 'seams' of unmineralized osteoid. Effectively, there is an increase in the osteoid-to-mineral ratio.
- There are specific and non-specific features that suggest the diagnosis of osteomalacia:
  - Non-specific
    - osteopenia
    - coarsened trabeculae, which are reduced in number
  - Specific
    - Lucent 'seams' of unossified osteoid in the cortex – Looser's zones or 'pseudofractures'. These are perpendicular to the cortex and incompletely traverse the bone unless associated with fracture. They tend to be symmetrical and are located on the concave side of the bone, e.g. the medial aspect of the proximal femur. They often have sclerotic margins.
    - Characteristic sites for Looser's zones:
      - axillary border of scapulae (Figure 3.28b, arrow)
      - ribs
      - inferior pubic ramus
      - proximal femur (medial)
      - ilium
      - acromion
- Unlike Paget's disease, in which incremental fractures occur along the outer cortical bone (convexity), Looser's zones occur along the inner margin (concavity).
- Periosteal new bone occurs on the cortical margin but is less exuberant than that seen in osteoporosis.
- Osteomalacia is also associated with pathological fracture through soft bone (Figure 3.28b).

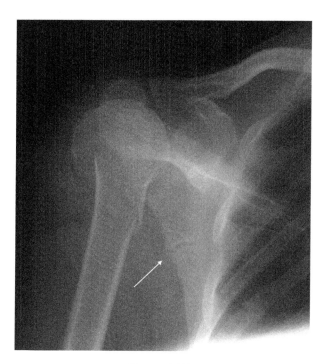

Figure 3.28b

Further reading

Adams JE. Renal bone disease: radiological investigation. *Kidney Int Suppl* 1999; **56**: S38–41.

Adams JE. Radiology of rickets and osteomalacia. In Feldman D, Glorieux FH, Pike W, eds., *Vitamin D*, 2nd edn. New York, NY: Elsevier, 2005; 967–94.

Pitt MJ. Rickets and osteomalacia. In Resnick D, Kransdorf MJ, eds., *Bone and Joint Imaging*, 3rd edn. Richmond, VA: Elsevier-Saunders, 2005; 563–75.

MSK Case 29

JOHN CURTIS

Clinical history
Wrist trauma in two different patients.

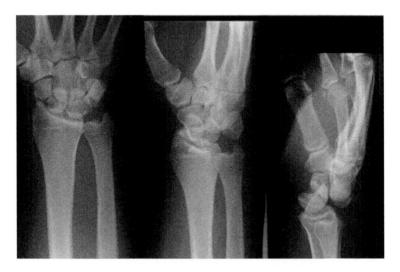

Figure 3.29a

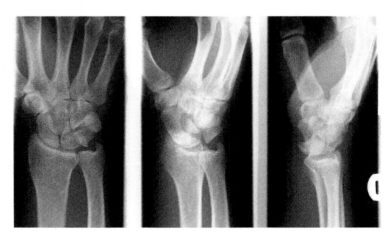

Figure 3.29b

Model answer
The frontal radiograph (Figure 3.29a) shows disruption of all the carpal arcs, and the lunate has a triangular shape. The lateral radiograph shows an empty distal concavity of the lunate with posterior displacement of the capitate. The capitate is displaced posteriorly with respect to the long axis of the radius. There is an associated fracture of the waist of the scaphoid. The appearances are those of a trans-scaphoid perilunate dislocation.

The frontal radiograph (Figure 3.29b) shows disruption of all the carpal arcs. The lunate has a triangular shape, with overlapping of the articular surfaces of the lunate-triquetrum and lunate-capitate. The lateral radiograph show volar dislocation of the lunate with rotation – the distal articular surface points in a volar direction. The capitate remains in alignment with the long axis of the radius. There is an associated fracture of the triquetrum but no scaphoid fracture. The appearances are those of lunate dislocation.

Questions

1. Which carpal bone is most frequently fractured?

Scaphoid fractures are the commonest injury caused by hyperextension. Most fractures (80%) occur through the scaphoid waist and may lead to avascular necrosis of the proximal pole. Avulsion fractures of the tuberosity occur with scapholunate ligament trauma.

Key points

- The lateral film provides most information about the nature of the injury. Never make the definitive diagnosis without referring to the lateral view. This is particularly important in real life, as well as in the exam!
- Look for combination injuries involving the radial styloid, scaphoid, proximal capitate, proximal hamate and ulnar styloid (Figure 3.29c).
- Perilunate dislocation is the commonest carpal dislocation. It is overlooked in 25% of cases despite being common in young sportsmen who fall on the outstretched hand. Perilunate and lunate dislocations should be regarded as injuries within a spectrum. Lunate dislocation is the final stage of perilunate injury.
- The lunate bone is the fulcrum of the proximal carpal row. Disruption of the Gilula carpal arcs (Figure 3.29d) should be looked for on the frontal film – this is usually manifest as a triangular shape to the lunate bone.

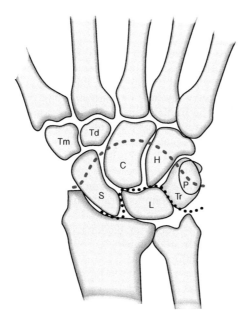

Figure 3.29c Lunate injuries are ligamentous (dotted line). Perilunate injuries are associated with fractures through the distal carpal bones (greater arc injury) (dashed line). Tm, trapezium; Td, trapezoid; C, capitate; H, hamate; S, scaphoid; L, lunate; Tr, triquetrum; P, pisiform. Modified after Kaewlai R, Avery LL, Asrani AV, *et al.*

Multidetector CT of carpal injuries: anatomy, fractures, and fracture-dislocations. *Radiographics* 2008; **28**: 1771–84.

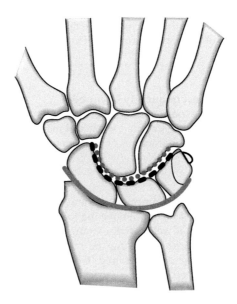

Figure 3.29d Gilula carpal arcs. Arc 1 (solid line), proximal surfaces of scaphoid, lunate, triquetrum; arc 2 (dashed line), distal surfaces of scaphoid, lunate, triquetrum; arc 3 (dotted line), proximal surfaces of capitate and hamate. Modified after Kaewlai R, Avery LL, Asrani AV, *et al*. Multidetector CT of carpal injuries: anatomy, fractures, and fracture-dislocations. *Radiographics* 2008; **28**: 1771–84.

- Carpal instability injuries comprise:
  - Stage I – rotatory subluxation of the scaphoid (scapholunate dissociation) (Figures 3.29e, 3.29f). Disruption of the scapholunate and radioscaphoid ligaments. There is a wide gap (Figure 3.29e, thick arrow) between the scaphoid and lunate bones ('Terry-Thomas' or 'Madonna' sign). There is foreshortening of the scaphoid on the frontal projection with a ring sign (Figure 3.29e, thin arrows) created by scaphoid rotation. The lateral projection shows no loss of alignment of the radius, lunate and capitate.
  - Stage II – perilunate dislocation – this is caused by hyperextension, ulnar deviation and carpal supination. As the volar ligaments disrupt, the capitate dislocates posteriorly, which is usually accompanied by either (1) fracture of the waist of the scaphoid or (2) complete scapholunate dissociation. The capitate is malaligned with the long axis of the radius.
  - Stage III – scapholunate–triquetrum ligament disruption. This results in separation of the triquetrum from the lunate
  - Stage IV – lunate dislocation (Figures 3.29b, 3.29g, 3.29h). This is the most severe injury and is primarily a result of posterior radiocarpal ligament disruption in addition to other injuries described. The capitate retains its alignment with the long axis of the radius. Figures 3.29g and 3.29h show a trans-scaphoid lunate dislocation with an associated triquetrum fracture (Figure 3.29h, arrow).

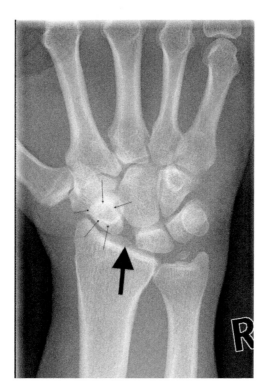

Figure 3.29e

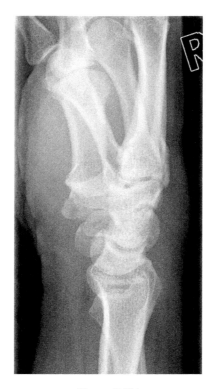

Figure 3.29f

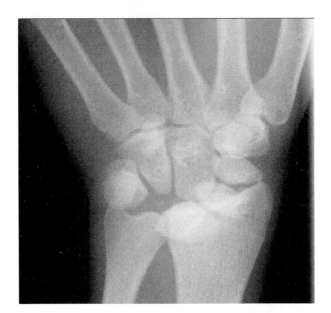

Figure 3.29g

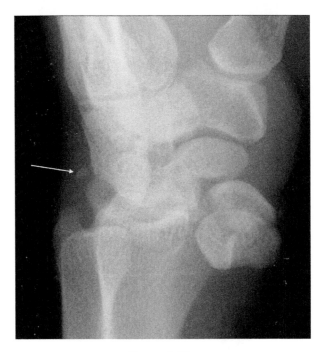

Figure 3.29h

Further reading

Gilula LA. Carpal injuries: analytic approach and case exercises. *AJR Am J Roentgenol* 1979; **133**: 503–17.

Goldfarb CA, Yin Y, Gilula LA, Fisher AJ, Boyer MI. Wrist fractures: what the clinician wants to know. *Radiology* 2001; **219**: 11–28.

Kaewlai R, Avery LL, Asrani AV, *et al.* Multidetector CT of carpal injuries: anatomy, fractures, and fracture-dislocations. *Radiographics* 2008; **28**: 1771–84.

Peh WCG, Galloway HR. Imaging of wrist injuries. In Vanhoenacker FM, Maas M, Gielen JL, eds., *Imaging of Orthopedic Sports Injuries*. Berlin: Springer, 2007; 201–24.

MSK Case 30

JOHN CURTIS

Clinical history
Elderly male with a cough.

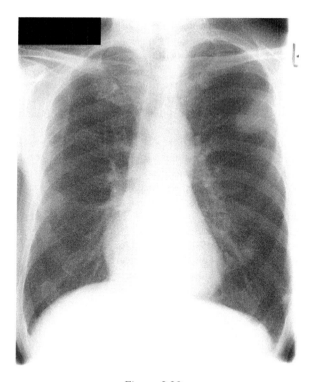

Figure 3.30a

Model answer
This frontal chest radiograph in an elderly male (Figure 3.30a) demonstrates a solitary expansile bony lesion involving the anterior aspect of the left third rib. It has the appearances of an aggressive lesion. There is a healed fracture of the posterolateral

aspect of the left tenth rib. No additional bony lesions. The heart and mediastinum are normal. Lungs clear. I would like to look at previous films, if available, to assess if this is long-standing. A bone scan would be useful in determining whether the lytic lesion is (1) osteoblastic and (2) solitary or multiple.

Questions

1. What are the differential diagnoses for this appearance?
- Plasmacytoma and, if multiple, myeloma. This is likely to be 'cold' on bone scintigraphy.
- Lytic metastasis – from bronchial, renal cell, breast or thyroid carcinoma.
- Fibrous dysplasia – no change over previous films.
- Brown tumour – look for other signs of hyperparathyroidism and surgical clips in the neck signifying parathyroidectomy.

2. What are the causes of expansile rib lesions in adults and children?
See below.

Key points

- Expansile rib lesions in an adult:
  - Myeloma or plasmacytoma.
  - Lytic metastases represent the commonest malignant rib lesions.
  - Chondrosarcoma is the commonest primary malignant bone tumour and is typically located near the costochondral junction.
  - Brown tumour of hyperparathyroidism – look for other signs of hyperparathyroidism, e.g. erosive osteolysis of distal clavicle, brown tumours in humerus.
  - Fibrous dysplasia – monostotic or polyostotic. Monostotic fibrous dysplasia is the commonest cause of an expansile rib lesion in children – typically a 'ground-glass' rib lesion. *Look at previous films.*
  - Paget's disease.
- *Always look below the diaphragm and in the neck region* – the presence of surgical clips in the retroperitoneum or neck may suggest previous renal cell or thyroid carcinoma respectively as the underlying primary malignant cause of the lytic bone lesion.
- Expansile rib lesions in a child:
  - Fibrous dysplasia – monostotic or polyostotic. Monostotic fibrous dysplasia is the commonest cause of an expansile rib lesion in children – typically a 'ground-glass' rib lesion. *Look at previous films.*
  - Lymphangiomatosis – well-defined lucent lesions affecting multiple ribs. Rare.
  - Simple bone cyst – solitary rib.
  - Enchondroma – with or without internal chondroid calcification.
  - Brown tumour of hyperparathyroidism – look for other signs of hyperparathyroidism, e.g. erosive osteolysis of distal clavicle, brown tumours in humerus.
  - Eosinophilic granuloma – lysis without sclerosis ± bevelled edges.
  - Ewing's sarcoma and primitive neuroectodermal tumour (Askin tumour).
  - Lymphoma.
- Keep looking at the film! In Figure 3.30b the chest radiograph demonstrates numerous 'cannonball' lung lesions. There is also lytic destruction of the right fifth rib. Use your lists for each radiographic abnormality to find the disease that fits with both abnormalities. In this case it was due to renal cell carcinoma, metastatic to the lungs and bone.

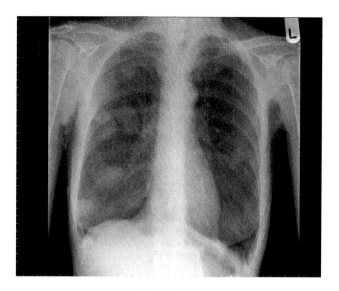

Figure 3.30b

Notes

The diagnosis in the case shown in Figure 3.30a was a solitary plasmacytoma, confirmed on CT-guided percutaneous biopsy.

Further reading

Glass RB, Norton KI, Mitre SA, Kang E. Pediatric ribs: a spectrum of abnormalities. *Radiographics* 2002; **22**: 87–104.

Guttentag AR, Salwen JK. Keep your eyes on the ribs: the spectrum of normal variants and diseases that involves the ribs. *Radiographics* 1999; **19**: 1125–42.

Levine BD, Motamedi K, Chow K, Gold RH, Seeger LL. CT of rib lesions. *AJR Am J Roentgenol* 2009; **193**: 5–13.

MSK Case 31

JOHN CURTIS

Clinical history
10-year-old girl with backache.

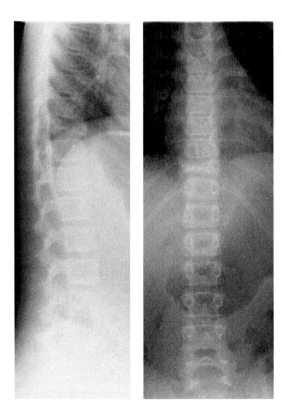

Figure 3.31a   Figure 3.31b

Model answer

The lateral radiograph (Figure 3.31a) shows virtually complete loss of the vertebral body height at T10 (vertebra plana). There is no involvement of the posterior elements and no evidence of kyphosis. There is increase in the disc space above and below T10. The frontal radiograph (Figure 3.31b) shows asymmetrical reduction in vertebral body height. The pedicles are intact and there is no compensatory scoliosis. The appearances are highly suggestive of eosinophilic granuloma (EG, also known as Langerhans cell histiocytosis, LCH).

Questions
1. **What are the other skeletal manifestations of EG?**
   - Aggressive lysis with or without a periosteal reaction.
   - Calvarial lytic lesions with a bevelled edge and a button sequestrum.
   - Diametaphyseal involvement of long bones.

- Resolution without treatment.
- Vertebral involvement may be solitary or multifocal. Spontaneous regression and healing is common.

2. **What are the other causes of vertebra plana?**
   The mnemonic for vertebra plana is MELT:
   M – myeloma, metastases (less likely than myeloma)
   E – eosinophilic granuloma
   L – lymphoma, leukaemia
   T – trauma, tuberculosis

Key points

- Eosinophilic granuloma (EG) is a term reserved for the localized form of LCH that involves only the skeleton or lung. EG of bone tends to involve children under 15 years of age, with an average age of onset of 10–14 years. Pulmonary involvement in children is part of a systemic disorder, which may regress with age, unlike in adults, when it tends to be isolated to lungs, associated with smoking in 95% and progressive.
- 10% of cases of EG with isolated bony involvement will go on to develop widespread involvement.
- Males are twice as commonly affected as females. It is uncommon in non-Caucasians.
- EG may present with pain and fracture or may be totally asymptomatic.
- Lytic, destructive lesions arise from the medulla with endosteal scalloping.
- Solitary lesions are more common than multiple lesions.
- In long bone involvement, the diaphyses and metaphyses are more frequently involved than epiphyses. Isolated epiphyseal involvement is rare – more typical is the involvement of the growth plate. It is very rare for there to be involvement distal to the knees and elbows.
- Skull vault lesions are 'punched out' and are typically devoid of sclerotic margins. Differing degrees of inner and outer table destruction frequently give rise to the impression of a 'hole within a hole' appearance and a bevelled edge to the lytic lesions (Figure 3.31c, arrow). No periosteal reaction in the skull.
- 'Floating teeth' are caused by expansile lytic change within the alveolar bone of the mandible.

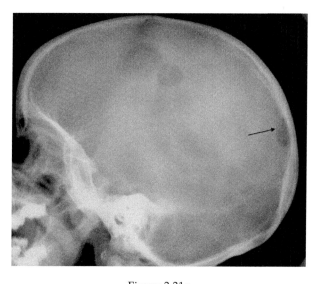

Figure 3.31c

Further reading

David R, Oria RA, Kumar R, *et al.* Radiologic features of eosinophilic granuloma of bone. *AJR Am J Roentgenol* 1989; **153**: 1021–6.

Hoover KB, Rosenthal DI, Mankin H. Langerhans cell histiocytosis. *Skeletal Radiol* 2007; **36**: 95–104

Stull MA, Kransdorf MJ, Devaney KO. Langerhans cell histiocytosis of bone. *Radiographics* 1992; **12**: 801–23.

MSK Case 32

JOHN CURTIS

Clinical history

Long-standing back pain in an elderly male.

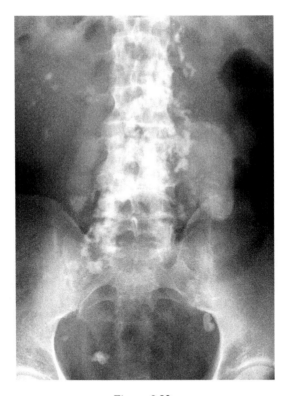

Figure 3.32a

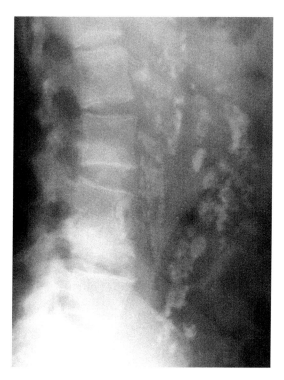

Figure 3.32b

Model answer

AP and lateral radiographs (Figures 3.32a, 3.32b). The lateral radiograph shows destruction of the L3/4 disc space with destruction and sclerosis of the end plates. There is probable ankylosis of the L3/4 disc space. No anterior wedging of L3 but there is loss of the normal lumbar lordosis. Both projections demonstrate bilateral calcified psoas abscesses, more marked on the left. There are numerous calcified mesenteric lymph nodes.

The appearances are those of previous tuberculous spondylitis of the lumbar spine (Pott's disease).

Questions
1. **What are the features of tuberculous osteomyelitis?**
   - Haematogenous spread of tubercle bacilli to bones of the extremities.
   - In long bones, infective focus tends to be epiphyseal in position.
   - In children, metaphyseal infection involves the growth plate and may cross into the epiphysis.
   - Initial radiology is similar to pyogenic osteomyelitis – osteolysis and periostitis. Presentation is delayed in tuberculous osteomyelitis, unlike pyogenic osteomyelitis, when presentation is usually prompt.

Key points
- Approximately 50% of all cases of skeletal TB involve the spine, mainly at the lower thoracic and upper lumbar regions. The commonest site is L1.
- Typically TB involves more than one vertebra.
- The anterior vertebral body is more commonly affected, because infection occurs by haematogenous spread via the venous plexus of Batson.

- There is destruction of the anterior vertebral body adjacent to the intervertebral disc. Subsequent destruction of the disc at this site allows infection to spread, involving multiple disc levels, so typical of TB spondylitis.
- Anterior subligamentous involvement may cause multiple levels to be involved with or without disc involvement.
- Disc destruction leads to narrowing of the disc space and anterior wedging, kyphosis and formation of a gibbus.
- Spread also occurs into the soft tissues, giving rise to psoas abscesses, which can extend into the groin.
- Calcification of a psoas abscess is virtually pathognomonic for TB spondylitis.
- TB rarely affects the posterior elements, unlike neoplastic disease.
- CT and MRI are useful in detecting early disease. MRI is useful in differentiating tuberculous from pyogenic spondylitis.
- Features suggestive of TB spondylitis, as opposed to pyogenic spondylitis, include:
  - multiple levels of involvement via subligamentous spread
  - thoracic spine involvement
  - indolent disc destruction
  - calcified paravertebral mass
  - absence of sclerosis
  - thin and smooth rim enhancement of abscess wall
  - hyperintense signal on T2-weighted images

Further reading

Burrill J, Williams CJ, Bain G, *et al*. Tuberculosis: a radiologic review. *Radiographics* 2007; **27**: 1255–73.

Engin G, Acunas B, Acunas G, Tunaci M. Imaging of extrapulmonary tuberculosis. *Radiographics* 2000; **20**: 471–88.

Harisinghani MG, McLoud TC, Shepard JA, *et al*. Tuberculosis from head to toe. *Radiographics* 2000; **20**: 449–70.

Jung NY, Jee WH, Ha KY, Park CK, Byun JY. Discrimination of tuberculous spondylitis from pyogenic spondylitis on MRI. *AJR Am J Roentgenol* 2004; **182**: 1405–10.

MSK Case 33

JOHN CURTIS

Clinical history

A 30-year-old male with painless hip swelling and reduced hip movement. Normal serum biochemistry.

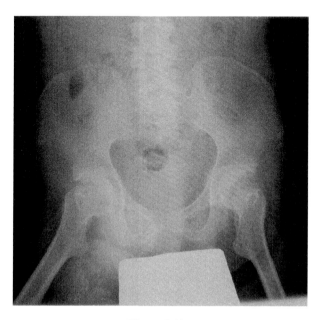

Figure 3.33a

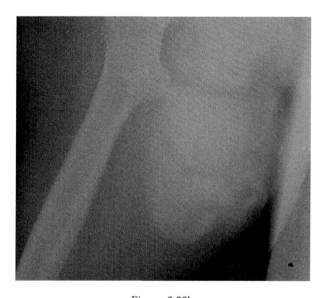

Figure 3.33b

Model answer

The pelvic and right thigh radiographs (Figures 3.33a, 3.33b) demonstrate multiple heterogeneous, lobulated, rounded calcified masses in the periarticular soft tissues of the inner right thigh. The mass lesions resemble calcified cysts with amorphous internal calcification. Given the normal biochemistry, this makes tumoral calcinosis the most likely diagnosis. The bone is normal, with no evidence of erosion.

The differential diagnosis includes calcification associated with renal failure.

Questions

1. **What are the differential diagnoses for this appearance?**
   - Identical appearance to tumoral calcinosis:
     - Chronic renal failure – associated with hyperparathyroidism and tends to improve after dialysis. It is sometimes called secondary tumoral calcinosis.
   - Similar appearance to tumoral calcinosis:
     - Dystrophic calcification – scleroderma, dermatomyositis (tends to be sheet-like).
     - Tumours – synovial sarcoma, chondrosarcoma, osteosarcoma, synovial osteochondromatosis.
     - Calcium pyrophosphate dihydrate deposition disease (CPPD).
     - Hypercalcaemia – hyperparathyroidism, hypervitaminosis D, milk alkali syndrome, sarcoidosis.
     - Hyperuricaemia – severe tophaceous gout.
     - Myositis ossificans.

Key points

- Tumoral calcinosis is an inherited disorder with equal sex incidence characterized by massive periarticular calcification. It is significantly more common in patients of African descent.
- Almost all patients have normal serum biochemistry, except for hyperphosphataemia in a minority. This feature distinguishes the cause of these appearances from chronic renal failure.
- Regions affected, in decreasing order of frequency:
  - hip
  - elbow
  - shoulder
  - foot
  - wrist
- Lesions are cystic with a white toothpaste-like material consisting of calcium hydroxyapatite crystals with amorphous calcium carbonate and calcium phosphate.
- Radiographically these lesions are typically multiple, amorphous, lobulated, cystic and located in the bursal regions of the extensor compartments around large joints.
- CT demonstrates the calcified mass lesions to advantage and provides an accurate location – around the hip it is located in the great trochanteric bursa. CT may show fluid–fluid levels. A gradient of calcification within lesions suggests a suspension of calcium in suspension.
- There is no erosion or bone destruction.
- Treatment is by surgical resection of the larger lesions and by medication to lower serum phosphate (acetazolamide and aluminium hydroxide). Fine needle aspiration.

Further reading

Banks KP, Bui-Mansfield LT, Chew FS, Collinson F. A compartmental approach to the radiographic evaluation of soft-tissue calcifications. *Semin Roentgenol* 2005; **40**: 391–407.

Olsen KM, Chew FS. Tumoral calcinosis: pearls, polemics, and alternative possibilities. *Radiographics* 2006; **26**: 871–85.

Images courtesy of Dr Julian Tuson, University Hospital Aintree, Liverpool.

MSK Case 34

JOHN CURTIS

Clinical history

Spot diagnosis in a young adult male.

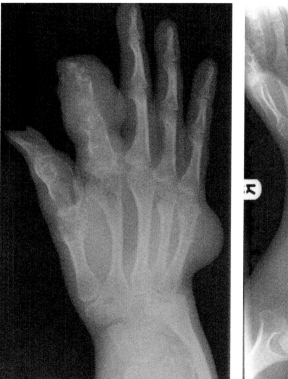

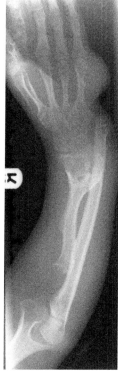

Figure 3.34a   Figure 3.34b

Model answer

This right-sided hand radiograph (Figure 3.34a) demonstrates soft tissue swelling of the thumb, index finger and little finger with well-defined, expansile lytic lesions in the diaphyses of the little finger metacarpal and the phalanges of the thumb and index finger. The forearm radiograph (Figure 3.34b) shows a shortened radius with a Madelung's-type deformity of the wrist (volar tilt of the radius with shortening of the radius). There is an expansile lesion of the distal radius with chondroid matrix calcification. No phleboliths seen. I would like to view previous films to assess any interval change and to see a radiograph of the other hand and forearm. (This was normal.)

The appearances are those of multiple enchondromas affecting one side of the body (Ollier's disease).

Questions

1. **What are the features of Madelung's deformity?**

   Growth arrest in the distal radial epiphysis results in radial bowing in a volar and ulnar direction. As a result the ulna is longer than the radius.

   The conditions that lead to a Madelung's-type deformity are diaphyseal aclasia (multiple exostoses), Ollier's disease and multiple epiphyseal dysplasia.

Key points

- Ollier's disease is rare and not inherited.
- It is characterized by multiple enchondromas located mainly in the diametaphyseal region in tubular bones of the hands and feet, almost always unilaterally. (NB: unilateral involvement in Maffucci's syndrome occurs in about 50%).
- Involved long bones are deformed and shortened. The iliac bone may be affected.
- Enchondromas are frequently complicated by pathological fractures and are characterized by expansile lucent lesions within the long bones, with or without chondroid matrix calcification.
- The risk of developing chondrosarcoma is about 25% by the age of 40 years. This risk is significantly increased in Maffucci's syndrome.
- Chondrosarcoma is suggested by (increased) pain, deep endosteal scalloping (more than two-thirds of cortical thickness), bone destruction, soft tissue mass, focal loss of matrix calcification, periosteal reaction and increased uptake on bone scanning.

Further reading

Flach HZ, Ginai AZ, Oosterhuis JW. Maffucci syndrome: radiologic and pathologic findings. *Radiographics* 2001; **21**: 1311–16.

Murphey MD, Flemming DJ, Boyea SR, *et al*. Enchondroma versus chondrosarcoma in the appendicular skeleton: differentiating features. *Radiographics* 1998; **18**: 1213–37.

Images courtesy of Dr Brian Eyes, University Hospital Aintree, Liverpool.

MSK Case 35

JOHN CURTIS

Clinical history
Young man aged 20 years with leg pain.

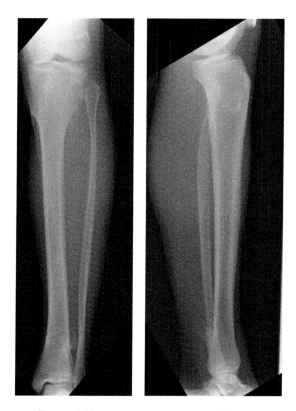

Figure 3.35a   Figure 3.35b

Model answer
AP and lateral radiographs of the tibia and fibula (Figures 3.35a, 3.35b) demonstrate bony exostoses arising from the distal and proximal ends of the tibia. The long axis of each exostosis (osteochondroma) points away from the joint. No fracture or soft tissue mass. No evidence of malignant transformation.

The appearances are those of hereditary multiple exostoses (HME) or diaphyseal aclasia. Other affected bones should be subjected to radiography. Previous films are important in assessing interval changes, especially if malignancy is considered.

Questions
1. **How is this condition inherited?**
   Autosomal dominant.
2. **What are the complications of this condition?**
   - Abnormal bone modelling leading to growth disturbance and malalignment.
   - Fracture.

- Vascular and neural compression. This may lead to popliteal artery aneurysm with femoral osteochondromas and peroneal nerve injury with fibular osteochondromas.
- Formation of bursa.
- Rib osteochondromas may cause haemothorax, and periarticular lesions may cause haemarthrosis.
- Malignant transformation – the cartilage cap becomes chondrosarcomatous in up to 5% of patients with multiple lesions (and in only 1% of those with solitary lesions).

Key points

- Osteochondromas or exostoses arise in any bone that is formed in cartilage. They are located in the metaphysis close to the growth plate and point *away* from the joint. The lesion, which comprises cortex and medulla, is connected to the native bone by a bony stalk. The cartilage cap is not visible on plain radiographs.
- Chondrosarcoma secondary to HME is very rare before 20 years of age and accounts for 8% of all chondrosarcomas
- Clinical and radiographic features of malignancy:
  - (increased) pain or a painless, hard and slowly enlarging mass
  - growth in a previously stable osteochondroma in an adult
  - irregularity to the surface of the osteochondroma
  - focal loss of bone density internally
  - adjacent bony destruction
  - calcified soft tissue mass

Further reading

Levine SM, Lambiase RE, Petchprapa CN. Cortical lesions of the tibia: characteristic appearances at conventional radiography. *Radiographics* 2003; **23**: 157–77.

Murphey MD, Choi JJ, Kransdorf MJ, Flemming DJ, Gannon FH. Imaging of osteochondroma: variants and complications with radiologic-pathologic correlation. *Radiographics* 2000; **20**: 1407–34.

MSK Case 36

Clinical history

Swollen, red and painless foot in a 40-year-old man.

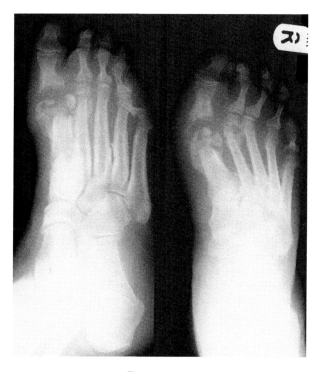

Figure 3.36a

Model answer

These are DP and oblique radiographs of the foot (Figure 3.36a), which demonstrate fractures of the first and second metatarsal heads with exuberant callus formation and periosteal reaction, fragmentation and distension of the first metatarsophalangeal (MTP) joint. There is digital vascular calcification between the first and second metatarsals. There is a degenerative arthropathy of the fifth metatarsophalangeal joint. There is an absence of gas in the soft tissues. The appearances are those of a Charcot's or neuropathic foot due to diabetes mellitus.

Questions

1. **What are the other causes of neuroarthropathy (Charcot's) joint?**
   - Syphilis (tabes dorsalis) – spine, hip, knee and rarely, ankle
   - Syringomyelia – shoulder, elbow and wrist
   - Alcoholism – MTP and interphalangeal joints of the foot
   - Myelomeningocele – ankle and intertarsal joints

2. **What are the radiological features that favour infection rather than neuroarthropathy?**
- Joint changes overlying skin ulceration
- Sclerotic sequestra and periosteal reactions

Key points

- Long-standing, poorly controlled diabetes mellitus is the commonest cause of a neuropathic (Charcot) joint and usually affects the foot and ankle (Figure 3.36b), although it may also affect the knee.
- Joint changes are typically seen in patients with a history of no trauma or minimal trauma.
- Atrophic neuroarthropathic change together with digital vascular calcification of the foot strongly suggests diabetes mellitus.
- Clinically patients may have a warm, red foot with reduced or absent pain sensation. Often there are ulcers and joint deformity.
- Neuroarthropathy begins in the mid foot – subluxation occurs in the second tarsometatarsal joint and then affects joints lateral to this. Metatarsophalangeal resorption is typical.
- Typical 'diabetic fractures' include subchondral fractures of the metatarsal heads, especially the second (Figure 3.36a), and avulsion fracture of the posterior calcaneal tubercle. Talocalcaneal fragmentation is also typical (Figure 3.36b).
- *Always* suspect a neuropathic joint in patients with Lisfranc fractures/dislocations (Figure 3.36c) in the absence of trauma.
- Infection and neuropathic arthropathy may coexist. MRI and white cell scintigraphy may be necessary to differentiate the two conditions.
- Lower extremity neuroarthropathy may also be seen in patients with:
  ○ leprosy
  ○ myelomeningocele
  ○ alcoholism leading to peripheral neuropathy
  ○ congenital insensitivity to pain (Riley–Day syndrome)
  ○ Charcot–Marie–Tooth disease (motor and sensory neuropathy)

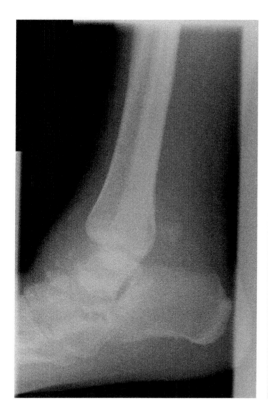
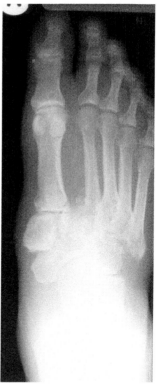

Figure 3.36b   Figure 3.36c

Further reading
Jones EA, Manaster BJ, May DA, Disler DG. Neuropathic osteoarthropathy: diagnostic dilemmas and differential diagnosis. *Radiographics* 2000; **20**: S279–93.

MSK Case 37

JOHN CURTIS

Clinical history
Twisting injury while skiing. Knee 'gives way'.

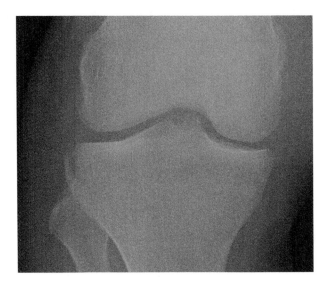

Figure 3.37a

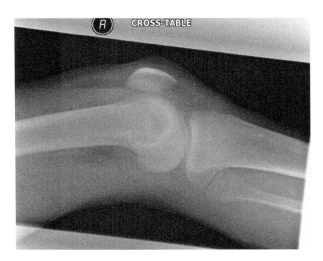

Figure 3.37b

Model answer
Frontal and lateral radiographs of the right knee (Figures 3.37a, 3.37b). The lateral radiograph shows a lipohaemarthrosis. There is a lucent line running parallel with the femoral shaft suggesting a fracture of the medial femoral condyle. The AP view

shows a small undisplaced vertical avulsion fracture at the lateral tibia just below the tibial plateau. The appearances are highly suggestive of a Segond fracture. This fracture is unstable and is associated with a tear of the anterior cruciate ligament and a tear of the lateral meniscus. In this case there is a suspected medial femoral condylar fracture. There is also a blood–fat interface superficial to the anterior border of the patella.

Possible questions
1. **What is the significance of a lipohaemarthrosis?**
   It implies a fracture of bone through the joint surface (i.e. intra-articular fracture). The horizontal-beam lateral knee radiograph depicts a blood–fat interface – the fat floats to the top above the blood.
2. **What further investigation is required?**
   MRI of the knee to search for internal ligamentous and meniscal damage and marrow oedema at the site of the avulsed cortical fragment. MRI will also confirm the fracture of the medial femoral condyle.

Key points
- A Segond fracture will cause anterolateral knee instability and is a consequence of severe varus strain and internal rotation during knee flexion. This injury may be seen in skiers and snowboarders. It is manifest as a cortical avulsion fracture of the proximal lateral tibia at the site of insertion of the middle third of the lateral capsular ligament.
- In varus stress the ACL acts as a restraining structure. As a consequence Segond fractures are associated with tears of the ACL in 75–100% of patients, and lateral meniscal tears in 66–75% of patients.

Notes
1. In this case MRI confirmed the presence of a lipohaemarthrosis secondary to a fracture of the medial femoral condyle (Figure 3.37c: FFE T2-weighted image). There was no evidence of ACL rupture or meniscal injury in this case.
2. The varus strain has resulted in the avulsion injury of the lateral tibia and a fracture of the medial femoral condyle. Without this fracture, it is highly likely that there would have been ACL disruption with or without meniscal injury.

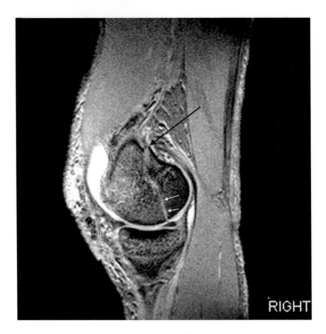

Figure 3.37c

Further reading

Campos JC, Chung CB, Lektrakul N, *et al*. Pathogenesis of the Segond fracture: ana-tomic and MR imaging evidence of an iliotibial tract or anterior oblique band avulsion. *Radiology* 2001; **219**: 381–6.

Crotty JM, Snow RD, Brogdon BG, DeMouy EH. Magnetic resonance imaging of trauma patterns in the knee. *Emerg Radiol* 1998; **4**: 237–44.

Goldman AB, Pavlov H, Rubenstein D. The Segond fracture of the proximal tibia: a small avulsion that reflects major ligamentous damage. *AJR Am J Roentgenol* 1988; **151**: 1163–7.

Matherne TH, Monu JUV, Schruff L, Neitzschman HR. Avulsions around the knee portend instability. *Emerg Radiol* 2005; **11**: 213–18.

Miller LS, Yu JS. Radiographic indicators of acute ligament injuries of the knee: a mechanistic approach. *Emerg Radiol* 2010; **17**: 435–44.

MSK Case 38

JOHN CURTIS

Clinical history
90-year-old female following a minor fall.

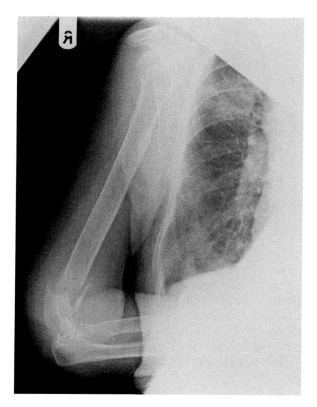

Figure 3.38a

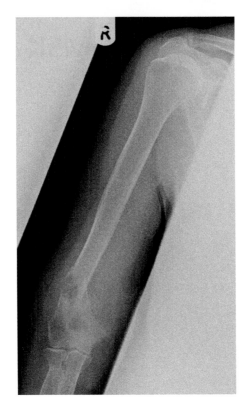

Figure 3.38b

Model answer

These are AP and lateral views of the right humerus (Figures 3.38a, 3.38b). There is a comminuted fracture in the distal humerus with displacement. The underlying bone is abnormal – there is a lytic lesion with permeation of bone. The appearances are those of a pathological fracture. There is a 3 cm mass in the right upper zone of the lung, likely to represent a primary bronchial neoplasm.

The unifying diagnosis is fracture through a bony metastasis secondary to carcinoma of the bronchus. An isotope bone scan and staging CT of the thorax are indicated.

Questions

1. **Which primary neoplasms commonly metastasize to bone?**
   - Lytic:
     - breast
     - bronchus
     - thyroid
     - kidney
   - Sclerotic:
     - breast
     - prostate
2. **Which bone metastases can be sclerotic?**
   - Prostate
   - Any adenocarcinoma
   - Breast
   - Carcinoid

- Bladder
- (Lymphoma)

3. **Which metastases are expansile and associated with a soft tissue mass?**
   - Kidney
   - Thyroid

4. **Which neoplasms are commonly responsible for metastases in children?**
   - Neuroblastoma
   - Lymphoma/leukaemia
   - Rhabdomyosarcoma
   - Ewing's sarcoma
   - Thyroid

Key points

- Metastases in bone may be caused by haematogenous, lymph spread or direct invasion by tumour. Long bones and bone-marrow-rich bones are more commonly affected than other sites.
  - haematogenous – e.g. vertebral venous plexus (of Batson) causing vertebral metastases.
  - lymph spread – e.g. renal carcinoma.
  - direct spread – e.g. Pancoast tumour with direct invasion of the ribs, rectal carcinoma invading the sacrum.
- *Important in the FRCR viva* – If you notice lytic metastases look for a possible underlying cause on the same film. Conversely, once you have detected a neoplasm look for metastases. *Do not forget myeloma and lymphoma as causes of lytic bone lesions.*
- Chest radiograph – look on the edge of the film for humeral metastases. In a patient with rib metastases, look for a mastectomy, or breast asymmetry in cases of breast carcinoma. Do not forget to look for surgical clips below the diaphragm that suggest nephrectomy for renal carcinoma or clips in the neck that suggest thyroidectomy (caution: a lytic lesion in the rib + surgical neck clips may represent parathyroidectomy and brown tumour).
- Expansile metastases suggest renal (Figure 3.38c) or thyroid carcinoma.
- Lytic metastases in the fingers are commonly caused by bronchial carcinoma (Figures 3.38d–3.38f). Expansile lytic lesions in the terminal phalanx are also caused by glomus tumours, enchondromas and implantation dermoid.

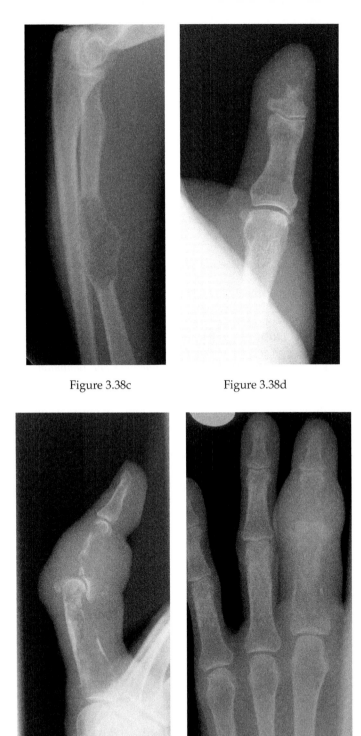

Figure 3.38c

Figure 3.38d

Figure 3.38e

Figure 3.38f

Further reading

Miller TT. Bone tumors and tumorlike conditions: analysis with conventional radiography. *Radiology* 2008; **246**: 662–74.

Resnick D. *Diagnosis of Bone and Joint Disorders*, 4th edn. Philadelphia, PA: Saunders, 2002; 3757, 3922–4.

Figures 3.38d–3.38f courtesy of Dr Brian Eyes, University Hospital Aintree, Liverpool.

MSK Case 39

JOHN CURTIS

Clinical history
Swelling of both hands.

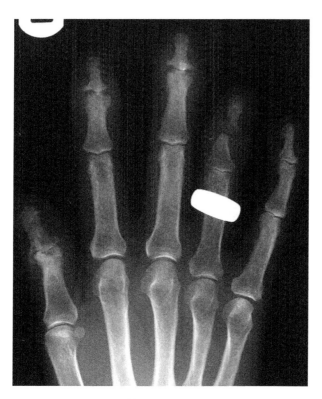

Figure 3.39a

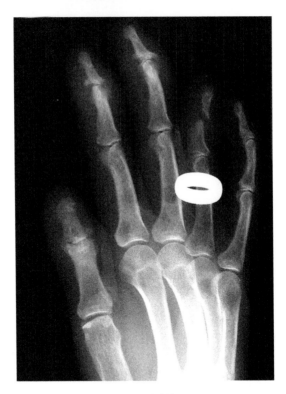

Figure 3.39b

Model answer

The hand radiographs (Figures 3.39a, 3.39b) demonstrate soft tissue swelling of the distal part of the thumb, distal index and middle fingers together with marginal erosions in the DIP joints and new bone formation ('mouse-ears') of the distal phalanges. No osteopenia. There is marked bone resorption of the distal portion of the middle phalanx of the ring finger ('pencil-in-cup' deformity). There are no osteophytes and no evidence of subchondral sclerosis. The appearances are those of psoriatic arthritis.

Questions

1. What is the differential diagnosis?

Erosive osteoarthritis. The distribution of changes is similar to psoriatic arthropathy but the absence of central erosions, osteophytes and subchondral sclerosis and the presence of marginal erosions and new bone formation makes psoriatic arthropathy most likely. Erosive osteoarthritis is much more common in middle-aged and elderly females (F : M = 12 : 1).

Key points

- Psoriatic arthropathy (PA) is a rheumatoid factor-negative inflammatory arthritis associated with psoriasis.
- PA is seen in about 10% of patients with psoriasis and may pre-date the skin changes in up to 15% of patients. In psoriasis nail changes (pitting, ridging, onycholysis and subungal keratosis) are more common in those patients who have PA.

- M = F, third to sixth decades. Rare in Africans and Chinese. HLA B27 positive in 80% of cases.
- PA is more prevalent in HIV infection.
- Various presenting types:
  - DIP joint involvement – classical 'distal arthritis' in 5–19% of cases
  - Symmetrical arthropathy similar in distribution to rheumatoid arthritis – ulnar styloid erosion in up to 25% of cases.
  - Asymmetrical arthritis mutilans (preceded by 'pencil-in-cup' deformities) in up to 5% of cases.
  - Psoriatic sacroiliitis and sponyloarthropathy occurring in 20–40% of cases.
- Pathologically similar to RA, with synovial inflammation, and fibrosis and new bone formation at joint margins ('mouse-ears') and at tendinous insertions. Asymmetrical (unlike RA)
- Psoriatic arthropathy in the hand/foot:
  - Characterized by destruction and proliferation of bone.
  - Hands are affected twice as often as feet.
  - No osteopenia (unlike RA). Asymmetrical soft tissue swelling.
  - Erosions marginal and irregular. DIP joints are the first joints to be affected.
  - DIP and PIP joint erosions and bone resorption (joint space narrowing not seen till later). Asymmetrical and oligoarticular. DIP involvement with or without PIP and MCP joint involvement.
  - 'Pencil-in-cup' joint deformity (Figure 3.39c) is characteristic of PA and is due to bony proliferation of the distal part of the joint (the 'cup') and resorption of the proximal part (the 'pencil'). Arthritis mutilans results.
  - Sausage digit – DIP and PIP joint involvement in the same digit with 'telescoping'.
  - Big toe – destruction of the IP joint with cartilage loss and new bone formation and sclerosis of the DP ('ivory phalanx') is virtually pathognomonic of PA.
  - Acro-osteolysis (uncommon), periosteal reactions.

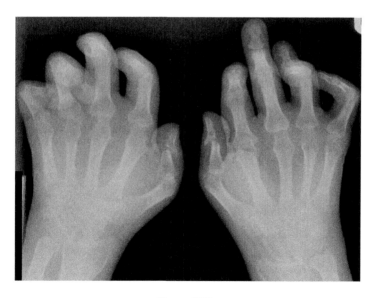

Figure 3.39c

Further reading

Chew FS, Roberts CC, Lalaji AP. *Musculoskeletal Imaging: a Teaching File*, 2nd edn. Philadelphia, PA: Lippincott Williams & Wilkins, 2006.

Helliwell PS, Taylor WJ. Classification and diagnostic criteria for psoriatic arthritis. *Ann Rheum Dis* 2005; **64**: ii3–8.

Ory PA, Gladman DD, Mease PJ. Psoriatic arthritis and imaging. *Ann Rheum Dis* 2005; **64**: ii55–7

Images courtesy of Dr Brian Eyes, University Hospital Aintree, Liverpool (Figures 3.39a, 3.39b), and Dr David Parker, Ysbyty Maelor, Wrexham (Fig 3.39c).

MSK Case 40

JOHN CURTIS

Clinical history

Painful hands in a 60-year-old female. History of severe postpartum haemorrhage 20 years previously.

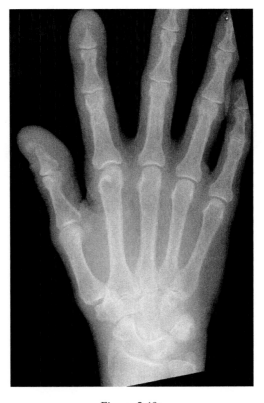

Figure 3.40a

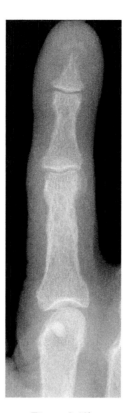

Figure 3.40b

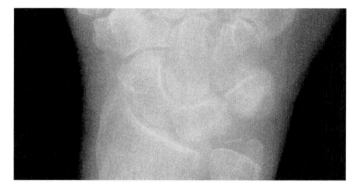

Figure 3.40c

Model answer

This is a DP radiograph of the right hand, with detail views of the index finger and wrist (Figures 3.40a–3.40c). There is osteopenia with coarsening of the trabecular pattern and linear lucency of the phalangeal cortices. There is subperiosteal resorption of the radial aspect of the phalanges, terminal tuft resorption and mid-phalangeal osteolysis of the terminal phalanges of the thumb, index finger and little finger. There is a juxta-articular erosion at the radial aspect of the DIP joint of the middle finger. There is calcification in the triangular fibrocartilage. There is a well-defined lytic lesion in the lunate, likely to be a brown tumour. The appearances are those of hyperparathyroidism. I would like to examine the distal forearm in search of a dialysis fistula. It is likely she has renal insufficiency as a result of renal shutdown following postpartum haemorrhage.

Questions

1. **What is the commonest cause of hyperparathyroidism in the UK?**

   Chronic renal failure. This causes vitamin D deficiency, resulting in hypocalcaemia, which in turn promotes increased activity of the parathyroid glands and excess parathyroid hormone production.

2. **What is the most convincing radiological sign that points to a diagnosis of hyperparathyroidism?**

   Subperiosteal resorption of the radial aspect of the phalanges is virtually pathognomonic of hyperparathyroidism.

Key points

- Hyperparathyroidism is a common examination film and may be seen in the viva and long case parts of the examination. There is a plethora of radiological signs, which make this condition ideal examination material.
- Hyperparathyroidism increases the osteoclast : osteoblast ratio, which leads to bone resorption. This is an attempt by the body to normalize the serum calcium in the face of chronically low levels of calcium.
- Hyperparathyroidism can be primary (hyperplasia, single or multiple adenomas and, rarely, carcinoma), secondary (chronic renal failure or malabsorption) or tertiary (long-standing secondary hyperparathyroidism)
- Brown tumours are seen to advantage in the hands and represent localized collections of fibrous tissue and giant cells. If necrotic, they may change into fluid-filled cysts. They are invariably associated with the other radiological manifestations of hyperparathyroidism (Figure 3.40d).
- Other radiological manifestations of hyperparathyroidism include:
  - pepper-pot skull
  - erosion of outer clavicles
  - medial tibial erosion
  - loss of lamina dura
  - osteosclerosis and osteopenia – 'rugger-jersey spine' of renal osteodystrophy
  - soft tissue calcification – cartilage, vascular
  - periosteal new bone formation
- Tip for the exam – let the examiner know that you know the diagnosis and its associations by looking at the wrist (and indicating to the examiner that you are doing so) for an arteriovenous dialysis fistula.

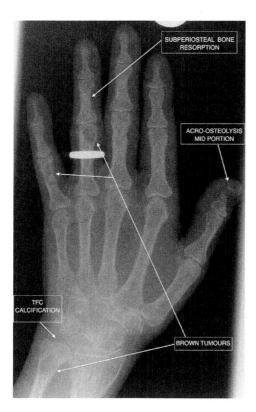

Figure 3.40d

Further reading

Chew FS, Huang-Hellinger F. Brown tumor. *AJR Am J Roentgenol* 1993; **160**: 752.

Eisenberg RL. Bubbly lesions of bone. *AJR Am J Roentgenol* 2009; **193**: W79–94.

Jetvic V. Imaging of renal osteodystrophy. *Eur J Radiol* 2003; **46**: 85–95.

Jones SN, Stoker DJ. Radiology at your fingertips: lesions of the terminal phalanx. *Clin Radiol* 1988; **39**: 478–85.

McDonald DK, Parman L, Speights VO. Best cases from the AFIP: primary hyperparathyroidism due to parathyroid adenoma. *Radiographics* 2005; **25**: 829–34.

Miller TT. Bone tumors and tumorlike conditions: analysis with conventional radiography. *Radiology* 2008; **246**: 662–74.

Tigges S, Nance EP, Carpenter WA, Erb R. Osteodystrophy: imaging findings that mimic those of other diseases, *AJR Am J Roentgenol* 1995; **165**: 143–8.

Wittenberg A. The rugger jersey spine sign. *Radiology* 2004; **230**: 491–2.

MSK Case 41

JOHN CURTIS

Clinical history
Painless swelling of both hands in a 40-year-old woman. Abnormal chest radiograph.

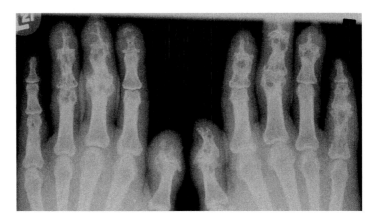

Figure 3.41a

Model answer
There are multiple well-defined 'punched out' lucent lesions in the phalanges of both hands without direct joint involvement (Figure 3.41a). The trabecular bone has a lace-like pattern, especially in the middle phalanges. There is destruction of the distal phalanx of the left thumb and marked cortical erosion of several distal phalanges. There is swelling of the soft tissues of the finger tips ('pseudoclubbing'). No periosteal reaction.

These are the classical appearances of osseous sarcoidosis. I would like to see the patient's chest radiograph to look for hilar lymphadenopathy and changes compatible with parenchymal sarcoidosis.

Questions
1. **List five additional causes of 'cyst-like' bone lesions of phalanges.**
   - Implantation dermoid
   - Glomus tumour
   - Gout (low-signal tophi on MRI)
   - Rheumatoid arthritis
   - Enchondroma

Key points
- Osseous involvement occurs in up to 13% of patients and is usually seen in association with systemic sarcoidosis, which takes a chronic course. Osseous sarcoidosis is unusual without skin involvement. *A chest radiograph should be requested when a diagnosis of osseous sarcoidosis is suspected.* This patient had bilateral hilar lymph node enlargement.

- Hands and feet (Figure 3.41b) are most often involved (middle and distal phalanges). Involvement of other bones is very rare.
- Migratory arthralgia without radiographic abnormality occurs in 10–40% of cases. Löfgren's syndrome is self-limiting and comprises the triad of erythema nodosum, arthralgia (classically involving the ankles) and mediastinal lymphadenopathy.
- Sarcoidosis is associated with myopathy and muscle nodules. Tendons and other soft tissues may be involved by nodules, which have a high signal on MRI (unlike gouty tophi, which have a low signal).
- Osseous lesions are often asymptomatic. Lesions are usually 'hot' on bone scintigraphy, which, like MRI, is more sensitive than radiography.
- Osteolytic lesions on radiography – articular spaces preserved, usually no periosteal reaction.
  - well-defined 'cystic' areas – not true cysts: 'punched-out' solid lesions caused by non-caseating granulomata; endosteal thinning of the cortex
  - lace-like trabecular pattern – multiple granulomata
  - extensive erosion of bone with fracture
- Diffuse vertebral sclerosis has been described in sarcoidosis. Acro-osteosclerosis described.
- MRI is much more sensitive than radiography in the detection of osseous and extraosseous lesions. Periosteal reactions, which are not visible radiographically, may be visualized at MRI.
- Treatment is with steroids. Improvement is possible, but severe changes are unlikely to improve.

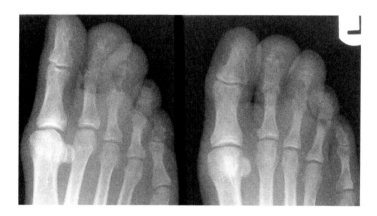

Figure 3.41b

Further reading

Chew FS. Radiology of the hands: review and self-assessment module. *AJR Am J Roentgenol* 2005; **184**: S157–68.

Koyama T, Ueda H, Togashi K, *et al*. Radiologic manifestations of sarcoidosis in various organs. *Radiographics* 2004; **24**: 87–104.

Moore SL, Teirstein AE. Musculoskeletal sarcoidosis: spectrum of appearances at mr imaging. *Radiographics* 2003; **23**: 1389–99.

Resnick D, Niwayama G. Sarcoidosis. In Resnick D, Niwayama G, eds., *Diagnosis of Bone and Joint Disorders*, 3rd edn. Philadelphia, PA: Saunders, 1995; 4333–52.

Yaghmai I. Radiographic, angiographic and radionuclide manifestations of osseous sarcoidosis. *Radiographics* 1983; **3**: 375–96.

Images courtesy of Dr Otto Chan, London.

MSK Case 42

JOHN CURTIS

Clinical history

Left hip pain and swelling in a 60-year-old woman. History of previous Girdlestone operation of the left hip.

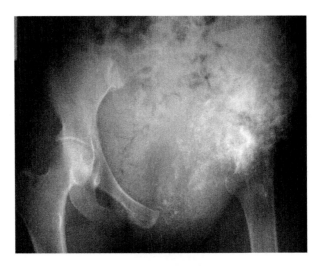

Figure 3.42a

Model answer

This AP radiograph (Figure 3.42a) demonstrates destructive replacement of the left superior and inferior pubic rami with an amorphous mass with 'ring and arc' chondroid calcification. The margins are ill-defined. There is evidence of a previous Girdlestone operation and there is surgical removal of the femoral head. The appearances are those of an aggressive malignant lesion, most likely a peripheral primary chondrosarcoma. Previous radiographs should be examined to determine any prior pelvic lesion to determine if this is a primary or secondary chondrosarcoma.

A chest radiograph (or CT thorax) and MRI of the pelvis are indicated for further evaluation.

Questions

1. **What is the difference between central and peripheral chondrosarcomas?**
   Central lesions arise from the medulla of the bone, without soft tissue mass lesions until the cortex is breached. Peripheral lesions arise in the cortical bone and are invariably associated with soft tissue mass lesions.
2. **What factors result in pelvic lesions presenting late?**
   Early lesions may cause little or no symptoms, usually with subtle or normal radiographic appearances. Pain, when present, progresses insidiously. Pelvic chondrosarcomas are typically well advanced by the time of presentation. CT is more sensitive in the detection of subtle chondroid matrix calcification and the peripheral soft tissue mass lesions.

Key points

- Chondrosarcoma is a malignant neoplasm that produces chondroid matrix calcification.
- Primary lesions arise de novo and represent the third most common primary malignant neoplasm of bone. (The commonest is myeloma, and the next most frequent is osteosarcoma.)
- Secondary lesions arise from pre-existing enchondromas or the cartilage caps of osteochondromas.
- Central lesions arise from the medulla, causing bony expansion. Peripheral lesions arise from the cortical bone or from enchondromas/osteochondromas and typically cause soft tissue mass lesions.
- Large central lesions may be seen with a soft tissue mass if the bone is eroded.
- Typical sites for peripherally sited chondrosarcoma include shoulder and pelvis.
- Centrally sited lesions typically occur in long bones, e.g. femur, humerus.
- The pelvis is a common site for chondrosarcoma (hip acetabulum) and a *rare site for solitary enchondroma*.
- In the pelvis, chondrosarcoma commonly involves the ilium and is often large at presentation.
- Chondrosarcomas may involve the ribs at the costochondral junction (Figure 3.42b). As with pelvic involvement, the rib is a common site for chondrosarcoma and a *rare site for solitary enchondroma*.
- In contrast the hands and feet are rare sites for chondrosarcomas but *very common sites for enchondromas*.
- Chondrosarcomas are also seen in the spine (usually thoracic) and involve the posterior elements and the head and neck region (skull base).

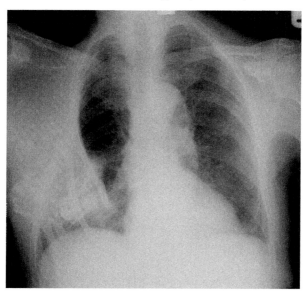

Figure 3.42b

Further reading

Littrell LA, Wenger DE, Wold LE, *et al*. Radiographic, CT, and MR imaging features of dedifferentiated chondrosarcomas: a retrospective review of 174 de novo cases. *Radiographics* 2004; **24**: 1397–409.

Murphey MD, Walker EA, Wilson AJ, *et al*. From the archives of the AFIP. Imaging of primary chondrosarcoma: radiologic–pathologic correlation. *Radiographics* 2003; **23**: 1245–78.

MSK Case 43

JOHN CURTIS

Clinical history

41-year-old woman, previously well, presents with insidious onset of pain and swelling of the wrist. No history of trauma.

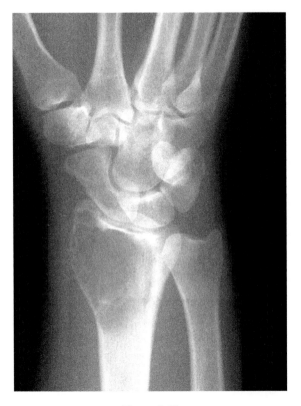

Figure 3.43

Model answer

In this wrist of an adult with a fused skeleton (Figure 3.43) there is an expanding, eccentric, lytic lesion arising from the subchondral portion of the distal radius. There is a wide zone of transition between the lesion and normal bone. On the radial side of the lesion there is early cortical erosion and there is a network of thin, delicate trabeculae traversing the lesion. There is no internal mineralization. The appearances are most likely to be due to giant-cell tumour of the radius.

Questions
1. **What are the differential diagnoses?**
   - Giant-cell reparative granuloma (usually obtain a history of trauma, cortex usually intact).

- Aneurysmal bone cyst (usually metaphyseal in an unfused skeleton).
- Chondromyxoid fibroma.
- Brown tumour of hyperparathyroidism (nothing in this patient's history to suggest renal failure).
- Angiosarcoma.
- Myeloma or expansile lytic metastasis, e.g. renal cell carcinoma.

Key points

- Giant-cell tumours (GCTs) represent 5% of all primary bone tumours. These tumours have a higher incidence in India and China. The cell of origin is probably a precursor of the osteoclast.
- Most GCTs are solitary and located at the subarticular regions of long bones in a fused skeleton in patients aged 20–50, and they are more common in females. GCTs in short bones tend to affect younger patients and may be multiple and prone to pathological fracture.
- Up to 70% of GCTs occur in the knee (distal femur > proximal tibia). The distal radius is the next most frequent site for GCTs. Proximal humerus and sacrum may also be involved. The spine is rarely involved.
- Radiographic appearances – subarticular, eccentrically expansile with a mixture of well-defined and poorly defined borders. The sharp border, when present, usually points towards the diaphysis. They are malignant in 20% and may be locally aggressive with cortical destruction, unlike in giant-cell reparative granuloma (GCRG), where the lesion is more benign and the cortex is intact. GCRG is associated with trauma, is more common in females, and is radiographically indistinguishable from GCT.
- CT and MRI help to determine the extent of the lesion but do not have any advantage over plain radiography in determining the diagnosis. On MRI, fluid levels may be seen with the lesion.

Further reading

Eisenberg RL. Bubbly lesions of bone. *AJR Am J Roentgenol* 2009; **193**: W79–94.

Miller TT. Bone tumors and tumorlike conditions: analysis with conventional radiography. *Radiology* 2008; **246**: 662–74.

Murphey MD, Nomikos GC, Flemming DJ, *et al.* From the archives of the AFIP. Imaging of giant cell tumor and giant cell reparative granuloma of bone: radiologic–pathologic correlation. *Radiographics* 2001; **21**: 1283–309.

MSK Case 44

JOHN CURTIS

Clinical history
This is a 4-year-old boy who has fallen from his bike.

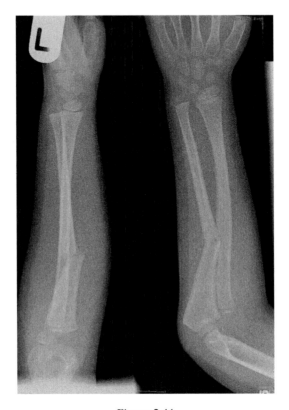

Figure 3.44

Model answer
There is a displaced fracture of the proximal third of the ulna with anterior disloca-tion of the radial head (Figure 3.44). There is a normal relationship of the capitellum with the anterior humeral line but there is interruption of the radio-capitellar line. This is a Monteggia fracture/dislocation (Bado type I).

Questions
1. **What is the Bado classification of Monteggia fractures?**

   Type I – fracture of proximal ulna + anterior dislocation of the radial head. There may be an associated wrist injury (65%).

   Type II – fracture of proximal ulna + posterior dislocation of the radial head (18%).

   Type III – fracture of proximal ulna close to the coronoid process + lateral disloca-tion of the radial head (16%).

Type IV – fracture of proximal ulna and radius at the same level + anterior dislocation of the radial head (1%).

2. **What complications may occur with Monteggia fractures?**
Radial nerve injuries in approximately 20% of cases.

Key points

- Monteggia fracture/dislocations are common in adults and rare in children and result from hyperpronation during a fall onto the outstretched hand.
- They are frequently overlooked in children – so *don't* miss them.
- The radial head dislocation can be picked up readily if there is any discontinuity of the radio-capitellar line. This is the line that should pass through the mid-axial radius and central third of the capitellum *on all projections*.
- Monteggia fracture/dislocation is a typical 'ring fracture' – the 'ring' being formed by the distal and proximal radio-ulnar joints and the ulna and radius bones. Galeazzi fractures are mid-distal radial fractures with distal radio-ulnar dislocation and are complicated by ulnar nerve injuries.
- Up to 50% of Monteggia fracture/dislocations can be overlooked on initial radiographs. For this reason always obtain a radiograph of the elbow and wrist in forearm trauma, using true AP and lateral projections of each joint.
- Isolated ulnar shaft fractures are rare – therefore always look for elbow dislocation. Note also that in children dislocated radial heads may occur without ulnar fractures because of the 'plastic' nature of children's bones.

Further reading

Ashlock SJ, Harris JH. West OC, Zelitt D. Acute elbow injuries. *Emerg Radiol* 1998; **5**: 416–37.

Barron D, Branfoot T. Imaging trauma of the appendicular skeleton. *Imaging* 2003; **15**: 324–40.

Gleeson AP, Beattie TF. Monteggia fracture–dislocation in children. *J Accid Emerg Med* 1994; **11**: 192–4.

Hunter TB, Peltier LF, Lund PJ. Radiologic history exhibit. Musculoskeletal eponyms: who are those guys? *Radiographics* 2000; **20**: 819–36.

John SD, Wherry K, Swischuk LE, Phillips WA. Improving detection of pediatric elbow fractures by understanding their mechanics. *Radiographics* 1996; **16**: 1443–60.

MSK Case 45

JOHN CURTIS

Clinical history
19-year-old female with gradual onset of dull shin pain.

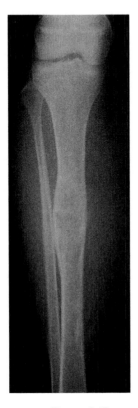 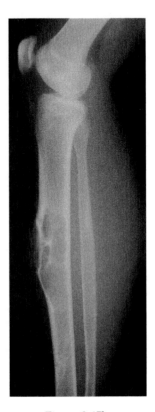

Figure 3.45a   Figure 3.45b

Model answer
The AP and lateral radiographs of the tibia and fibula (Figures 3.45a, 3.45b) show a well-defined, tubular, expansile, multiloculated lytic lesion in the medulla of the tibial diaphysis. There is endosteal scalloping within the tibia (especially medial) and a proportion of the lytic lesions have a sclerotic rim. It has a soap-bubble appearance. There is no periosteal reaction or soft tissue swelling. The diagnosis is between an adamantinoma, osteofibrous dysplasia and fibrous dysplasia.

Questions
1. **What other conditions may cause multiloculated lytic lesions in the tibial diaphysis?**
   - Non-ossifying fibroma – eccentric.
   - Fibrous dysplasia – young age, ground-glass matrix.

- Osteofibrous dysplasia – younger age, involves the anterior tibial diaphysis in 90% of cases. More benign course with spontaneous regression. This condition is indistinguishable from adamantinoma radiologically.

Key points

- Adamantinoma is a rare, low-grade malignant epithelial tumour of bone, so called because it resembles adamantinoma of the jaw histologically.
- It affects young patients, 20–50 years of age (females younger, males older).
- 80% of cases occur in the anterior tibial diaphysis – in 27% of cases there is a multi-focal tibial lesion and in 10% of these cases there is a coexisting satellite fibula lesion.
- MRI is the best imaging tool for determining tumour extent.
- Typically it acts as a low-grade indolent malignancy but occasionally it may be aggressive – either locally or with distant metastases to lung, bone, lymph nodes, liver and pericardium.
- Aggressiveness is seen more commonly in young males who present with pain.

Further reading

Camp MD, Tompkins RK, Spanier SS, Bridge JA, Bush CH. Best cases from the AFIP: adamantinoma of the tibia and fibula with cytogenetic analysis. *Radiographics* 2008; **28**: 1215–20.

Eisenberg RL. Bubbly lesions of bone. *AJR Am J Roentgenol* 2009; **193**: W79–94.

Levine SM, Lambiase RE, Petchprapa CN. Cortical lesions of the tibia: characteristic appearances at conventional radiography. *Radiographics* 2003; **23**: 157–77.

Miller TT. Bone tumors and tumorlike conditions: analysis with conventional radiography. *Radiology* 2008; **246**: 862–74.

O'Donnell P. Evaluation of focal bone lesions: basic principles and clinical scenarios. *Imaging* 2003; **15**: 298–323.

Images courtesy of Dr Otto Chan, London.

MSK Case 46

JOHN CURTIS

Clinical history
Painful finger in a 24-year-old man.

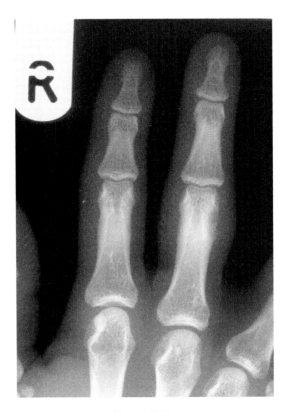

Figure 3.46a

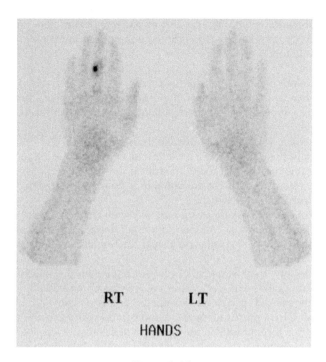

Figure 3.46b

Model answer

There is global soft tissue swelling in the region of the proximal phalanx of the middle finger (Figure 3.46a). There is a well-defined cortical lucent lesion approximately 5 mm diameter in the ulnar aspect of the distal metaphysis. No cortical destruction or periosteal reaction. An isotope bone scan (Figure 3.46b) demonstrates marked focal increased tracer activity corresponding to the lytic lesion. The most likely diagnosis is osteoid osteoma.

Questions

1. **What are the differential diagnoses?**
   - Intracortical Brodie's abscess
   - Intracortical haemangioma
2. **What are the differences between an osteoid osteoma and osteoblastoma?**
   Histologically, there is no difference. Radiologically, osteoblastomas are larger, are more expansile with less surrounding sclerosis. Osteoblastomas are less likely to cause pain and are less responsive to salicylates than osteoid osteomas. Unlike osteoid osteomas, osteoblastomas grow progressively and occasionally may undergo malignant change. Osteoblastomas are usually located in flat bones or vertebrae.

Key points

- Osteoid osteoma is a benign osteoblastic neoplasm accounting for 12% of such lesions. It characteristically contains a central vascular area with surrounding bony sclerosis. This manifests on radiographs as a rim of sclerosis, which surrounds a lucent nidus.
- Average age of presentation 20 years. Males affected more than females (3 : 1).
- Uncommon in non-white populations.

- Pain is a universal symptom, and 75% of patients obtain relief with salicylates, which inhibit prostaglandins, thought to be important in maintaining the vascularity of the lesion.
- Distribution:
  - 50% of lesions occur in femur or tibia
  - 10–15% hand – distal and proximal phalanges (metacarpals – very rare)
  - 10% spine – typically neural arch (patients often have painful scoliosis)
  - 10% foot
  - intra-articular lesions usually involve the hip
- Radiologically, the lesions have a lucent nidus with surrounding cortical sclerosis. Sometimes this may be marked with cortical thickening. Lesions tend to be less than 1 cm; lesions over 1.5 cm are *unlikely* to be osteoid osteomas. Occasionally there is no surrounding sclerosis.
- Intra-articular osteoid osteomas are more difficult to diagnose. Sclerosis is absent or subtle. Joint effusion is common, often accompanied by periarticular osteopenia. Occasionally periarticular periosteal reaction occurs. Bone scan may show global joint uptake.
- Bone scintigraphy may be useful in cases of high clinical suspicion with normal or subtle radiographs and can localize the area for CT or MRI scanning. It can be useful for the excised specimen to ensure its complete removal.
- Thin-section CT is optimal for lesion demonstration (and is better than MRI). CT demonstrates a lucent nidus in the epicentre of sclerosis. Occasionally a calcified matrix may be found in the nidus. Dynamic CT may show nidus enhancement.
- MRI shows the nidus and sclerosis along with bone marrow oedema. Nidus – low signal on T1, intermediate to high signal on T2 depending on degree of nidus matrix calcification. Marked nidus enhancement with gadolinium.
- Excision of the nidus is curative – surgical or by interventional radiological techniques (thermal ablation or excision).
- Osteoblastomas are similar histologically but are less painful, tend not to respond to salicylates and are larger than osteoid osteomas.

Further reading

Chai JW, Hong SH, Choi JY, *et al*. Radiologic diagnosis of osteoid osteoma: from simple to challenging findings. *Radiographics* 2010; **30**: 737–49.

Kransdorf MJ, Stull MA, Gilkey FW, Moser RP. From the archives of the AFIP: osteoid osteoma. *Radiographics* 1991; **11**: 671–96.

JOHN CURTIS

Clinical history

Post-injury and progress films following reduction of an elbow dislocation in a 10-year-old boy.

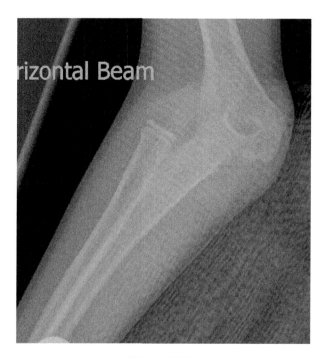

Figure 3.47a

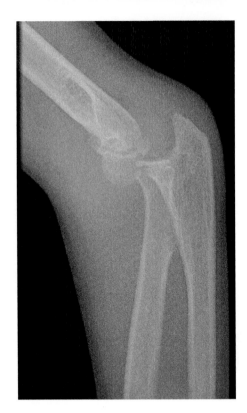

Figure 3.47b

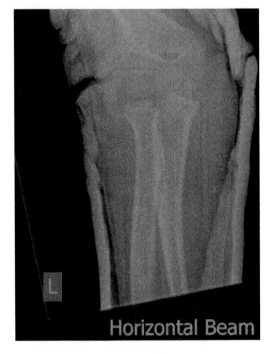

Figure 3.47c

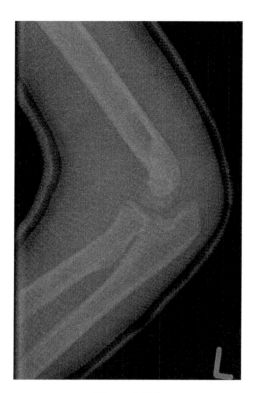

Figure 3.47d

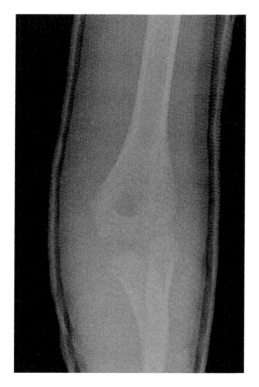

Figure 3.47e

Model answer
The initial AP and lateral radiographs of the elbow (Figures 3.47a, 3.47b) demonstrate a posterior dislocation of the elbow with an associated joint effusion. The trochlear epiphysis is not yet formed. The medial epicondyle epiphysis is not seen at the normal position and is avulsed, lying within the joint between the ulna and humerus. This is best seen on the lateral film and is confirmed on the post-reduction films (Figures 3.47d, 3.47e), which demonstrate persistent displacement of the epiphysis within the posterior joint.

Questions
1. **What is the mechanism of this injury?**
   Hyperextension injury with valgus stress – avulsion of the medial epicondyle epiphysis caused by contraction of the forearm flexor muscles. Occasionally violent flexion at the elbow may produce a similar injury.
2. **What would you do next?**
   Communicate this result to the orthopaedic team for prompt internal fixation of the medial epicondyle epiphysis.

Key points
- There are four distal humeral epiphyses, one radial and one ulnar epiphysis, and *knowing the order in which they appear is extremely important*. Always search for the medial (internal) epicondyle, and remember that in almost every case the *medial epicondyle epiphysis appears before the trochlea*.
- The order of appearance of ossification of the epiphyses is as follows (CRITOE):

C	capitellum	1 year
R	radial head	4 years
I	internal (medial) epicondyle	7 years
T	trochlea	10 years
O	olecranon	10 years
E	external (lateral) epicondyle	11 years

- The medial epicondyle epiphysis is the bony origin of the flexor muscles of the forearm and is likely to be avulsed during hyperextension-valgus injuries. They are often associated with elbow dislocations, when the avulsed medial epicondyle epiphysis becomes trapped in the joint after reduction.
- Always look for the trochlea. If it is present, always search for the medial epicondyle and, if it is absent from its normal position, suspect avulsion. Even if the trochlea is not present look for the medial epicondyle epiphysis in its usual site. When in doubt, radiograph the opposite side.

Further reading
Ashlock SJ, Harris JH, West OC, Zelitt D. Acute elbow injuries. *Emerg Radiol* 1998; **5**: 416–37.

John SD, Wherry K, Swischuk LE, Phillips WA. Improving detection of pediatric elbow fractures by understanding their mechanics. *Radiographics* 1996; **16**: 1443–60.

Images courtesy of Dr Gurdeep Mann, Alder Hey Children's Hospital, Liverpool.

MSK Case 48

JOHN CURTIS

Clinical history
A 20-year-old man with pain and swelling of the jaw.

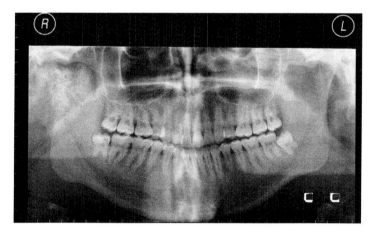

Figure 3.48a

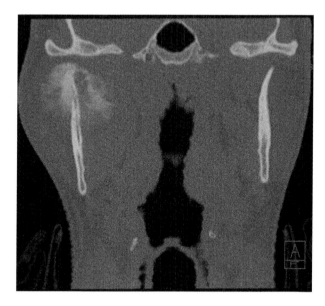

Figure 3.48b

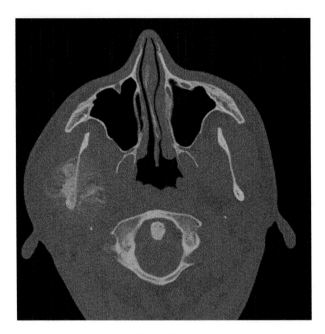

Figure 3.48c

Model answer

The orthopantomogram (OPG, Figure 3.48a) demonstrates a large calcified lesion overlying the upper right mandible. The mandibular condyle and ramus are not clearly seen. I would like to carry out a CT scan of the jaw.

This demonstrates a large calcified mass replacing the condylar and sub-condylar portions of the right mandible (Figures 3.48b, 3.48c). There is a sunburst periosteal reaction, which encircles the long axis of the mandibular ramus. The most likely diagnosis is osteosarcoma of the mandible (gnathic osteosarcoma). The sun-ray effect is due to radiating tumour 'spicules' within a soft tissue mass.

Questions

1. **What investigations would you do next?**

   An MRI of the head and neck region is required to determine the soft tissue extent of the tumour, and to assess the presence or absence of lymphadenopathy (Figures 3.48d, 3.48e). A bone scan is required to assess for the presence of multifocal or metastatic lesions. A CT scan of the thorax is required to search for pulmonary metastases.

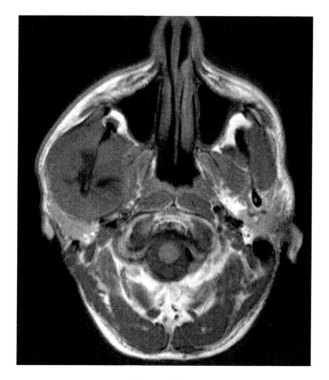

Figure 3.48d

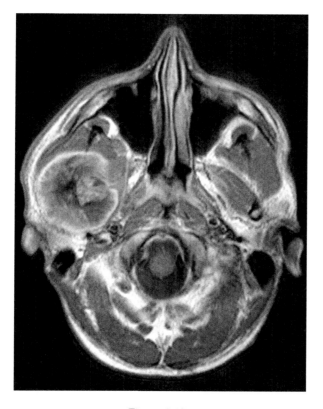

Figure 3.48e

2. **What other tumours involve the mandible?**

- Carcinomas that originate in the oral cavity and locally invade bone.
- Myeloma – multiple 'punched-out' lesions in the region of the angle, ramus and molar teeth.
- Metastases – primary tumour origins include lung, kidney, thyroid, stomach, prostate and breast.
- Sarcomas other than osteosarcomas – fibrosarcoma, Ewing's sarcoma (onion-skin periosteal reaction often absent in the jaw).

Key points

- Osteosarcomas in the mandible account for approximately 9% of all osteosarcomas. They may be osteolytic or osteoblastic (or mixed) and are termed gnathic osteosarcomas. Histologically they are predominantly chondroblastic.
- Gnathic osteosarcomas are distinct from conventional osteosarcomas. Patients have an older age of onset and there is a reduced incidence of extraskeletal metastases. However, they have the same radiological features as conventional lesions.
- In general, osteosarcomas may cause sunburst, hair-on-end and Codman's triangle type periosteal reactions. Occasionally lamellated or disorganized periosteal reactions may occur.
- Permeative patterns of destruction, soft tissue mass lesions and cortical destruction imply that the lesion is aggressive.
- CT is ideal for looking at the mineralized osteoid within the soft tissue mass.
- MRI is ideal for looking at the extent of marrow and soft tissue infiltration and extraskeletal spread.
- A metastasis to the mandible is four times more common than a metastasis to the maxilla. The commonest primary tumours are lung, kidney, thyroid, prostate and stomach.

Further reading

Dunfee BL, Sakai O, Pistey R, Gohel A. Radiologic and pathologic characteristics of benign and malignant lesions of the mandible. *Radiographics* 2006; **26**: 1751–68.

Murphey MD, Robbin MR, McRae GA, *et al.* The many faces of osteosarcoma. *Radiographics* 1997; **17**: 1205–31.

Rana RS, Wu JS, Eisenberg RL. Pattern of the month: periosteal reaction. *AJR Am J Roentgenol* 2009; **193**: W259–72.

Images courtesy of Dr Huw Lewis-Jones, University Hospital Aintree, Liverpool, and Dr Rebecca Hanlon, University Hospital Aintree, Liverpool.

Clinical history
Shoulder pain in a 40-year-old female who does not smoke.

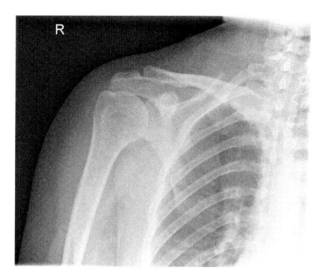

Figure 3.49a

Model answer
There is a well-defined spherical opacity projected over the medial right clavicle and lung apex (Figure 3.49a). No bone or joint abnormality. Further investigation with MRI is advised, including the cervical spine to determine the cause of the shoulder pain.

Questions
1. **What is the most likely diagnosis in a non-smoker?**
   Schwannoma or neurofibroma.

Key points
- Always look at the lungs on a shoulder radiograph. Make sure that this is one of your first actions.
- Do not overlook pneumothoraces, rib and vertebral destruction or mass lesions in the lung or mediastinum.
- A schwannoma is a slow-growing nerve sheath tumour that arises from spinal or intercostal nerves. In the thorax these tumours are well defined and spherical (small lesions) or ovoid (large lesions).
- On MRI, schwannomas are isointense with muscle on T1-weighted images and hyperintense to muscle on T2-weighted images. Large lesions exhibit heterogeneous enhancement with gadolinium and smaller lesions more homogeneous enhancement.
- Bony erosions signify slow-growing lesions and suggest benignity.

- It may be difficult to differentiate neurofibromas from schwannomas. If the originating nerve is identified, an eccentric position of the tumour with respect to the nerve suggests a schwannoma.
- Schwannomas are more likely than neurofibromas to be heterogeneous.
- Neurofibromas affect patients 20–30 years of age and are solitary in 90% of cases. In 10% of cases there is an association with neurofibromatosis, in which the lesions tend to be bigger.
- Schwannomas affect patients 20–40 years of age. Most lesions are solitary.

Notes

In this case the diagnosis was neurofibromatosis (Figure 3.49b). The lesions seen on MRI are neurofibromas.

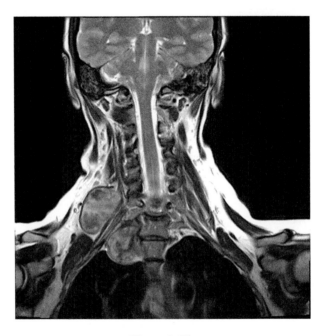

Figure 3.49b

Further reading

Lin J, Martel W. Cross-sectional imaging of peripheral nerve sheath tumors: characteristic signs on CT, MR imaging, and sonography. *AJR Am J Roentgenol* 2001; **176**: 75–82.

Tateishi U, Gladish GW, Kusumoto M, *et al*. Chest wall tumors: radiologic findings and pathologic correlation. Part 1. Benign tumors. *Radiographics* 2003; **23**: 1477–90.

Neuroradiology Case 1

REKHA SIRIPURAPU

Clinical history
A 31-year-old female presents with a three-week history of right-sided neck mass.

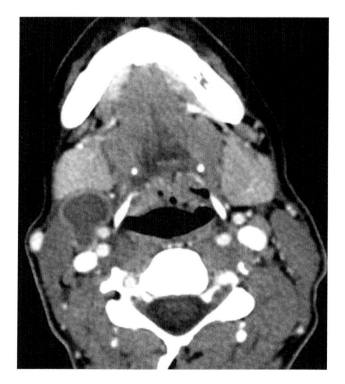

Figure 4.1a

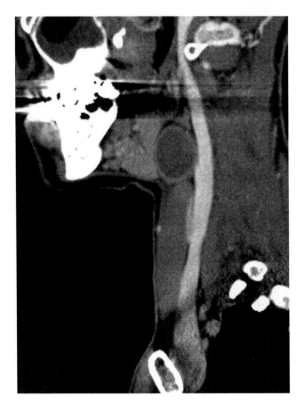

Figure 4.1b

Model answer

These are selected images from a contrast-enhanced CT scan of the neck with axial and sagittal reformats (Figures 4.1a, 4.1b). There is a well-defined low-density lesion with peripheral rim enhancement in the right upper neck immediately posterior to the submandibular gland and between the sternocleidomastoid muscle and carotid space. No enlarged lymph nodes are evident on the images available.

The differential considerations include a second branchial cleft cyst, a level 2a suppurative lymph node and a level 2a necrotic metastatic node. Although the location and age favours a branchial cleft cyst, the peripheral enhancement is unusual, unless infected. A necrotic metastatic lymph node remains in the differential. I would suggest urgent ENT referral, correlation with risk factors, inflammatory markers and fine needle aspiration (FNA) or biopsy for further evaluation.

Questions

1. **What are the different types of branchial cleft cysts (BCC) and their common location?**
   First BCC – periauricular or periparotid.
   Second BCC – posterior to submandibular gland, anteromedial to sternocleido-mastoid muscle and anterolateral or lateral to carotid space.
   Third BCC – posterior cervical space.
   Fourth BCC – as a sinus tract from the left pyriform sinus.
2. **What space is a common location for second branchial cysts to occur?**
   The submandibular space.
3. **What is the primary that most commonly causes necrotic nodal metastases?**
   Head and neck squamous cell carcinoma.

4. What is the other primary that should be considered for a cystic metastasis in this location?

Papillary thyroid carcinoma.

Key points
- Anomalies of the second branchial cleft can range from a fistula to a cyst.
- The second branchial cyst can occur anywhere along a second branchial fistula tract, from the pharyngeal wall of the palatine tonsil to the anteromedial aspect of the sternocleidomastoid muscle. They can also be found anywhere in the craniocaudal direction from the oropharynx down to the supraclavicular fossa.
- The second branchial cleft cyst represents about 95% of all branchial cleft cysts.
- Surgical excision is the treatment of choice for these lesions if they do not resolve. Recurrent swelling may be due to infection/inflammation. Picibanil sclerotherapy (OK432) has been used with great success and is offered as the treatment of choice in some centres.

Notes
This is a pathologically proven case of a branchial cleft cyst.

Further reading
Hudgins PA, Gillison M. Second branchial cleft cyst: not!! *AJNR Am J Neuroradiol* 2009; **30**: 1628–9.

Koeller KK, Alamo L, Adair CF, Smirniotopoulos JG. Congenital cystic masses of the neck: radiologic–pathologic correlation. *Radiographics* 1999; **19**: 121–46.

Neuroradiology Case 2

REKHA SIRIPURAPU

Clinical history

A 30-year-old man presents with worsening daily orthostatic headaches.

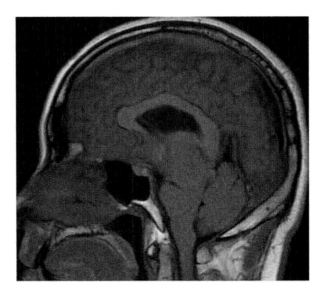

Figure 4.2a

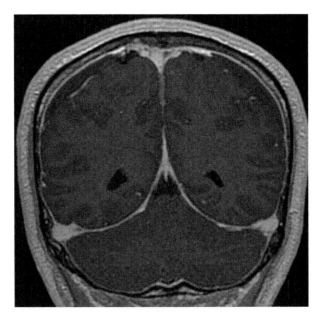

Figure 4.2b

Model answer

These are selected sagittal T1-weighted and post-contrast coronal T1-weighted MR images (Figures 4.2a, 4.2b). The sagittal image shows abnormal descent of the brainstem and corpus callosal splenium, flattening of the pons, effacement of suprasellar cistern with the chiasm draped over the sella, low-lying tonsils and prominent dural venous sinuses. The post-contrast coronal image shows bilateral subdural collections and diffuse smooth pachymeningeal thickening and enhancement.

The constellation of findings is consistent with intracranial hypotension. FLAIR and gradient echo would distinguish subdural hygromas from haematomas. Previous trauma or procedural history would be helpful to exclude secondary causes. I would like to arrange an MR spine or CT myelogram to look for evidence of CSF leak.

Questions

1. **What is the aetiology of intracranial hypotension (IH)?**
   IH is caused by leakage of CSF from the subarachnoid space. IH is either primary/spontaneous or secondary to iatrogenic manipulation and breaching of the dura, such as following a lumbar puncture or cranial/spinal surgery. Spontaneous IH is believed to occur due to a combination of weakness in the dural sac and trivial trauma. There is an association between spontaneous IH and a heterogeneous group of connective tissue disorders that includes Marfan's syndrome.
2. **What is the classic clinical hallmark?**
   Postural or orthostatic headache that is exacerbated by standing and relieved by lying.
3. **What is your management plan?**
   MR spine or CT myelography may be useful to identify a site of CSF leak. Epidural blood patch is performed as treatment.

Key points

- The opening CSF pressure is usually low, but can be normal or low-normal. This can occur if the leak is intermittent or when there are variable flow rates.
- The vast majority of spontaneous CSF leak occurs at the level of the thoracic spine.
- Brain MRI features include abnormal descent of the brainstem, flattening of the pons, compression of ventricles, effacement of suprasellar cistern with the chiasm draped over the sella, low-lying tonsils, pituitary engorgement, prominent dural venous sinuses, bilateral subdural collections and diffuse smooth pachymeningeal thickening and enhancement.
- Spinal MRI features of IH include spinal pachymeningeal enhancement and extradural fluid collections.

Further reading

Forghani R, Farb RI. Diagnosis and temporal evolution of signs of intracranial hypotension on MRI of the brain. *Neuroradiology* 2008; **50**: 1025–34.

Moyeri NN, Henson JW, Schaefer PW, Zervas NT. Spinal dural enhancement on magnetic resonance imaging associated with spontaneous intracranial hypotension. *J Neurosurg* 1998; **88**; 912–18.

Neuroradiology Case 3

REKHA SIRIPURAPU

Clinical history

A 50-year-old female presents with nausea and dizziness.

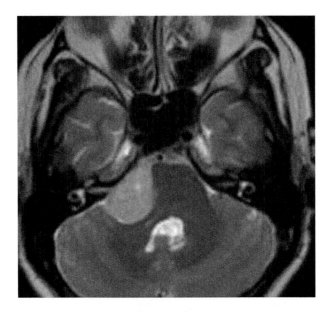

Figure 4.3a

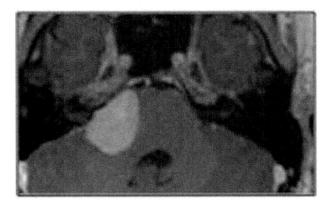

Figure 4.3b

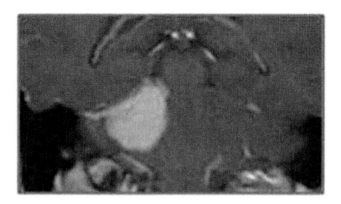

Figure 4.3c

Model answer

These are selected axial T2-weighted, axial T1-weighted post-contrast and coronal T1-weighted post-contrast images (Figures 4.3a–4.3c). There is a large right cerebello-pontine angle cistern mass that is neither associated with enlargement of nor extends into the internal auditory canal (IAC). It is slightly hyperintense to grey matter on the T2-weighted sequence and shows homogeneous enhancement with a dural tail. There is no enhancement in the IAC. There is significant mass effect on the fourth ventricle, with compression of the right middle cerebellar peduncle and intrinsic high T2-weighted signal change. Given the absence of IAC involvement and the presence of a dural tail, the appearances are most suggestive of a cerebellopontine angle meningioma. I will inform the clinician of the findings urgently, in view of the mass effect.

Questions

1. **Is a dural tail pathognomonic of meningioma?**
   No. The presence of a dural tail is a feature of meningioma and can be seen in up to 72% of cases but it is not pathognomonic of the condition. Other lesions such as dural metastases (breast, prostate) and granulomatous diseases (such as tuberculosis and sarcoidosis) may also show a dural tail.
2. **What are the most common locations for intracranial meningioma?**
   The most common locations in descending order are parasagittal dura, convexities, sphenoid wing, CP angle cistern, olfactory groove and the planum sphenoidale.
3. **What is the commonest location for a spinal meningioma?**
   In descending order of frequency: thoracic > cervical > lumbosacral.

Key points

- Meningiomas are more common in females than males.
- Meningiomas arise from the cap cells in the arachnoid layer.
- On CT, meningiomas are either iso- or hyperdense to brain parenchyma. The lesion may be associated with hyperostosis or bone destruction. Calcification is common in meningioma. The tumour typically shows homogeneous contrast enhancement.
- In adults, spinal meningiomas are the second most common spinal tumours.
- Previous exposure to therapeutic ionizing radiation is a risk factor for the development of meningiomas.

Further reading

Grossman RI, Yousem DM. *Neuroradiology: the Requisites*, 2nd edn. St Louis, MO: Mosby, 2003; 98–105.

Newton HB, Jolesz FA, eds. *Handbook of Neuro-oncology Neuroimaging*. New York, NY: Academic Press, 2008; 3–4, 13–14, 31.

Neuroradiology Case 4

REKHA SIRIPURAPU

Clinical history

A 32-year-old female presents with complex partial seizures.

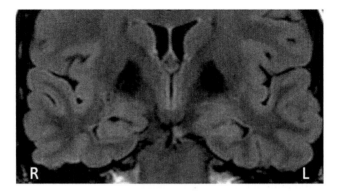

Figure 4.4

Model answer

Coronal FLAIR image of the temporal lobes (Figure 4.4) shows that the left hippocampus is slightly smaller than the right. There is subtle FLAIR high signal intensity within the left hippocampus with loss of internal architecture. The left temporal horn is slightly more prominent than the right. No cortical abnormality on the presented section.

The findings are consistent with left hippocampal sclerosis.

Questions

1. **List a few causes of temporal lobe epilepsy**.

   Mesial temporal sclerosis, cavernoma, cortical dysplasia, neoplasms such as astrocytoma, dysembyroplastic neuroepithelial tumours (DNET) and ganglioglioma.

2. **What is the imaging modality of choice for mesial temporal sclerosis, and what are the findings?**

   High-resolution (3D volume acquisition) T1- and T2-weighted MRI of the temporal lobes without contrast in the coronal and axial planes.

   Hyperintense T2/FLAIR signal and atrophy of the hippocampus with loss of internal architecture is the characteristic finding. Secondary signs include ipsilateral fornix and mamillary body atrophy and enlarged temporal horn.

   Other abnormalities include white matter atrophy in the parahippocampal gyrus and increased T2 signal in the anterior temporal white matter.

Key points

- Temporal lobe epilepsy is one of the commonest causes of medically refractory epilepsy. Mesial temporal sclerosis (MTS) is the most common abnormality found in temporal lobe epilepsy, and it is bilateral in 20% of cases.
- MTS was originally a pathological diagnosis, before the advent of MRI. Pathologically it consists of neuronal loss to a varying degree, macroscopic atrophy, gliosis and reorganization.
- HS can be bilateral (symmetrical or asymmetrical) or unilateral.
- This form of epilepsy has a good outcome with surgical treatment in 70–80% of patients.

Further reading

Grossman RI, Yousem DM. *Neuroradiology: the Requisites*, 2nd edn. St Louis, MO: Mosby, 2003; 447–9.

Osborn AG. *Diagnostic Imaging: Brain.* Salt Lake City, UT: Amirsys, 2004; I (10): 50–3.

Neuroradiology Case 5

REKHA SIRIPURAPU

Clinical history

A 64-year-old woman presents with headaches following trivial trauma.

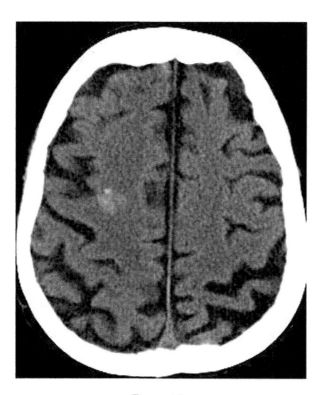

Figure 4.5a

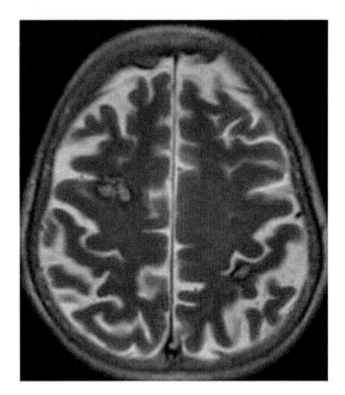

Figure 4.5b

Model answer

These are axial images from a non-contrast-enhanced CT brain scan and a T2-weighted MRI Scan (Figures 4.5a, 4.5b). On the CT scan, there is a hyperdense lesion in the posterior frontal lobe without mass effect or oedema. The hyperdensity could represent blood products or calcification.

The T2-weighted MR shows two well-defined lesions, one of which corresponds to the CT finding. Both show a central region of high T2-weighted signal surrounded by a hypointense rim.

I would like to correlate the findings with a gradient echo sequence to look for blooming. The findings are consistent with cavernous malformation (cavernous angioma).

Questions

1. **How do patients with cavernous malformation present?**

   Patients most commonly present with seizures and haemorrhage. Other presentations include progressive or transient neurological deficits, headaches, asymptomatic or an incidental finding.

2. **What are characteristic imaging findings?**

   Cavernoma, or cavernous angioma, or cavernous malformation, is of high density on non-contrast CT. The high density may represent blood, calcification or a combination of both. The lesion does not exert a mass effect. However, acute lesions can demonstrate adjacent oedema. Cavernomas are angiographically occult, and conventional catheter angiography has no role in diagnosis.

MR findings are characteristic. T1- and T2-weighted signal intensity is variable and depends on the type of blood products present. Subacute bleeds typically demonstrate high signals on T1- and T2-weighted scans. Cavernous angiomas typically have a low T2-weighted rim, representing haemosiderin. The gradient echo sequence may highlight other lesions that are not apparent on the T1- or T2-weighted sequences. They are commonly seen associated with a developmental venous anomaly (DVA).

Key points

- Equal sex distribution.
- Usual age at presentation second to fifth decade.
- Familial cavernomas are inherited in an autosomal dominant manner with incomplete penetrance.
- The typical imaging features of a cavernoma can be obscured by recent haemorrhage, and in these cases repeat follow-up imaging with MRI is advisable.
- Up to 54% of cases have multiple lesions, usually seen in familial cases and following radiotherapy.

Further reading

Grossman RI, Yousem DM. *Neuroradiology: the Requisites*, 2nd edn. St Louis, MO: Mosby, 2003; 231–4.

Porter PJ, Willinsky RA, Harper W, Wallace MC. Cerebral cavernous malformation: natural history and prognosis after clinical deterioration with or without haemorrhage. *J Neurosurg* 1997; **87**: 190–7.

Neuroradiology Case 6

REKHA SIRIPURAPU

Clinical history

A 65-year-old female presents acutely with altered consciousness. Report the CT first.

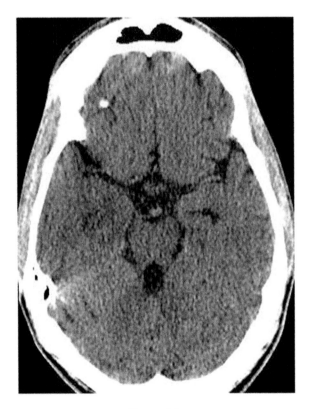

Figure 4.6a

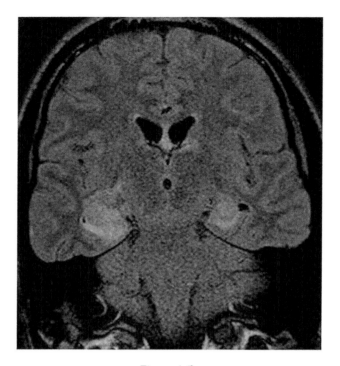

Figure 4.6b

Model answer

This is a single image from a non-contrast-enhanced axial CT of the brain (Figure 4.6a). There is a region of low density in the right medial temporal lobe with efface-ment of the right temporal horn. The differential diagnoses include encephalitis, neoplasm and ischaemia. If the patient is still in the CT scanner, I will ask for a con-trast-enhanced CT scan to look for focal enhancement. The patient will require an MRI for further characterization of the lesion. Other investigations that are required include an EEG and lumbar puncture.

This is a coronal FLAIR MR image of the brain (Figure 4.6b). This shows bilateral asymmetric high signal intensity in the mesial temporal lobes, more prominent on the right. High signal intensities are also seen in the fornices and left frontal cor-tex. The findings are highly suggestive of herpes simplex viral (HSV) encephalitis. I would call the referring clinician immediately to convey the findings.

Questions

1. **What is the imaging modality of choice and what are typical findings?**

   MR is the imaging modality of choice, as outcome depends on early diagnosis. Bilateral asymmetrical T2/FLAIR high signal intensity in the temporal lobes, infer-ior frontal lobes and cingulate region, with progressive mass effect with or with-out restricted diffusivity, is typical. Bilateral symmetrical and unilateral T2/FLAIR high signal in the temporal regions and in the insular cortex can also be seen.

   Gyriform enhancement may be visualized, but this varies with severity and stage of disease.

2. **Which structures in the temporal lobes does HSV have a predilection for?**

   The hippocampus and parahippocampal region.

3. **What is the pathogenesis of herpes encephalitis?**

   Commonly, the agent is HSV type 1 in adults and HSV type 2 in neonates. In adults, about one-third of infections are due to primary infection and the remain-der are due to reactivation.

Key points

- Encephalitis is inflammation of brain tissue. Severe encephalitis can cause cerebral oedema and intracranial haemorrhage.
- Viral encephalitis occurs either through dissemination in the bloodstream or from retrograde neuronal extension. HSV encephalitis is believed to be due to retrograde neuronal extension via cranial nerves I (olfactory) or V (trigeminal).
- The CT findings can be normal in HSV encephalitis, and a normal CT does not exclude the disease. The finding of typical HSV changes on CT is an indication of severe disease and represents a poor prognostic sign.
- Atrophy of the regions involved occurs in the chronic phase.

Further reading

Grossman RI, Yousem DM. *Neuroradiology: the Requisites*, 2nd edn. St Louis, MO: Mosby, 2003; 288–90.

Neuroradiology Case 7

REKHA SIRIPURAPU

Clinical history

Headaches and recurrent falls.

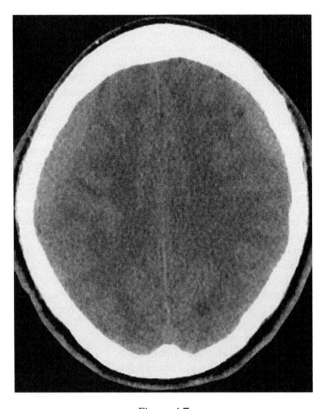

Figure 4.7

Model answer

This axial non-contrast CT image of the brain (Figure 4.7) shows bilateral displacement of the cortical surface and grey/white matter interface away from the calvarium, more prominent in the right frontal region. The findings are consistent with bilateral isodense subdural collections, right larger than left. There is mass effect, with effacement of cortical sulci. I would assess the remainder of the examination, in particular looking for brain herniation. I will inform the referring clinician urgently and suggest neurosurgical referral.

Questions

1. **Where does the fluid lie in a subdural collection?**
   The fluid accumulates between the dura and arachnoid space.
2. **Can an acute subdural be isodense?**
   Yes, isodense acute subdurals have been reported in patients with significant anaemia or disseminated intravascular coagulopathy. Tears in the arachnoid membrane can also lead to decreased density from CSF dilution.
3. **How do you define acute, sub-acute and chronic subdural collections?**
   The blood products can be:
   - up to three days old in the acute phase
   - between three days and three months old in the sub-acute phase
   - more than three months old in the chronic phase
4. **Which patient groups are at high risk for bilateral subdurals?**
   Elderly patients with recurrent falls, shunted hydrocephalus and intracranial hypotension.

Key points

- Subdural collections do not cross the midline.
- Subdurals can cross suture lines.
- Subdural blood can track along the tentorium. This is difficult to appreciate in the axial plane, but is better visualized in the coronal plane on CT.

Futher reading

Grossman RI, Yousem DM. *Neuroradiology: the Requisites*, 2nd edn. St Louis, MO: Mosby, 2003; 248–52.

Neuroradiology Case 8

REKHA SIRIPURAPU

Clinical history
An 18-year-old male presents with seizures.

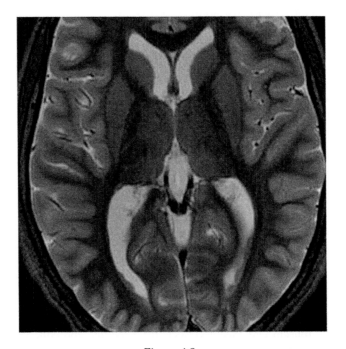

Figure 4.8a

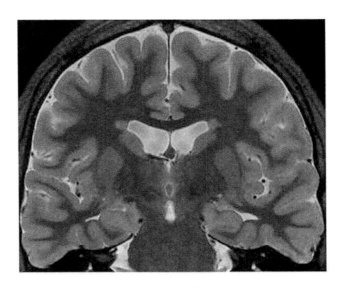

Figure 4.8b

Model answer

These are selected axial and coronal T2-weighted images of the brain at the level of the basal ganglia (Figures 4.8a, 4.8b). There are bilateral symmetric nodular subependymal lesions at the occipital horns and frontal horns superior to the caudate nuclei. These are isointense to the grey matter on the available sequence. I would like to confirm that these lesions have identical signal to grey matter on other sequences.

No other abnormality is seen. In particular, the mesial temporal lobes are unremarkable. The findings are consistent with subependymal grey matter heterotopia.

Questions

1. **What is the most common type of heterotopia?**
   The most common type of heterotopic grey matter is the subependymal nodular type. Subependymal heterotopia can be isolated or associated with other anomalies of the brain.
2. **What is the clinical presentation of isolated nodular heterotopia?**
   Patients with isolated nodular heterotopia typically have normal neurological examination and normal early development. They present with the onset of epilepsy, usually during the second decade of life.
3. **Is there a genetic predisposition?**
   Yes, some cases are X-linked or autosomal recessive.

Key points

- Heterotopia is normal grey matter in abnormal locations.
- Heterotopia is a migrational disorder.
- There are three groups: subependymal, focal subcortical and band heterotopia.
- There is no contrast enhancement of the heterotopia.
- Other malformations/abnormalities can be associated with grey matter heterotopias. Common entities include schizencephaly, corpus callosal abnormalities and Dandy–Walker malformation.

Further reading

Barkovich AJ. Morphologic characteristics of subcortical heterotopias: MR imaging study. *AJNR Am J Neuroradiol* 2000; **21**: 290–5.

Kornienko VN, Pronin IN. *Diagnostic Neuroradiology*. Berlin: Springer, 2009; 39, 49, 415, 585.

Neuroradiology Case 9

REKHA SIRIPURAPU

Clinical history

A 43-year-old female presents with headaches.

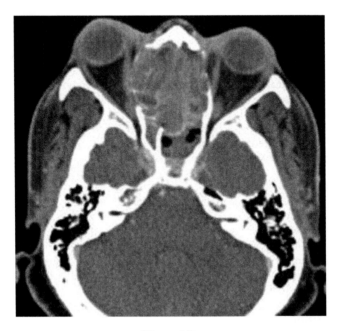

Figure 4.9a

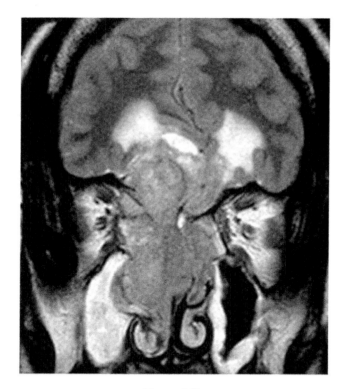

Figure 4.9b

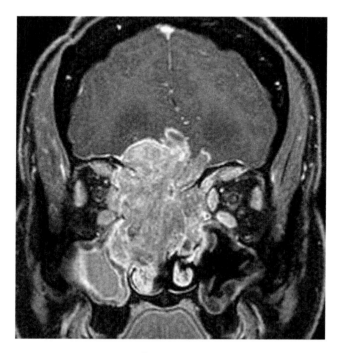

Figure 4.9c

Model answer

The contrast-enhanced axial CT of the head (Figure 4.9a) shows a large enhancing mass centred within the ethmoid sinuses and nasal cavity, extending into the right orbit. I am suspicious of encroachment of the lamina papyracea and would like to assess the bone windows in several planes for bony destruction.

Coronal T2-weighted and post-contrast coronal T1-weighted images (Figures 4.9b, 4.9c) show the mass extending beyond the orbital contours into the right orbit. There is a small amount of soft tissue in the left orbit. Superiorly, the mass can be seen extending into the anterior cranial fossa. There is bifrontal high signal on T2 and low signal on T1 adjacent to the mass, consistent with oedema at these sites. The anterior cerebral arteries are displaced to the left by this mass. A cyst at the tumour–brain interface is also seen. Inferiorly there is encroachment of the right maxillary infundibulum. The imaging appearances are consistent with an aggressive neoplasm. The differentials include esthesioneuroblastoma (olfactory neuroblastoma), squamous cell carcinoma, sinonasal neuroendocrine carcinoma (SNEC) and sinonasal undifferentiated carcinoma (SNUC). I am suspicious of encroachment of the lamina papyracea and would like to assess the bone windows in several planes for bony destruction. The patient will require a staging CT to look for evidence of distant metastasis.

Questions

1. What is an olfactory neuroblastoma?

It is a rare malignant neoplasm of neuroectodermal origin that arises from the olfactory epithelium in the cribriform region, the upper third of nasal septum and along the superior and supreme nasal turbinates. The incidence is bimodal, with a peak at 11–20 years and a second peak at 50–60 years. CT and MR show a homogeneous mass with moderate to marked enhancement. These tumours are of intermediate signal intensity on T1-weighted imaging and intermediate to high signal intensity on T2-weighted imaging. The presence of peritumoral cysts capping the intracranial portion of the tumour strongly suggests a diagnosis of olfactory neuroblastoma. Undifferentiated sinonasal carcinoma is a differential on imaging.

2. What is a sinonasal undifferentiated carcinoma?

This is a rare, aggressive tumour composed of sheets of undifferentiated cells. These tumours are distinguished from the more well-differentiated olfactory neuroblastoma by the lack of a neurofibrillary background on light microscopy. They are often advanced at presentation, with a propensity for early metastatic disease. SNUC occurs in the same anatomical location as olfactory neuroblastoma and would be hard to differentiate on imaging.

On MRI, they are large lesions that are isointense to skeletal muscle on T1-weighted imaging, and isointense to intermediate signal on T2-weighted imaging. They enhance heterogeneously with gadolinium.

Key points

- Esthesioneuroblastoma is the former name for olfactory neuroblastoma.
- Metastases can occur in approximately one-third of patients.
- Radiologically it is important to try and assess invasion of tumour into the brain parenchyma or if the tumour has remained extra-axial when the lesion has breached the anterior cranial fossa. This alters surgical management significantly.

Further reading

Mafee MF, Valvassori GE, Becker M. Sinonasal pathology. In *Imaging of the Head and Neck*, 2nd edn. Stuttgart: Thieme, 2005; 434–6.

Raghavan P, Phillips DC. Magnetic resonance imaging of sinonasal malignancies. *Top Magn Reson Imaging* 2007; **18**: 259–67.

Som PM, Curtin HD. *Head and Neck Imaging*, 4th edn. St Louis, MO: Mosby, 2002; 285–90.

Neuroradiology Case 10

REKHA SIRIPURAPU

Clinical history
A 48-year-old female presents with headaches.

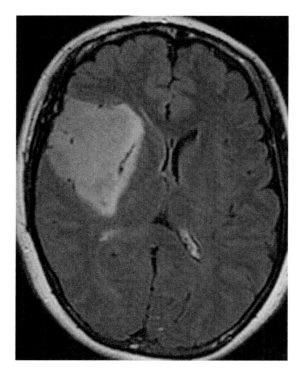

Figure 4.10a

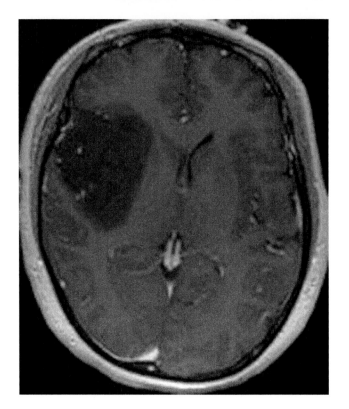

Figure 4.10b

Model answer

These are selected axial MRI brain images at the level of the basal ganglia (Figures 4.10a, 4.10b). The axial FLAIR sequence shows a wedge-shaped area of increased signal intensity in the right MCA territory. The lesion does not enhance with intravenous contrast. There are enhancing vessels in the periphery of the mass. There is mass effect with compression of the right lateral ventricle and midline shift. The differential diagnoses include a low-grade primary neoplasm and an acute infarct. Diffusion-weighted imaging (DWI) would help differentiate between the two diagnoses. An acute infarct would demonstrate restricted diffusivity, and I would correlate with clinical history as to the timing of events.

Given the clinical symptoms of headaches and no suggestion of an acute presentation, a low-grade primary neoplasm is favoured.

Questions

1. **What further imaging might help distinguish tumour from infarct?**
   Follow-up imaging will not show the expected temporal evolution of an infarct. MR perfusion and spectroscopy may be useful.
2. **What features on MR are associated with higher-grade gliomas?**
   - Irregular margins with heterogeneous enhancement.
   - Necrosis – areas of low T1 and high T2 signal without enchancement.
   - Acute haemorrhage.
   - Calcification is rare in glioblastoma multiforme (GBM).
3. **What is the peak incidence of gliomas?**
   Fifth to sixth decades.

4. **Is there a gender predilection?**
   Gliomas are more common in men than women, with a ratio of approximately 1.5 male to 1 female.

Key points
- Gliomas are the most common primary brain tumours in adults.
- In adults, gliomas occur predominantly in the supratentorial regions.
- In children, gliomas occur predominantly in the infratentorial regions.
- Low-grade gliomas include astrocytomas, oligodendrogliomas and mixed oligoastrocytomas.
- Low-grade gliomas on MR usually demonstrate low T1-weighted signal and high T2/FLAIR signal, and they do not enhance with intravenous contrast.

Notes
In this case the diagnosis was a low-grade glioma.

Further reading
Grossman RI, Yousem DM. *Neuroradiology: the Requisites*, 2nd edn. St Louis, MO: Mosby, 2003; 128–30.

Neuroradiology Case 11

REKHA SIRIPURAPU

Clinical history
A 48-year-old woman presents with visual problems.

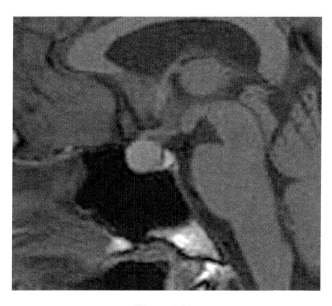

Figure 4.11a

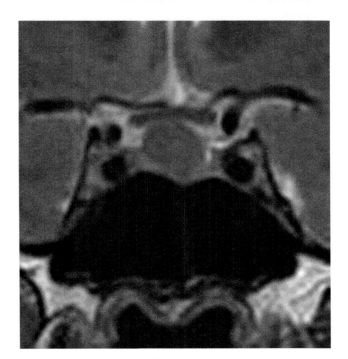

Figure 4.11b

Model answer

These are sagittal T1-weighted and coronal T2-weighted images of the sella (Figures 4.11a, 4.11b). There is a sellar mass extending into the suprasellar cistern. This lesion cannot be separated from the pituitary gland. The mass is of high signal intensity on T1-weighted sequence and isointense to grey matter on T2-weighted sequence. The mass extends into the suprasellar cistern and compresses the optic chiasm. The posterior pituitary bright spot and visualized portions of cavernous sinuses and intracavernous segment of the internal carotid arteries appear unremarkable. Given the high T1-weighted signal intensity, the differential considerations are Rathke's cleft cyst, haemorrhagic macroadenoma, and less likely a craniopharyngioma. I would like to perform a dynamic contrast-enhanced MRI of the pituitary gland to further characterize the lesion.

Questions

1. **What are the imaging features of Rathke's cleft cyst?**

   Typical Rathke's cleft cysts appear as non-enhancing well-demarcated intrasellar lesions between the anterior and posterior pituitary lobes.

   The cysts can have a homogeneously hyperintense T1-weighted signal due to high protein concentration, and a hypointense T2-weighted signal. The T1-weighted signal can be variable, ranging from hypointense to hyperintense depending on the biochemical content, especially the protein concentration. Usually the cysts are similar signal to CSF on MRI.

2. **What feature would help distinguish Rathke's cleft cyst from haemorrhagic adenoma?**

   A fluid–fluid level within the lesion is extremely useful to differentiate an adenoma from a Rathke's cleft cyst. In the latter condition, haemorrhage and consequent fluid–fluid level have not been described.

3. How can patients present?

Visual abnormalities (optic chiasm compression), diabetes insipidus, headaches and hormonal dysfunction.

Key points

- Rathke's cleft cysts are derived from Rathke's pouch.
- Craniopharyngiomas have solid and cystic components with calcification. The lack of calcification and solid components will help distinguish Rathke's cleft cyst from craniopharyngiomas.
- Craniopharyngiomas are WHO grade 1, and two histologic subtypes have been recognized: adamantinomatous and papillary.
- Surgery is the treatment of choice for symptomatic Rathke's cleft cyst lesions.

Further reading

Bonneville F, Cattin F, Marsot-Dupuch K, *et al.* T1 signal hyperintensity in the sellar region: spectrum of findings. *Radiographics* 2006; **26**: 93–113.

Neuroradiology Case 12

REKHA SIRIPURAPU

Clinical history

A 23-year-old female presents with chronic fatigue.

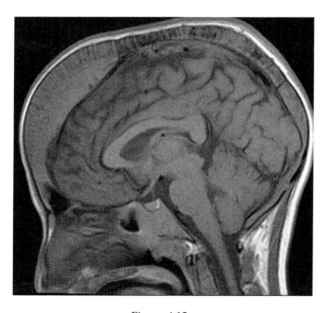

Figure 4.12a

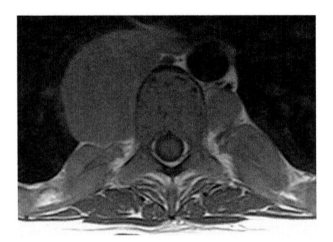

Figure 4.12b

Model answer

The sagittal T1-weighted image of the brain (Figure 4.12a) shows a widened diploic space, most prominent in the frontal bone, with a large extradural soft tissue mass displacing the frontal lobe. There is 'hair on end' appearance of diploic trabeculae.

Abnormal soft tissue is seen in the sphenoid sinus. The visualized brain parenchyma is unremarkable.

The axial T1-weighted image of the spine at the thoracic level (Figure 4.12b) shows multiple large paraspinal and rib masses. There is abnormal low signal intensity of the marrow of the vertebral body with subtle anterior epidural soft tissue. These findings are suggestive of extramedullary haematopoiesis and consistent with thalassaemia. Haemoglobin protein electrophoresis should confirm the diagnosis. Liver and cardiac T2* imaging can be performed to quantify iron deposition in these organs.

Questions
1. **What is thalassaemia?**
   Thalassaemia is a hereditary anaemia resulting from mutations that affect the synthesis of the globin chains in haemoglobin. It is typically seen in Mediterranean countries. Alpha- and beta-thalassaemias are so called because of defects in their respective globin chains.
2. **What are the radiographic features of thalassaemia?**
   The radiographic features of thalassaemia are mostly due to marrow hyperplasia. Markedly expanded marrow space leads to various skeletal manifestations predominantly affecting the spine, skull, facial bones and ribs. Posterior paravertebral, mediastinal, or presacral masses represent sites of extramedullary haematopoiesis. Epidural extension of soft tissue may also be seen in thalassaemia patients and may cause cord compression.
3. **What are the causes of low T1 marrow signal intensity in a patient with thalassaemia?**
   - Marrow hyperplasia secondary to chronic anaemia.
   - Iron deposition from repeated transfusions without proper chelation.
   - Increased iron deposition can occur even in untransfused patients with thalassaemia intermedia due to increased gastric iron absorption.
4. **What are the non-skeletal manifestations of thalassaemia?**
   Splenomegaly, gallstones and haemosiderosis (liver and pancreas).

Key points

- Adult haemoglobin is a tetramer made up of two alpha and two beta chains. Defective production of one type of chain results in accumulation of the other. This results in ineffective erythropoiesis and reduced erythrocyte lifespan.
- The accumulation of excess haemoglobin chains leads to abnormalities in the erythrocyte cell membrane, resulting in increased red cell destruction by the reticuloendothelial system (particularly the spleen). This, combined with the poor oxygen-carrying capacity of the individual erythrocytes and ineffective erythropoiesis, results in tissue hypoxia. As a result erythropoietin is released by the kidney to compensate, resulting in bone marrow expansion.
- The main cause of death in chronically transfused thalassaemia patients is from cardiac iron overload.
- T2*-weighted imaging is used to quantify liver and cardiac iron deposition. This imaging modality is therefore useful in prognostication and can influence management.

Further reading

Chan YL, Tse HY. Imaging in thalassemia. *J HK Coll Radiol* 2002; **5**: 155–61.

Tunaci M, Tunaci A, Engin G, *et al.* Imaging features of thalassemia. *Eur Radiol* 1999; **9**: 1804–9.

Neuroradiology Case 13

REKHA SIRIPURAPU

Clinical history
A 19-year-old female presents with abnormal behaviour followed by decrease in consciousness.

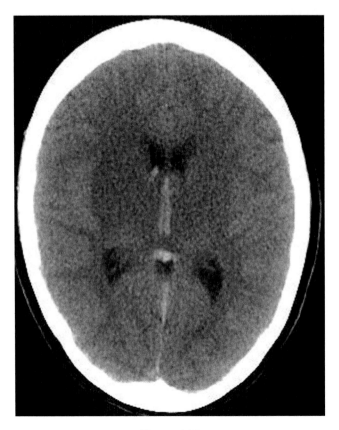

Figure 4.13

Model answer
This is a single image of a non-contrast CT brain at the level of the basal ganglia (Figure 4.13). It shows abnormal low density involving the basal ganglia and thalami with loss of the grey–white matter differentiation. The internal cerebral veins and possibly the straight sinus appear abnormally dense. The findings are highly suspicious for deep venous thrombosis. I will proceed with a CT venogram to confirm and assess the full extent of suspected cerebral venous thrombosis. MR and contrast-enhanced MR venogram is also another option. This is a neurological emergency, and I would call the referring physician to convey the findings.

Questions

1. **What constitutes the cerebral deep venous system? What are the draining territories?**

   The deep cerebral venous system includes the vein of Galen, the internal cerebral veins, and their tributaries; the Rosenthal vein (basal vein) and its tributaries; the medullary and subependymal veins, which drain the hemispheric white matter. The deep system drains the inferior frontal lobe; most of the deep white matter of the frontal, temporal and parietal lobes; the corpus callosum; the upper brainstem; the basal ganglia; and the thalamus.

2. **What are the different non-invasive modalities for assessing the cerebral venous system?**

   - CT venography. Fast, readily available, accurate and good spatial resolution. Use of ionizing radiation in CT venography has limited use in pregnant patients and children. Contrast allergy and renal impairment are other contraindications.
   - Time of flight (TOF) MR venography. Can be used in pregnant patients, and provides better assessment of brain parenchymal changes with additional cross-sectional MR imaging. MRV is limited by flow-related artefacts, equivocal findings and contraindications in patients with pacemakers and ferromagnetic devices.
   - Phase-contrast MR venography. Advantages and disadvantages are similar to those of TOF.
   - Contrast-enhanced MR venography. This is the most accurate of the MR techniques. It allows better depiction of dural sinuses and small veins, and has fewer flow-related artefacts. Its disadvantages are contraindication to gadolinium in renal impairment and contrast allergy.

Key points

- Venous thrombosis and infarcts should be borne in mind when patients present with infarcts in atypical locations that do not conform to arterial territories and intraparenchymal haemorrhage.
- Cerebral venous thrombosis is one of the possible causes of multiple intraparenchymal haemorrhages.
- Venous thrombosis accounts for 1% of strokes.
- Thrombectomy may be used in patients who deteriorate despite adequate anticoagulant treatment.

Further reading

Leach JL, Fortuna RB, Jones BV, Gaskill-Shipley MF. Imaging of cerebral venous thrombosis: current techniques, spectrum of findings, and diagnostic pitfalls. *Radiographics* 2006; **26**: S19–43.

Rodallec MH, Krainik A, Feydy A, *et al*. Cerebral venous thrombosis and multidetector CT angiography: tips and tricks. *Radiographics* 2006; **26**: S5–18.

Neuroradiology Case 14

REKHA SIRIPURAPU

Clinical history
A 21-year-old male presents with seizures.

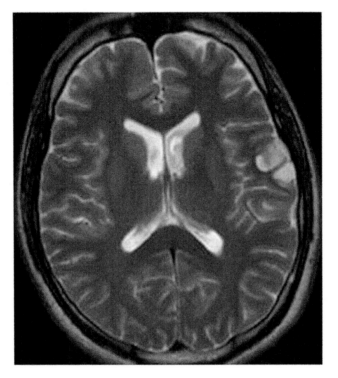

Figure 4.14a

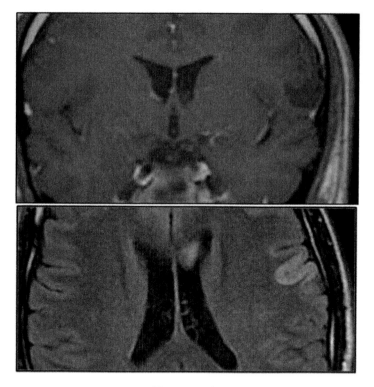

Figure 4.14b

Model answer

The image from an axial T2-weighted MRI scan (Figure 4.14a) shows a well-defined wedge-shaped peripheral/cortical-based left inferior frontal lesion. This lesion shows a high signal intensity that is similar to CSF and is associated with subtle scalloping/remodelling of the inner table of the skull. The contrast-enhanced coronal T1-weighted image (Figure 4.14b, top) shows no enhancement. No surrounding oedema.

The axial FLAIR image at a higher level (Figure 4.14b, bottom) shows abnormal cortical high signal intensity. The constellation of appearances and correlation with the seizure symptoms in a young patient are highly suggestive of a low-grade neoplasm such as dysembryoplastic neuroepithelial tumour (DNET). Other considerations such as ganglioglioma and neuroepithelial cyst are considered less likely.

Questions
1. **What are the most common sites for DNET?**
   Temporal (50–62%) and frontal (31%) are the most common.
2. **What does scalloping of inner table imply?**
   A very slow-growing process.
3. **Is there a gender predilection?**
   There is a male predominance.
4. **Name an important association.**
   Focal cortical dysplasias have been reported in over 50% of cases.

Key points

- DNETs are mainly seen in the paediatric population, associated with intractable seizures.
- They are generally benign lesions, although rare cases of malignant transformation have been reported in the literature.
- Calcification can be seen in 20% of cases.

Further reading

Fernandez C, Girard N, Paredes AP, *et al.* The usefulness of MR imaging in the diagnosis of dysembryoplastic neuroepithelial tumour in children: a study of 14 cases. *AJNR Am J Neuroradiol* 2003; **24**: 829–34.

Grossman RI, Yousem DM. *Neuroradiology: the Requisites*, 2nd edn. St Louis, MO: Mosby, 2003; 139.

Neuroradiology Case 15

REKHA SIRIPURAPU

Clinical history

A 79-year-old man presents with memory problems.

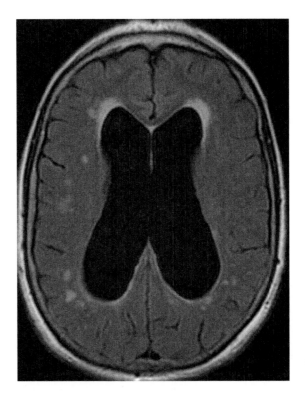

Figure 4.15a

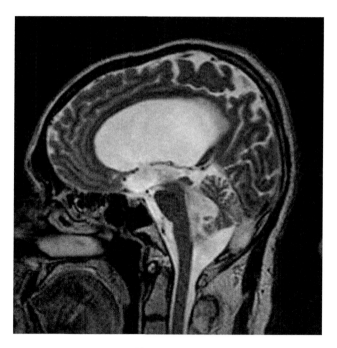

Figure 4.15b

Model answer

The axial FLAIR sequence (Figure 4.15a) shows disproportionate and marked enlargement of the lateral ventricles with prominent bifrontal periventricular high signal intensity suggestive of transependymal CSF oedema. There are also multiple foci of high signal within the deep white matter. The cortical sulci are compressed. The T2-weighted sagittal sequence (Figure 4.15b) demonstrates corpus callosal thinning.

I will assess the other ventricles, look for an aqueductal flow void and exclude an obstructive cause. In the absence of an obstructive lesion, and with an appropriate clinical scenario of gait apraxia, urinary incontinence and dementia, the appearances are suggestive of normal pressure hydrocephalus (NPH). .

Questions

1. What are the imaging findings in idiopathic NPH?

The classic radiological feature is ventricular enlargement, which is out of proportion to either normal-appearing or compressed sulci at the vertex. There should be no macroscopic obstruction to CSF flow.

Other features include enlargement of the temporal horns of the lateral ventricles not entirely attributable to hippocampus atrophy, sparing of the parahippocampal fissure, thinned corpus callosum and an aqueductal or fourth ventricular flow void on MRI.

Other supportive brain imaging findings include:

- Radionuclide cisternogram showing delayed clearance of radiotracer over the cerebral convexities after 48–72 hours. However, this is not specific for NPH.
- SPECT-acetazolamide challenge showing decreased periventricular perfusion that is not altered by acetazolamide.

2. What are the causes of secondary NPH?

Secondary NPH can be due to subarachnoid haemorrhage, meningitis, prior surgery and previous traumatic brain injury.

Key points
- NPH is difficult to diagnose. The diagnosis of idiopathic NPH is made using a combination of clinical, imaging and physiological criteria.
- Treatment is surgical. Ventricular shunting may improve symptoms.
- MRI is the imaging modality of choice.

Further reading
Grossman RI, Yousem DM. *Neuroradiology: the Requisites*, 2nd edn. St Louis, MO: Mosby, 2003; 375–7.
Relkin N, Marmarou A, Klinge P, Bergsneider M, Black PM. Diagnosing idiopathic normal pressure hydrocephalus. *Neurosurgery* 2005; **57**: S4–16.

Neuroradiology Case 16

REKHA SIRIPURAPU

Clinical history
A 59-year-old male presents with right-sided neck mass and otalgia.

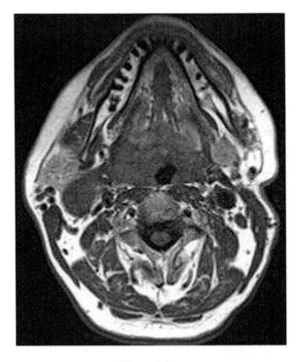

Figure 4.16a

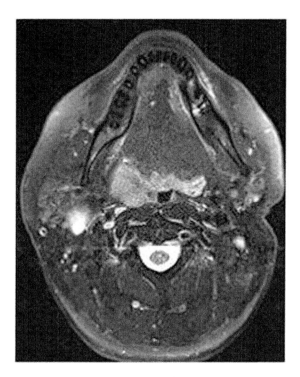

Figure 4.16b

Model answer

Non-contrast axial T1-weighted and fat-suppressed T2-weighted images at the level of the mandible (Figures 4.16a, 4.16b) show an abnormal isointense T1-weighted and hyperintense T2-weighted soft tissue mass centred in the right lateral oropharyngeal wall and palatine tonsil. Anteriorly, the mass extends to the right tongue base. Posteriorly, a fat plane is visualized with the longus colli muscle and carotid sheath. Medially, there is mass effect on the oropharyngeal airway. There is also increased signal on T2-weighted fat-suppressed images across the entire tongue base, which may be part of the same process. However, lingual tonsillar hypertrophy could have a similar appearance. An enlarged right neck-level 2A node is demonstrated. The lesion does not extend to the lingual cortex of the mandible, and the marrow signal is preserved.

The imaging findings are consistent with an oropharyngeal malignancy. The differentials include squamous cell carcinoma, minor salivary gland tumour and lymphoma. I would like to assess the rest of the MRI to assess the extent of disease. In addition, the patient will require a staging CT scan of the head, neck, chest and abdomen for assessment of both local and distant disease.

Questions

1. **What is the most common source of occult primary tumours that present as cervical lymphadenopathy alone?**
   Tonsillar carcinoma.
2. **Why is tumour size important in oropharyngeal malignancies?**
   Staging is based on size criteria.
3. **What is the cause of secondary otalgia in this patient?**
   Referred pain due to tumour involvement of structures (oropharynx in this case) that are innervated by the glossopharyngeal nerve.

Key points

- The differential diagnosis of secondary otalgia (referred otalgic pain) is wide. Other non-neoplastic causes include TMJ disorders, Eustachian tube dysfunction, Eagle's syndrome and neuralgia (cause unknown).
- Tonsillar carcinomas are often poorly differentiated and present with lymph node metastases.
- Small lesions are difficult to diagnose on cross-sectional imaging, as normal tonsils can be asymmetric.
- Local spread of tonsillar carcinoma includes base of tongue, soft palate and lateral pharyngeal wall.

Further reading

Grossman RI, Yousem DM. *Neuroradiology: the Requisites*, 2nd edn. St Louis, MO: Mosby, 2003; 653–9.

Neuroradiology Case 17

REKHA SIRIPURAPU

Clinical history

A 24-year-old woman is not rousable after a renal transplant.

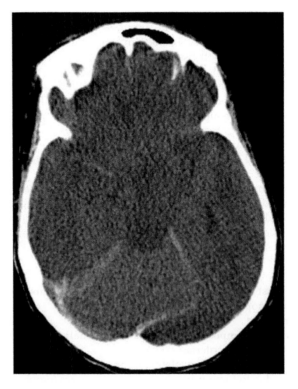

Figure 4.17a

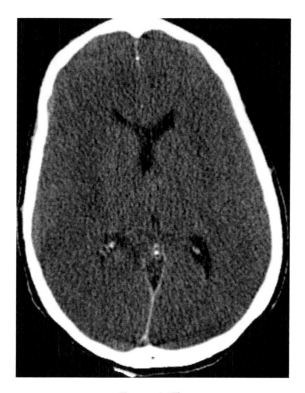

Figure 4.17b

Model answer

Non-contrast CT sections of the brain (Figures 4.17a, 4.17b) show sulcal effacement as well as high density in the tentorium bilaterally and the falx. There is diffuse abnormal low density of the supratentorial brain parenchyma with loss of grey–white differentiation and effacement of the basal cisterns. The cerebellum appears relatively hyperdense. I would like to discuss the case with the clinicians to determine if there were any hypotensive episodes during surgery or cardiopulmonary resuscitation. This 'pseudosubarachnoid' appearance is strongly suggestive of diffuse hypoxic encephalopathy and is a marker of poor prognosis.

Questions

1. **What is the pseudosubarachnoid sign?**
   A pseudosubarachnoid sign refers to brain CT findings of high-density areas along the basal cisterns, the Sylvian vallecula/fissure, the tentorium cerebelli or the cortical sulci in patients with severe brain oedema, though no SAH is seen at autopsy or lumbar puncture.

2. **What is the pathophysiology?**
   The mechanism for the development of a pseudosubarachnoid sign has not been elucidated fully. A few hypotheses have been put forward. Severe brain oedema may compress the dural sinuses, compromising the venous drainage from the brain and resulting in engorgement of the superficial veins, which stand out against the oedematous low-attenuated brain parenchyma, mimicking an SAH. Narrowing or disappearance of hypoattenuated CSF space due to oedematous brain may also be a contributing factor.

Key points

- Hypoxic–ischaemic encephalopathy is a rare entity.

• It is a very difficult diagnosis to make, but radiologists should be aware of this entity.

Further reading

Given CA, Burdette JH, Elster AD, Williams DW. Psuedo-subarachnoid haemorrhage: a potential imaging pitfall associated with diffuse cerebral oedema. *AJNR Am J Neuroradiol* 2003; **24**: 254–6.

Gutierrez LG, Rovira A, Portela LA, Leite C da C, Lucato LT. CT and MR in non-neonatal hypoxic–ischemic encephalopathy: radiological findings with pathophysiological correlations. *Neuroradiology* 2010; **52**: 949–76.

Neuroradiology Case 18

REKHA SIRIPURAPU

Clinical history
A 39-year-old female presents with left facial numbness.

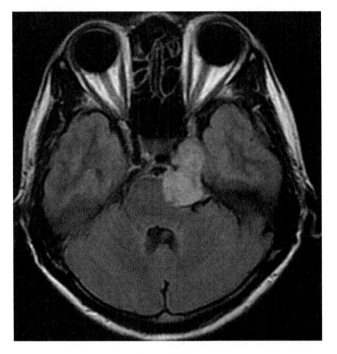

Figure 4.18a

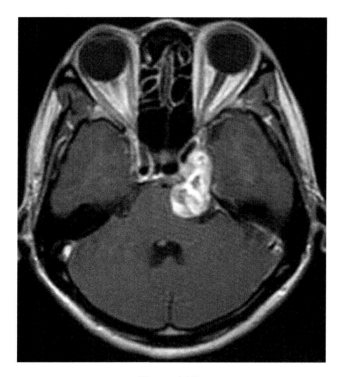

Figure 4.18b

Model answer

Axial FLAIR and contrast-enhanced axial T1-weighted sections (Figures 4.18a, 4.18b) show a well-defined extra-axial mass extending from the prepontine cistern, through Meckel's cave and into the cavernous sinus on the left. The mass demonstrates heterogeneous enhancement. There is mass effect and indentation of the left pons without intrinsic high signal intensity on FLAIR. Within the left cavernous sinus, the mass partially surrounds and displaces the left internal carotid artery (ICA). The ICA calibre is not reduced. No other extra-axial mass is demonstrated. The most likely diagnosis is trigeminal schwannoma. Perineural spread of tumour along the trigeminal nerve by, for example, an adenoid cystic carcinoma and meningioma are both differential diagnoses but considered less likely. I would like to review the rest of the imaging to delineate the extent of the tumour and exclude perineural spread of tumour, as well as to detect coexisting tumours. The latter is important, because schwannomas can be part of the neurofibromatosis 2 syndrome.

Questions

1. **What are the sites of origin of trigeminal schwannomas?**

   Trigeminal schwannomas can arise anywhere along the pathway from the pons to Meckel's cave to the cavernous sinus, and in the skull base foramina, i.e. superior orbital fissure (V1), rotundum (V2) and ovale (V3).

2. **What are the MR imaging characteristics?**

   These lesions are isointense to pons on T1-weighted images, hypointense or isointense (more cellular) or hyperintense (less cellular) on T2-weighted images, and nearly always enhance. Homogeneous enhancement is seen in around 70% of cases. Less common features of schwannoma include calcification, cystic change and haemorrhage.

3. **What is neurofibromatosis 2?**

An autosomal dominant disorder where the patient develops multiple schwannomas, meningiomas and ependymomas (acronym: MISME).

Key points

- Schwannomas arise from Schwann cells (Schwann cells are glial cells of the peripheral nervous system), and differ pathologically from neuromas/neurofibromas.
- Schwannomas are usually benign tumours, and malignant schwannomas of the trigeminal nerves are rare.
- Trigeminal tumours usually present clinically with 'burning' facial pain. Dysfunction of the muscles of mastication may be a late feature as the tumour enlarges.
- If there is extension of tumour into the cavernous sinus, cranial nerves III, IV and VI would likely be compressed.
- In cases where there is concern for perineural spread of tumour, and the clinical signs point to the trigeminal nerve, the divisions of the trigeminal nerve should be assessed and closely interrogated.

Further reading

Grossman RI, Yousem DM. *Neuroradiology: the Requisites*, 2nd edn. St Louis, MO: Mosby, 2003; 105–8.

Stone JA, Cooper H, Castillo M, Mukherji SK. Malignant schwannoma of the trigeminal nerve. *AJNR Am J Neuroradiol* 2001; **22**: 505–7.

Wippold FJ, Lubner M, Perrin RJ, Lämmle M, Perry A. Neuropathology for the neuroradiologist: Antoni A and Antoni B tissue patterns. *AJNR Am J Neuroradiol* 2007; **28**: 1633–8.

Neuroradiology Case 19

Clinical history
A 58-year-old male presents with right neck swelling.

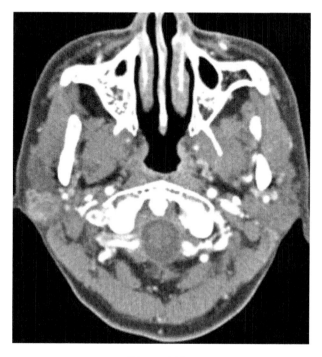

Figure 4.19a

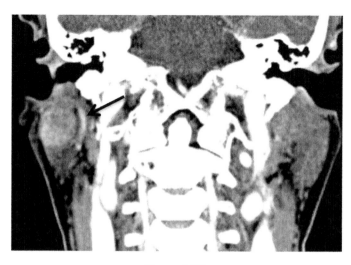

Figure 4.19b

Model answer

These are selected images from a contrast-enhanced neck CT with axial and coronal reformats, on soft tissue windows (Figures 4.19a, 4.19b). A heterogeneously enhancing well-defined solid mass is seen within the superficial lobe of the right parotid gland. The retromandibular vein (black arrow) is separate from the mass. The rest of the right and the left parotid gland are unremarkable. No enlarged lymph nodes are present. The appearances are suggestive of a neoplasm, and the differentials include benign lesions (such as pleomorphic adenoma) and malignant neoplasms (such as mucoepidermoid carcinoma and adenoid cystic carcinoma). I would like to review the rest of the imaging to detect features of malignancy such as lymph node enlargement and invasion of adjacent structures. The patient should have ultrasound-guided fine needle aspiration of the lesion.

Questions

1. **What imaging characteristics distinguish benign from malignant parotid neoplasms?**

   In benign tumours the edges are described as discrete, whereas in malignant neoplasms they are indistinct, fading into the surrounding gland. Invasion of adjacent structures and nodal seeding are indicators of malignancy. In reality, it is difficult to distinguish between a benign lesion and a low-grade malignancy in a well-defined small parotid mass. FNA or excision is required for diagnosis. Imaging is useful for localization and pre-surgical planning, as this can affect the surgical approach.

2. **How do you locate the intraparotid facial nerve on CT?**

   The facial nerve plane is extrapolated as a line connecting the stylomastoid foramen to a point just lateral to the retromandibular vein.

Key points

- 70–80% of salivary gland tumours occur in the parotid gland.
- Adenoid cystic carcinoma is the second most common malignant salivary gland tumour.
- Affects women > men.
- Adenoid cystic carcinoma has a predilection for perineural spread.
- Histologic subtypes:
  - commonest – cribriform pattern
  - best prognosis – tubular
  - worst prognosis – solid
- Facial nerve paralysis is associated with poor prognosis.

Notes

This well-defined lesion was shown on pathology to be an adenoid cystic carcinoma.

Further reading

Harnsberger RH. *Handbook of Head and Neck Imaging*, 2nd edn. St Louis, MO: Mosby, 1995; 60–74.

Witt RL. Major salivary gland cancer. *Surg Oncol Clin N Am* 2004; **13**: 113–27.

Neuroradiology Case 20

REKHA SIRIPURAPU

Clinical history
A 17-year-old male presents with deafness.

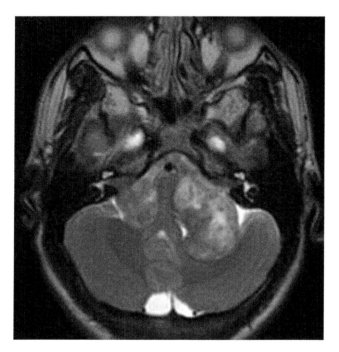

Figure 4.20a

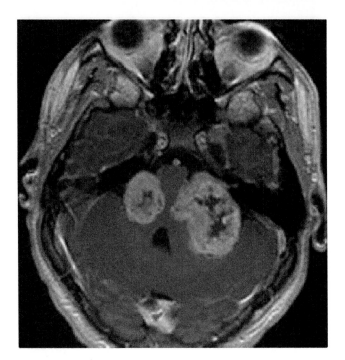

Figure 4.20b

Model answer

Axial T2-weighted and contrast-enhanced T1-weighted images at the level of the internal auditory canal (IAC) (Figures 4.20a, 4.20b) show large bilateral IAC masses extending into the cerebellopontine angle cisterns. On the right, the mass is isointense on the T2-weighted sequence and shows slightly heterogeneous contrast enhancement. On the left, the mass shows higher signal intensity on the T2-weighted sequence and heterogeneous enhancement. There is severe compression of the brainstem, with intrinsic high T2-weighted signal intensity. The post-contrast section also shows a possible enhancing nodule at the anterior aspect of Meckel's cave on the left. The appearances are suggestive of bilateral vestibular schwannomas and a possible left trigeminal schwannoma, consistent with neurofibromatosis type 2 (NF2). Given the degree of brainstem compression, I will call the referring clinician to inform him/her of the findings.

Questions

1. **What is the radiological hallmark of NF2?**
   Bilateral vestibular schwannomas.
2. **What are the other neoplasms seen in NF2?**
   Meningioma, gliomas and intramedullary ependymomas. These tumours can occur at a younger age and are commonly multiple.
3. **What other cranial nerves can be involved?**
   Schwannomas can develop in cranial nerves III to XII but are most commonly seen in CN VIII. Hypoglossal nerve schwannoma is a very rare cause of hypoglossal palsy.
4. **What is the inheritance pattern for NF2?**
   Autosomal dominant with full penetrance.

Key points

- NF2 is a less common disorder than NF1.

- Mnemonic for NF2 is MISME: Multiple Inherited Schwannomas, Meningiomas, Ependymomas.
- NF2 is diagnosed clinically. Diagnostic criteria (modified from Evans DG. Neurofibromatosis 2. *Genet Med* 2009; **11**: 599–610):
  1. bilateral vestibular schwannomas; *or*
  2. a first-degree relative with NF2 *and* either unilateral vestibular schwannoma or any two of the following: meningioma, schwannoma, glioma, neurofibroma, cataract (posterior sublenticular opacity); *or*
  3. unilateral vestibular schwannoma *and* any two of meningioma, schwannoma, glioma, neurofibroma, cataract; *or*
  4. multiple meningiomas *and* either unilateral schwannoma or any two of schwannoma, glioma, neurofibroma, juvenile cataract.

Further reading

DeAngelis LM. Brain tumors. *N Eng J Med* 2001; **344**: 114–23.

Ferner RE. Neurofibromatosis 1 and neurofibromatosis 2: a twenty first century perspective. *Lancet Neurol* 2007; **6**: 340–51.

Rodriguez D, Poussaint TY. Neuroimaging findings in neurofibromatosis type 1 and 2. *Neuroimaging Clin N Am* 2004; **14**: 149–70.

Neuroradiology Case 21

REKHA SIRIPURAPU

Clinical history

A 32-year-old male presents with fever, headaches and abnormal behaviour.

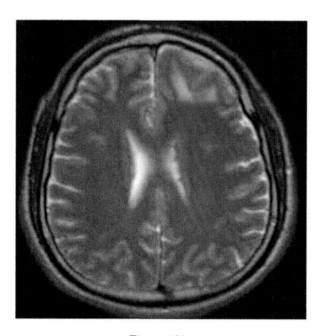

Figure 4.21a

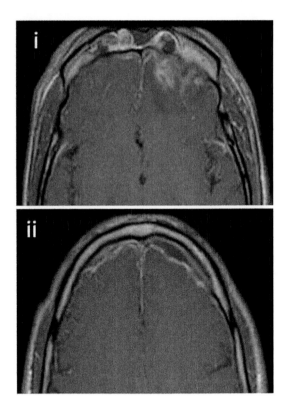

Figure 4.21b

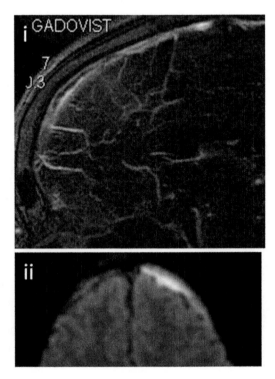

Figure 4.21c

Model answer

These are selected images from axial T2-weighted, contrast-enhanced axial T1-weighted, sagittal contrast-enhanced MIP and diffusion-weighted sequences from an MR study. The axial T2-weighted sequence (Figure 4.21a) shows abnormal high signal intensity in the left frontal lobe. Contrast-enhanced axial images (Figure 4.21b) show abnormal enhancement within the frontal lobe and bilateral rim-enhancing extra-axial collections, consistent with cerebritis and bilateral subdural empyemas, more prominent on the left. There is abnormal enhancement of the frontal sinuses, suggestive of frontal sinusitis.

The contrast-enhanced venogram (Figure 4.21c, i) shows a filling defect within the superior sagittal sinus consistent with venous thrombosis. The diffusion-weighted image (Figure 4.21c, ii) shows high signal intensity in the left frontal collection. I would correlate with the corresponding ADC map, which, if low, shows restricted diffusion. This finding would suggest the presence of purulent material.

The diagnosis is bilateral frontal subdural empyemas, left frontal cerebritis and superior sagittal sinus thrombosis secondary to frontal sinusitis. No evidence of a brain abscess is seen.

This is a neurological emergency. I will call the referring clinician to convey the findings and advise urgent neurosurgical referral. I would like to review the remaining images to assess the size of the empyema as well as to exclude thrombus within the other deep intracranial veins.

Questions

1. **What is the pathophysiology of subdural empyema?**
   Subdural empyema can be due to:
   - spread from an infected sinus through direct bony erosion
   - intracranial spread from infected venous thrombophlebitis
   - haematogenous spread from a distant source
   - iatrogenic/traumatic causes
   - direct spread from meningitis
2. **What is a subdural collection?**
   A collection in the subdural space, which is the potential space between the dura mater and arachnoid mater.
3. **What is the differential for a rim-enhancing subdural collection?**
   Chronic subdural haematoma and subdural empyema can be very difficult to distinguish from each other. Clinical features are extremely important, and diffusion-weighted imaging can be very helpful.
4. **What is the likely management in this case?**
   Intravenous antibiotic therapy with surgical drainage of the empyema, debridement of necrotic bone, if present, and input from otolaryngologists for frontal sinus surgery/drainage to locate the source of infection. Other supportive medical treatment may be required if there are ongoing clinical symptoms, i.e. seizures.

Key points

- The frontal sinus does not begin to pneumatize until the age of six. Children under this age will not suffer from frontal sinusitis.
- Isolated frontal sinusitis is rare – it tends to be associated with sinus infections at other sites.
- In infants and children, subdural empyema most often results as a complication of meningitis rather than paranasal sinus disease.
- MRI with contrast is the modality of choice for evaluation of celebritis.
- Lumbar puncture is contraindicated in suspected subdural empyema because of the risk of brain herniation.

Further reading

Goldberg AN, Oroszlan G, Anderson TD. Complications of frontal sinusitis and their management. *Otolaryngol Clin N Am* 2001; **34**: 211–25.

Greenlee JE. Subdural empyema. *Curr Treat Options Neurol* 2003; **5**: 13–22.

Osborn MK, Steinberg JP. Subdural empyema and other suppurative complications of paranasal sinusitis. *Lancet Infect Dis* 2007; **7**: 62–7.

Neuroradiology Case 22

REKHA SIRIPURAPU

Clinical history

A 39-year-old HIV-positive man presents with behavioural changes.

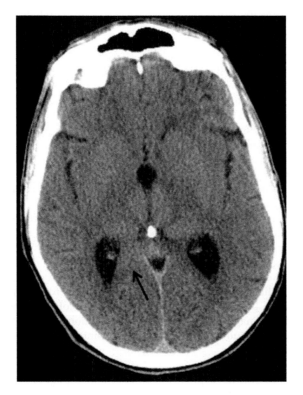

Figure 4.22a

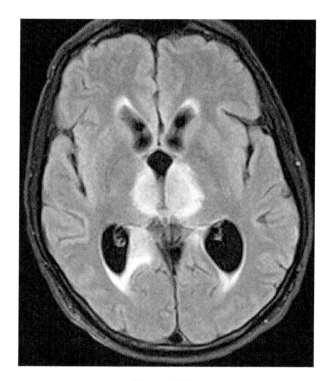

Figure 4.22b

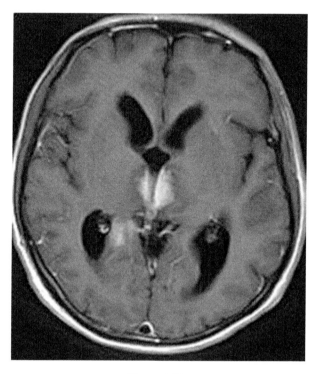

Figure 4.22c

Model answer

The non-contrast-enhanced CT (Figure 4.22a) shows subtle bilateral thalamic hyperdensity. There is asymmetry of the splenium of the corpus callosum with subtle hyperdensity in the right side.

The axial FLAIR image (Figure 4.22b) confirms the CT findings of a bilateral thalamic mass with right splenial signal change. There is compression of the third ventricle and consequent dilatation of the lateral ventricles with periventricular high signal suggestive of transependymal CSF seepage.

The gadolinium-enhanced axial T1-weighted study (Figure 4.22c) shows homogeneous enhancement in the thalami and the right splenium. The appearances are consistent with a neoplasm, most likely lymphoma. Thalamic glioma is a less likely differential diagnosis. Given the obstructive hydrocephalus, urgent neurosurgical referral is advised.

Questions

1. **What is the relevance of HIV status in this case?**
   Immunocompromised patients are at increased risk for developing primary CNS lymphoma (PCNSL). Primary CNS lymphoma in an HIV-seropositive patient is an AIDS-defining condition. The age at presentation is earlier (fourth decade) in patients with AIDS but the cell type (B cell) is similar to non-HIV-associated CNS lymphoma. The imaging appearance of cerebral lymphoma in the immunocompromised can differ markedly from immunocompetent individuals. Cerebral lymphoma in immunocompetent people tends to be a homogeneous mass that is hyperdense on CT and enhances avidly with contrast. Cerebral lymphoma does not tend to undergo cystic degeneration and necrosis in the immunocompetent. In immunocompromised people, the disease can present with multifocal cystic degenerative lesions. Non-enhancing cerebral lymphoma is uncommon.

2. **Why is the mass hyperdense on CT, and what would you expect on diffusion-weighted imaging (DWI)?**
   Hyperdensity on CT is explained by dense cellularity and high nuclear-to-cytoplasmic ratio. The mass would show restricted diffusivity on DWI.

3. **Which other patients are at increased risk of developing lymphoma?**
   Patients with rheumatoid arthritis, SLE, sarcoidosis, Sjögren's syndrome, chronic immunosuppression post-transplantation are all at increased risk of developing PCNSL.

4. **How is the diagnosis confirmed?**
   A histology specimen is required. It is important to withhold steroids prior to the biopsy, as these can result in a non-diagnostic specimen.

Key points

- Primary CNS lymphoma is limited to the CNS without systemic involvement. As well as affecting the brain, it can affect the leptomeninges, eyes or spinal cord.
- PCNSL is a subtype of non-Hodgkin's lymphoma. The majority is of the B-cell type, with approximately 3% T-cell type.
- PCNSL lesions are usually associated with a moderate amount of oedema and mass effect.
- PCNSL can affect any age group. In patients with AIDS, the median age for developing PCNSL is 36–38 years.

Notes

This is a biopsy-proven case of primary CNS lymphoma.

Further reading

Thurnher MM, Donovan Post MJ. Neuroimaging in the brain in HIV-1-infected patients. *Neuroimaging Clin N Am* 2008; **18**: 93–117.

Gavrilovic IT, Abrey LE. Primary central nervous system lymphoma. *Curr Oncol Rep* 2004; **6**: 388–95.

Neuroradiology Case 23

REKHA SIRIPURAPU

Clinical history

A 72-year-old woman presents with headache and right ophthalmoplegia.

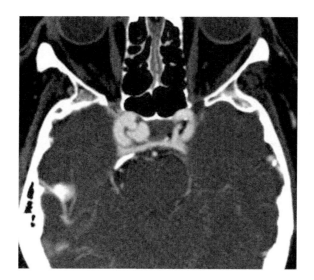

Figure 4.23a

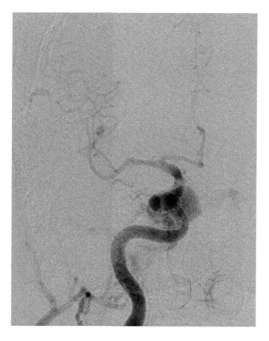

Figure 4.23b

Model answer

The single axial image from a CT angiogram (Figure 4.23a) shows abnormality in the cavernous segment of the right internal carotid artery (ICA), with an aneurysm arising from its medial wall. Compared to the contralateral side, there is greater contrast filling of the sinus and ipsilateral deep veins, consistent with a diagnosis of caroticocavernous fistula.

The single image from the frontal view of a right carotid angiogram (Figure 4.23b) shows early filling of the right cavernous sinus consistent with a caroticocavernous fistula. This fistula is likely to be between the ICA aneurysm and the cavernous sinus. The aneurysm seen on CT is not well demonstrated on the angiographic image but I would review all the other images to delineate it. Venous outflow is predominantly into the inferior petrosal sinus, inferiorly towards the pterygoid plexus, and across the intercavernous anastomosis to the contralateral cavernous sinus. I would like to review the rest of the CT and angiographic images to delineate anatomy, to look for synchronous aneurysms, and for treatment planning. The lesion may be amenable to endovascular treatment, and the case will need to be discussed with both the interventional neuroradiologist and the neurosurgeon.

Questions

1. **What are the types of caroticocavernous fistula (CCF)?**
There are two types, direct (type A) and indirect (types B to D). Direct communication between the cavernous ICA and cavernous venous sinus is called a direct fistula. The causes include trauma, iatrogenic, spontaneous rupture of a cavernous carotid aneurysm (as in this patient), atherosclerosis in the elderly and underlying vascular dysplasias and collagen abnormalities. Other associations include pregnancy, surgery and sinusitis.

An indirect fistula or a dural arteriovenous fistula is a shunt between meningeal branches of the cavernous ICA (type B), ECA (type C) or both ICA/ECA (type D) and the cavernous venous sinus. The cause of indirect fistulas is unkown, and venous thrombosis has been implicated in their aetiology.

2. **What are the clinical features?**
Pulsatile exophthalmos, orbital bruit, pain, chemosis and ophthalmoplegia.

Key points

- CCFs can be classified in several ways, based on their cause, their haemodynamic properties and their anatomy.
- The gold standard for diagnosis of a CCF is selective cerebral angiography, which can provide information about flow and venous drainage.
- Direct CCFs are typically high-flow fistulas.
- Indirect CCFs are usually low-flow fistulas.
- Endovascular repair is the typical treatment of CCFs. In a few cases surgical repair may be an option.

Further reading

Biondi A. Intracranial aneurysms associated with other lesions, disorders or anatomic variations. *Neuroimaging Clin N Am* 2006; **16**: 467–82.

Grossman RI, Yousem DM. *Neuroradiology: the Requisites*, 2nd edn. St Louis, MO: Mosby, 2003; 500–1.

Ringer AJ, Salud L, Tomsich TA. Carotid cavernous fistulas: anatomy, classification and treatment. *Neurosurg Clin N Am* 2005; **16**: 279–95.

Neuroradiology Case 24

Clinical history

A 53-year-old woman presents with acute right-sided weakness.

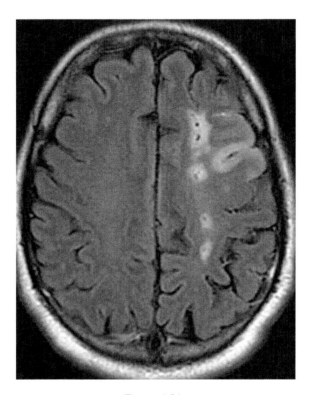

Figure 4.24a

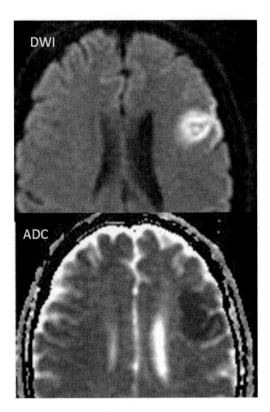

Figure 4.24b

Model answer

The axial FLAIR image (Figure 4.24a) shows abnormal cortical high signal intensity in the left frontal lobe. There is also high signal intensity on diffusion-weighted imaging (DWI), with corresponding low signal on the apparent diffusion coefficient (ADC) map (Figure 4.24b), in keeping with restricted diffusion. This is consistent with an acute left MCA territory infarct.

In addition, there are multiple other high-signal FLAIR intensities in the left centrum semiovale oriented in a linear fashion. This gives a 'rosary' or 'string of pearls' appearance and is very concerning for internal watershed ischaemia in the left MCA territory, which is likely to be from severe ICA disease. I will advise urgent assessment of the carotid arteries.

Questions

1. **Name some non-ischaemic causes of restricted diffusion.**

   Abscess, empyema, neoplastic causes such as primary CNS lymphoma, medulloblastoma, epidermoid cyst, status epilepticus, hypoglycaemia and Creutzfeldt–Jacob disease.

2. **What is a watershed region? What is a watershed infarct?**

   A watershed area is a region in the body that receives dual supply from distal branches of two different arterial systems. There is often anastomosis of the two arterial systems at this point. It is the most distal part of both arterial systems, where the perfusion pressure is lowest. Therefore, if there is impairment of flow in *both* vessels (e.g. in hypotension or, in this case, stenosis of the parent vessel of both vessels), the watershed area is vulnerable to ischaemia/infarction. Conversely, if only *one* vessel is occluded/stenosed, the watershed area is relatively protected from the effects of this occlusion/stenosis.

3. **What is meant by internal watershed infarcts?**
An internal watershed infarct can involve the junction between the deep and superficial arterial system of the MCA in the corona radiata.
4. **What is meant by cortical watershed infarcts?**
Cortical watershed infarcts occur between the cortical territories, such as between the ACA and MCA.

Key points
• Severe internal carotid disease is associated with watershed infarcts. Classically, severe ICA disease is thought to predispose to infarction by reducing perfusion to the watershed regions. More recent evidence suggests that emboli from unstable plaques may also contribute to the infarcts. There are some data to suggest that microemboli travel preferentially to the watershed regions.

Further reading
Grossman RI, Yousem DM. *Neuroradiology: the Requisites*, 2nd edn. St Louis, MO: Mosby, 2003; 174–95.

Krapf H, Widder B, Skalej M. Small rosarylike infarctions in the centrum ovale suggest hemodynamic failure. *AJNR Am J Neuroradiol* 1998; **19**: 1479–84.

Momjian-Mayor I, Baron JC. The pathophysiology of watershed infarction in internal carotid artery disease: review of cerebral perfusion studies. *Stroke* 2005; **36**: 567–77.

Neuroradiology Case 25

REKHA SIRIPURAPU

Clinical history
A 20-year-old female with neurofibromatosis type 1 (NF1) presents with blurring of vision.

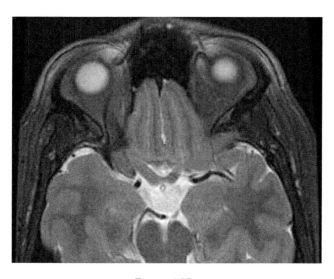

Figure 4.25a

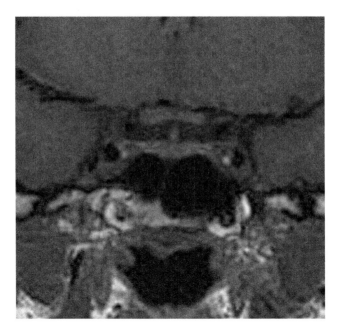

Figure 4.25b

Model answer

The axial T2-weighted image at the level of the optic chiasm (Figure 4.25a) shows slight enlargement of the right side of the chiasm and the right optic nerve anteriorly. This is confirmed on the coronal T1-weighted image (Figure 4.25b). In a patient with NF1, and with the given clinical history, this would be very concerning for an optic pathway glioma. I will arrange for a contrast-enhanced study to evaluate this lesion further.

Questions

1. **What is the association between NF1 and optic pathway glioma?**
   Of all patients with an optic pathway glioma, about one-third have NF1, and, of all tumours in this region, 40–70% occur in NF1 patients and appear to have a more benign biologic behaviour. NF1-associated tumours affect the optic nerve and chiasm with nearly equal prevalence, preserve the optic nerve shape, can extend beyond the optic pathway, and are usually not cystic.
2. **What are the imaging findings?**
   On T1-weighted sequences they are isointense to hypointense. On T2-weighted sequences they are hyperintense or isointense and show solid near-homogeneous enhancement; or, if necrosis is present, then there is a central non-enhancing zone.

Key points

- NF1 comprises 90% of all cases of neurofibromatosis and has an autosomal dominant inheritance.
- The differential diagnosis for this MRI appearance in a patient without NF1 is optic nerve sheath meningioma (ONSM). However, ONSM does not enlarge the optic chiasm and is usually associated with hyperostosis. ONSM compresses the optic nerve, unlike the optic nerve glioma, which expands it.
- Optic pathway gliomas are the commonest CNS tumours in a patient with NF1.
- Optic pathway gliomas, as the name suggests, can involve any part of the optic pathway: optic nerves, optic chiasm, optic tracts, lateral geniculate bodies, optic radiation and occipital lobes.

- MRI is the modality of choice: high-resolution axial and coronal T1-weighted sequences including fat-saturation and fast spin echo inversion recovery sequences. These latter two sequences can help assess involvement of the optic nerve.

Further reading

Barbagallo JS, Kolodzieh MS, Silverberg NB, Weinberg JM. Neurocutaneous disorders. *Dermatol Clin* 2002; **20**: 547–60.

Koeller KK, Rushing EF. Pilocytic astrocytoma: radiologic–pathologic correlation. *Radiographics* 2004; **24**: 1693–708.

Rodriguez D, Poussaint TY. Neuroimaging findings in neurofibromatosis type 1 and 2. *Neuroimaging Clin N Am* 2004; **14**: 149–70.

Neuroradiology Case 26

HAN WEI AW-YEANG

Clinical history

Student found unconscious at home in winter.

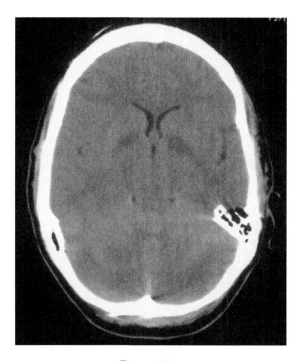

Figure 4.26a

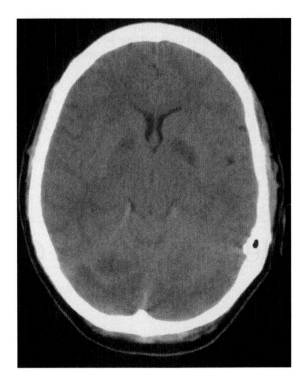

Figure 4.26b

Model answer

On the unenhanced CT (Figures 4.26a, 4.26b) there are symmetrical low-attenuation areas in the lentiform nuclei, more specifically in the globus pallidus bilaterally. No other abnormality is apparent in the remainder of the visualized brain parenchyma. With the clinical history above, carbon monoxide poisoning is a possibility.

The other causes of basal ganglia infarction include global hypoperfusion (near-drowning, strangling, cardiopulmonary arrest) methanol toxicity, cyanide poisoning, osmotic myelinolysis, hypoglycaemia, lactic acidosis and cocaine/heroin overdose.

Questions

1. **Why are the basal ganglia particularly vulnerable to ischaemic insults?**
   The basal ganglia are supplied by deep perforating branch end arteries (i.e. there is little or no collateral circulation), making them vulnerable to ischaemic/hypo-perfusion events.

2. **What sequelae are likely from the injury above?**
   There is likely to be global hypoperfusion, and this may result in cerebral oedema and coning.

Key points

- The basal ganglia are a group of subcortical nuclei with complex interconnections and complex vascular supply mainly from the anterior circulation.
- Infarcts affecting the basal ganglia are known as striatocapsular infarcts.
- Other uncommon neurometabolic causes of basal ganglia infarcts are Wilson's disease, Hallervorden–Spatz disease, Leigh's disease and mitochondrial myopathy.

Further reading

Kornienko VN, Pronin IN. *Diagnostic Neuroradiology*. Berlin: Springer, 2009; 151.

Osborn A, Tong K. *Handbook of Neuroradiology: Brain and Skull*. St Louis, MO: Mosby, 1996; 52–3, 568–9.

Tisch S, Silberstein P, Limousin-Dowsey P, Jahanshahi M. The basal ganglia: anatomy, physiology and pharmacology. *Psychiatr Clin N Am* 2004; **27**: 757–99.

von Kummer R, Bourquain H, Bastianello S, *et al*. Early prediction of irreversible brain damage after ischemic stroke at CT. *Radiology* 2001; **219**: 95–100.

Neuroradiology Case 27

HAN WEI AW-YEANG

Clinical history
A 22-year-old female presents with headaches and weakness of both hands.

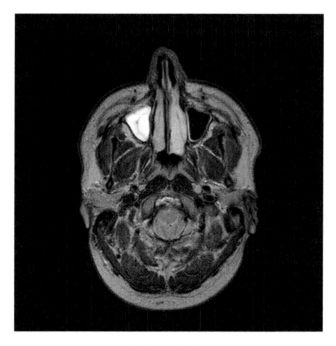

Figure 4.27a

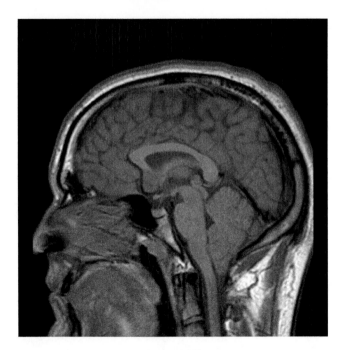

Figure 4.27b

Model answer

There are two images (Figures 4.27a, 4.27b). The first is from an axial T2-weighted MRI brain study and the second is a sagittal midline T1-weighted image.

The sagittal T1-weighted image demonstrates inferior herniation of the cerebellar tonsil. I would like to measure the distance the tip of the cerebellar tonsil extends below the level of the foramen magnum (the level of the foramen magnum is defined by a line running from the clivus to the basi occiput). The axial T2-weighted image shows effacement of the anterior subarachoid space. The cerebellar tonsil has peg-shape morphology. Incidental fluid in the right maxillary sinus is noted.

I would like to look for associated findings of syringohydromyelia and hydrocephalus.

The findings are consistent with a Chiari I malformation. The referring clinician will need to be informed of the clinical findings, and the patient will need referral to the neurosurgeons for consideration of decompressive surgery.

Questions

1. **How many types of Chiari malformations are currently classified?**

   There are four types of Chiari malformations:
   - Type I is usually diagnosed in adulthood and is characterized by herniation of the cerebellar tonsils through the foramen magnum.
   - Type II usually presents in the paediatric population and is due to the caudal displacement of fourth ventricle, medulla and cerebellum into the spinal canal. Type II Chiari malformations are almost always associated with at least a partially absent falx (leading to interdigitation of the central gyri on cross-sectional imaging) and a myelomeningocele.
   - In addition to the cerebellar herniation, the rare types III and IV Chiari malformations are associated with an encephalocele and cerebellar hypoplasia/ agenesis respectively.

   (NB: The term Arnold–Chiari malformation is usually reserved for type II Chiari malformation.)

2. What degree of herniation of the cerebellar tonsil is clinically significant?

The cerebellar tonsils have a range of downward displacement from the foramen magnum, depending on the age of the patient. The cerebellar tonsils vary in position normally with age. Generally in the first decade the tonsils protrude below the foramen magnum by < 6 mm, second to third decade < 5 mm, fourth to eighth decade < 4 mm, ninth decade < 3 mm.

Key points

- The most common symptoms of Chiari malformation are headaches and pain usually in the occipital and upper cervical region.
- Other associated bony anomalies are atlanto-occipital assimilation, platybasia, basilar invagination, a retroflexed dens and fused cervical vertebrae.
- Although the commonest cause of a Chiari type I malformation is congenital, there are also acquired causes: lumboperitoneal shunting, repeated lumbar punctures, lumbar drainage.
- Syringohydromyelia is associated in 30–70% of cases, located usually in the cervical to upper thoracic region.

Further reading

Speer MC, Enterline DS, Mehltretter L, *et al.* Chiari type I malformation with or without syringomyelia: prevalence and genetics. *J Genet Couns* 2003; **12**: 297–311.

Tubbs RS, Lyerly MJ, Loukas M, Shoja MM, Oakes WJ. The pediatric Chiari I malformation: a review. *Childs Nerv Syst* 2007; **23**: 1239–50.

Neuroradiology Case 28

HAN WEI AW-YEANG

Clinical history

A patient presents to the emergency department with headaches. Query cause.

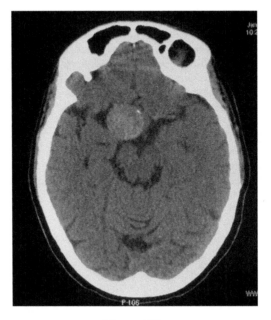

Figure 4.28a

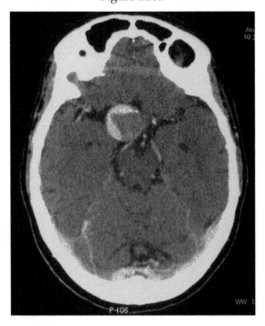

Figure 4.28b

Model answer

Pre- and post-contrast selected axial images through the brain are shown (Figures 4.28a, 4.28b).

The pre-contrast image shows that there is a large circular mixed-density lesion located in the interpeduncular cistern. The lesion is isodense peripherally. More centrally there are areas of slight increased density. There is also a tiny focus of high density, which may be due to calcification.

The post-IV-contrast image shows intense enhancement in part of the lesion. I would further evaluate the remainder of the examination to confirm my suspicions that this lesion represents a partially thrombosed aneurysm of the circle of Willis (CoW). I would also like to look for other synchronous lesions and would assess for any evidence of associated acute subarachnoid haemorrhage.

The findings on this examination would warrant immediate contact with the referring clinician to inform him/her of the results. This patient requires immediate referral to the nearest neurosurgical unit.

Questions

1. **What types of intracranial aneurysms do you know?**
   There are saccular or berry aneurysms. Other types are fusiform, dissecting, infectious, traumatic and oncotic aneurysms.
2. **What is the most common genetic abnormality associated with intracranial aneurysms?**
   Autosomal dominant polycystic kidney disease. Patients with polycystic kidney disease are also more likely to develop multiple aneurysms.
3. **Where do most CoW aneurysms occur?**
   The commonest location is the anterior communicating artery (30%) and the next commonest is at the origin of the posterior communicating artery (25%).

Key points

- Saccular aneurysms typically arise from the arterial bifurcations, usually at the convexity of the curve.
- The non-saccular aneurysms arise at non-branching sites along the vessel.
- Large aneurysms can contain thrombus and organized clots, just as in this case. They can be a source of distal emboli.
- Arterial hypertension is a significant risk factor. It predisposes to the development of multiple aneurysms and increases the likelihood of rupture.
- Connective tissue disorders associated with intracranial aneurysms: Marfan's syndrome, type 4 Ehlers–Danlos.
- Inflammatory disorders associated with intracranial aneurysms: systemic lupus erythematosus, Takayasu's disease, giant-cell arteritis.

Further reading

Bonneville F, Sourour N, Biondi A. Intracranial aneurysms: an overview. *Neuroimaging Clin N Am* 2006; **16**: 371–82.

Schievink WI. Intracranial aneurysms. *N Engl J Med* 1997; **336**: 28–40.

Yanaka K, Nagase S, Asakawa H, *et al*. Management of unruptured cerebral aneurysms in patients with polycystic kidney disease. *Surg Neurol* 2004; **62**: 538–45.

Images courtesy of Dr Ravi Adapala, Arrowe Park Hospital, Wirral.

Neuroradiology Case 29

HAN WEI AW-YEANG

Clinical history
Postural headaches.

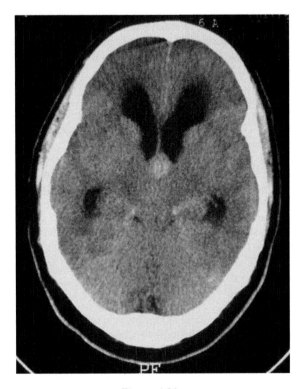

Figure 4.29a

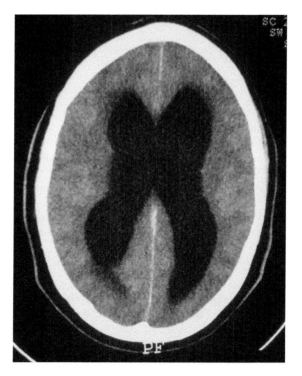

Figure 4.29b

Model answer

Two unenhanced selected axial CT images through the brain (Figures 4.29a, 4.29b) show a well-defined, hyperdense, oval lesion located at the foramina of Monro. There is gross hydrocephalus and sulcal effacement. There is subtle low attenuation adjacent to the anterior frontal horns suggestive of transependymal oedema. The appearances are consistent with a colloid cyst which is causing obstructive hydrocephalus and severely raised intracranial pressure. The referring clinician needs to be informed of the results immediately, as the patient is at risk of death and urgent surgery is required.

Questions

1. **What type of headaches do colloid cysts present with, and what is the mechanism of these headaches?**
   Colloid cysts classically present with paroxysmal headaches. Colloid cysts are pedunculated tumours and have a ball-valve effect at the foramina of Monro. They can suddenly cause blockage, and this effect can vary due to change in position from lying to standing up.

2. **What is the typical signal of colloid cysts on T1-weighted MRI, and why?**
   They are typically hyperintense, as they usually contain cholesterol. However, the cyst content can vary and thus the signal can vary.

3. **What is the typical signal of colloid cysts on MRI diffusion-weighted imaging?**
   Slight restriction on DWI when compared to CSF but less than an epidermoid.

4. **Do colloid cysts enhance?**
   Mild peripheral enhancement is normal. Internal enhancement suggests a solid lesion.

5. **Would the density of the colloid cyst on CT or the signal characteristics of the lesion on MRI affect treatment?**

A hyperdense colloid cyst is likely to have more solid contents and to be harder to drain. Cysts with high T2 signal may be easier to drain than those with low T2 signal.

Key points

- Colloid cysts account for 0.5–1% of all intracranial mass lesions.
- They arise from the anterior roof of the third ventricle.
- There is a slight male predominance, especially in the third to fourth decade of life.
- Neurosurgical approach can be via an open approach, transcallosal or transcortical, or via the endoscopic route.
- Colloid cysts vary in size from 0.3 to 4 cm, and they are slow-growing lesions.
- Colloid cysts are usually hyperdense on CT but may be iso- or hypodense. They can have calcification, but this is rare.

Further reading

Maeder PP, Holtås SL, Basibüyük LN, *et al*. Colloid cysts of the third ventricle: correlation of MR and CT findings with histology and chemical analysis. *AJNR Am J Neuroradiol* 1990; **11**: 575–81.

Osborn AG. *Diagnostic Imaging: Brain*. Salt Lake City, UT: Amirsys, 2004; I (7): 9–10.

Purdy RA, Kirby S. Headaches and brain tumors. *Neurol Clin N Am* 2004; **22**: 39–53.

Wilms G, Marchal G, Van Hecke P, *et al*. Colloid cysts of the third ventricle: MR findings. *J Comput Assist Tomogr* 1990; **14**: 527–31.

Images courtesy of Dr Ravi Adapala, Arrowe Park Hospital, Wirral.

Neuroradiology Case 30

HAN WEI AW-YEANG

Clinical history
A teenager presents with weakness in the legs.

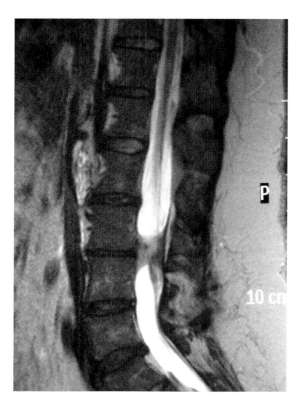

Figure 4.30a

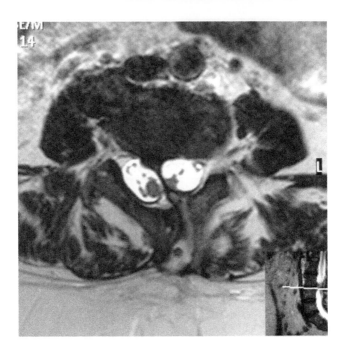

Figure 4.30b

Model answer

These are T2-weighted sagittal and axial images of the lumbar spine (Figures 4.30a, 4.30b). There is a low-signal band dividing the spinal canal and lower spinal cord. The appearance is consistent with diastematomyelia of the spinal cord with an osteo-cartilaginous band. Each hemicord appears to have its own dural sac.

The conus medullaris is not clearly seen on these images but there is a significant chance that it is situated below L2. I would look for associated abnormalities like scoliosis, myelomeningocele, spinal lipomas, syringohydromyelia, hemivertebrae, butterfly vertebrae and spina bifida.

Questions

1. **Is there a gender predilection for this condition?**
   Yes, females are affected more than males.
2. **Which level of the spinal cord is the most commonly affected?**
   The lumbar level.
3. **How frequently are osteocartilaginous bands seen in diastematomyelia?**
   In 40% of cases.
4. **Do the vertebral segmentation abnormalities occur above or below the diastematomyelia?**
   These occur at the level of the diastematomyelia.
5. **Why is there an associated abnormality of the bony spine?**
   The development of the notochord influences the development of the vertebral bodies.

Key points

- Diastematomyelia is also known as split cord malformation. The spinal cord splits into two portions, either symmetrically or asymmetrically. Each hemicord has its own central spinal canal.

- The level of the spinal cord which is affected is as follows, in decreasing order of frequency: lumbar > thoracic > cervical.
- The spur/band that splits the cord forms from cartilage, with a variable number of ossification centres. Thus the spur can be variable in appearance, depending on the amount of cartilage and bone present.
- The spur can be bone, cartilage or fibrous tissue.
- Ossified spur: high signal on T1-weighted and low signal on T2-weighted sequences due to internal marrow signal.
- Non-ossified spur: isointense to mildly hyperintense compared to CSF on T1-weighted, and low on T2-weighted sequences.

Further reading
Barkovich AJ. *Pediatric Neuroimaging*, 4th edn. Philadelphia, PA: Lippincott Williams & Wilkins, 2005; 744–52.

Naidich TP, Harwood-Nash DC. Diastematomyelia: hemicord and meningeal sheaths; single and double arachnoid and dural tubes. *AJNR Am J Neuroradiol* 1983; **4**: 633–6.

Neuroradiology Case 31

HAN WEI AW-YEANG

Clinical history
An adult with asthma presents with frontal headaches.

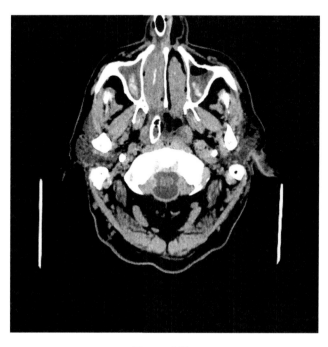

Figure 4.31a

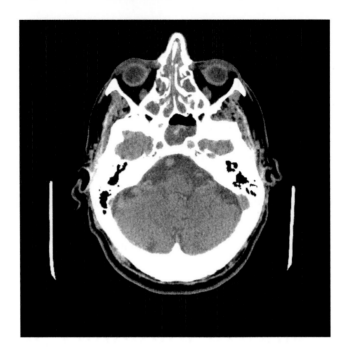

Figure 4.31b

Model answer

These are selected axial non-contrast CT head images (Figures 4.31a, 4.31b). There is complete opacification of the right maxillary antrum and ethmoid complexes bilaterally. The left maxillary antrum and sphenoid sinus show air–fluid levels. The sphenoid sinus and both maxillary antra have areas of high density. There is no expansion of the sinuses, and the pterygopalatine fat planes appear preserved. The bony margins appear intact but I would confirm this by assessing the bony windows and would pay particular attention to the lamina papyracea and skull base for dehiscence.

These findings suggest allergic fungal sinusitis. The differential diagnoses include sinonasal polyposis or mucoceles that also contain multiple mycetomas or desiccated secretions.

Questions

1. **Is there a difference between allergic fungal sinusitis (AFS) and invasive fungal sinusitis?**

   Fungal sinusitis is classified into *invasive* and *non-invasive* fungal sinusitis. Allergic fungal sinusitis falls into the sub-classification of non-invasive sinusitis occurring in immunocompetent patients with atopy. The other subgroup is fungal ball.

   Invasive fungal sinusitis is less common, and is sub-classified into three subgroups: acute necrotizing, chronic invasive and granulomatous invasive.

   Acute necrotizing and chronic invasive fungal sinusitis occur in immunocompromised patients including transplant recipients and diabetics.

2. **What is the cause of high-attenuation areas in fungal sinusitis?**

   The high attenuation in allergic fungal sinusitis is likely due to a combination of heavy metals (iron and manganese), calcium, and inspissated secretions that are often found in fungal elements.

3. **What is the treatment of AFS?**

   Surgical clearance of disease. The goal of treatment is to prevent recurrence.

Key points

- Allergic fungal sinusitis usually occurs in patients with atopy.
- Patients are immunocompetent.
- Diagnosis of AFS is by histopathology with no evidence of mucosal fungal invasion and exclusion of other fungal sinusitis disorders.

Further reading

Gamba JL, Woodruff WW, Djang WT, Yeates AE. Craniofacial mucormycosis: assessment with CT. *Radiology* 1986; **160**: 207–12.

Manning SC, Merkel M, Kriesel K, Vuitch F, Marple B. Computed tomography and magnetic resonance diagnosis of allergic fungal sinusitis. *Laryngoscope* 1997; **107**: 170–6.

Mukherji SK, Figueroa RE, Ginsberg LE, *et al.* Allergic fungal sinusitis: CT findings. *Radiology* 1998; **207**: 417–22.

Neuroradiology Case 32

HAN WEI AW-YEANG

Clinical history

Spontaneous headache.

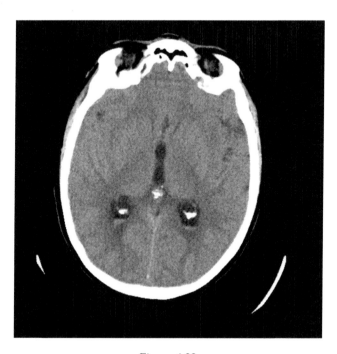

Figure 4.32

Model answer

The axial unenhanced brain CT (Figure 4.32) shows dense fluid layering in the occipital horns of the lateral ventricles. Appearances are consistent with acute subarachnoid haemorrhage (SAH). I would like to look closely at the rest of the available imaging for a cause of the haemorrhage, such as a circle of Willis aneurysm or an arteriovenous malformation.

The patient will need urgent referral to the nearest neurosurgical centre.

Questions

1. **What are the causes of SAH?**
   The causes of SAH are trauma, ruptured cerebral aneurysm, perimesencephalic haemorrhage, arteriovenous malformation, bleeding disorder, use of anticoagulants, idiopathic, and rarely bleeding into brain tumours.
2. **An oculomotor (third) nerve palsy may indicate bleeding from which artery?**
   The posterior communicating artery. A posterior communicating artery aneurysm may also cause a third nerve palsy.
3. **What are the factors that increase the likelihood of an aneurysm rupturing?**
   Factors that increase the risk include the size and location of the aneurysm. Aneurysms located in the posterior cerebral circulation have a higher risk of rupturing than those located in the anterior cerebral circulation.
4. **What are the CT signs of subarachnoid blood?**
   - Dense fluid layering in the dependent parts of the CSF spaces.
   - Dense fluid outlining the cerebral gyri.
   - Dense fluid outlining the tentorium.

Key points

- Subarachnoid haemorrhage is most commonly due to trauma. Of non-traumatic causes, ruptured cerebral aneurysm constitutes 80–85% of these cases.
- The incidence of SAH is higher in women than in men (3 : 2) and increases with age.
- Traumatic SAH from closed head injuries tends to overlie the convexities, while SAH from ruptured aneurysm tends to be in the basal cisterns.
- Traumatic SAH from closed head injuries can be due to vascular injuries or parenchymal contusions.

Further reading

Suarez JI, Tarr RW, Selman WR. Aneurysmal subarachnoid hemorrhage. *N Engl J Med* 2006; **354**: 387–96.

van Gijn J, Kerr RS, Rinkel GJ. Subarachnoid haemorrhage. *Lancet* 2007; **369**: 306–18.

Neuroradiology Case 33

HAN WEI AW-YEANG

Clinical history
A patient presents to the emergency department with headaches.

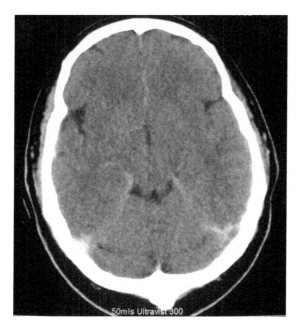

Figure 4.33a

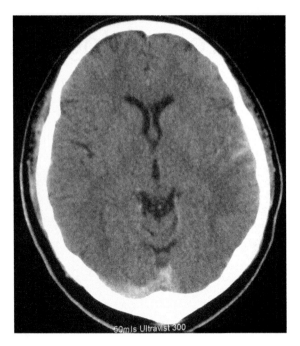

Figure 4.33b

Model answer

These are two selected post-contrast axial CT images through the brain (Figures 4.33a, 4.33b). There is a filling defect within the left transverse sinus. There are linear high densities within the sulci of the left temporal region. The appearances are consistent with a thrombus in the left transverse sinus that is associated with a subarachnoid haemorrhage. I would like to review the rest of the imaging to look for the extent of the thrombus and the presence of infarction, as well as to assess the severity of the subarachnoid bleed. The patient should ideally be treated at a specialist neurological centre.

Questions

1. **What causes the empty delta sign or the reverse delta sign on a post-contrast CT?**
   The delta sign results from a high density of dural enhancement that surrounds luminal thrombus within the superior sagittal sinus. The so-called 'pseudo-delta' sign on unenhanced CT is caused by blood surrounding the superior sagittal sinus in cases of subdural haemorrhage.
2. **What are the common false-positive MRI signs of a sinus thrombus?**
   Asymmetrical arachnoid granulations, congenital hypoplasia of one of the transverse sinuses, time-of-flight artefacts (slow flow or complex flow pattern) or fat in the sinuses.
3. **Which cerebral venous sinus is most often involved?**
   The superior sagittal sinus.
4. **Which MR sequence is the most sensitive for thrombus detection?**
   FLAIR (fluid attenuated inversion recovery) sequences are more sensitive than PD (proton density), which in turn are more sensitive than T2-weighted sequences.

Key points

- Figure 4.33c is a T1-weighted coronal MR image of a left-sided transverse sinus thrombus. Note the high signal in the sinus. The five commonest causes of T1 high signal are thrombus/blood, fat, posterior pituitary, melanoma metastasis, gadolinium.

- The presence of a high-attenuation superior sagittal sinus on a non-contrast-enhanced CT may sometimes suggest thrombosis (although this sign is not always reliable – it is particularly difficult in the young). If clinically suspicious, suggest a contrast-enhanced CT if this sign is present.
- The order of frequency of dural sinus involvement is: sagittal > transverse > sigmoid > deep venous system > cavernous sinus
- Cerebral deep venous thrombosis is rare in comparison to cerebral dural sinus thrombosis.
- There are many causes of cerebral venous thrombosis. The important causes are: pregnancy, dehydration, oral contraceptives, trauma, tumour, haematological disorders (polycythaemia, sickle cell disease, leukaemias), infections (meningitis, encephalitis, subdural empyemas)
- An important complication of dural venous thrombosis is cerebral venous infarction due to increased venous hypertension leading to decrease in cerebral blood flow and reduced cerebral blood perfusion. Classically, venous infarcts are associated with parenchymal haemorrhage.

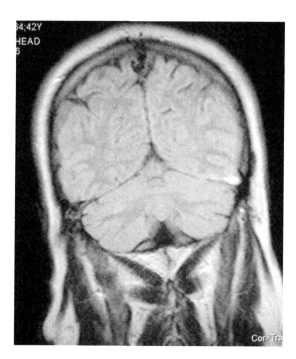

Figure 4.33c

Further reading

Ganeshan D, Narlawar R, McCann C, Lewis-Jones H, Curtis J. Cerebral venous thrombosis: a pictorial review. *Eur J Radiol* 2010; **74**: 110–16.

Linn J, Pfefferkorn T, Ivanicova K, *et al.* Noncontrast CT in deep cerebral venous thrombosis and sinus thrombosis: comparison of its diagnostic value for both entities. *AJNR Am J Neuroradiol* 2009; **30**: 728–35.

Selim M, Caplan LR. Radiological diagnosis of cerebral venous thrombosis. *Front Neurol Neurosci* 2008; **23**: 96–111.

Images courtesy of Dr Ravi Adapala, Arrowe Park Hospital, Wirral.

Neuroradiology Case 34

HAN WEI AW-YEANG AND JESSIE AW

Clinical history
An adult presents with urinary incontinence.

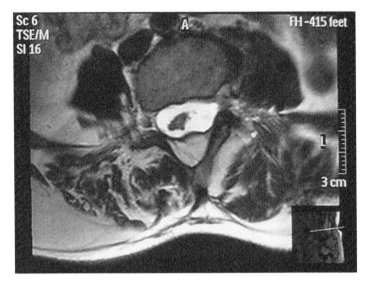

Figure 4.34a

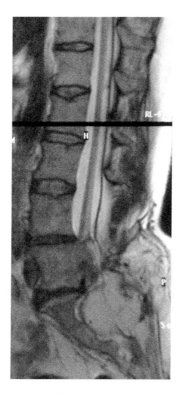

Figure 4.34b

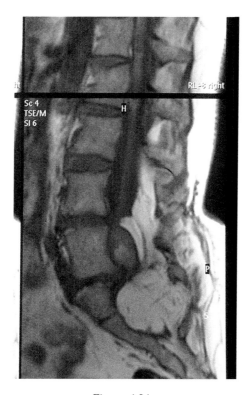

Figure 4.34c

Model answer

These are axial T2-weighted and sagittal T1- and T2-weighted images from an MRI of the lumbar spine (Figures 4.34a–4.34c).

The sagittal T1- and T2-weighted images demonstrate deficiency of the posterior elements of the sacrum and probably the posterior elements of L4 and L5. The thecal sac is contained in the spinal canal on these selected images. The findings are consistent with spina bifida.

The sagittal T1- and T2-weighted images show the cord terminating at the L4/5 level. The axial T2-weighted image shows the conus, which appears triangular, displaced anteriorly and to the right, most probably representing the placode. The findings represent a neural cord defect: a low-lying and tethered cord.

At S1/2 level there is a large lobulated lesion, which is high-signal on T1- and T2-weighted sequences. It appears to be in continuity with the thickened epidural fat from L3 to L5 level and with the overlying subcutaneous tissue. The appearance is in keeping with a large spinal lipoma, most probably representing a lipomyelocele as there does not appear to be any herniation of the thecal sac through the defect.

In summary, there is a spina bifida with a low-lying tethered cord and a lipomyelocele.

Questions

1. **At what level does the conus normally terminate in a child?**
   The conus should normally terminate at the L1–2 level. If the conus lies below this level then is it low-lying.
2. **How frequently is there an associated lipomeningocele?**
   Up to 70%.
3. **What are the other causes of tethered cord syndrome besides spinal lipoma?**
   Thickened filum terminale, diastematomyelia and meningocele.

Key points

- Spinal dysraphism is an umbrella term encompassing a heterogeneous group of complex spinal anomalies which have in common abnormalities of midline closure of the osseous structures, paraspinal soft tissues and neural tissues.
- The neural placode is an open spinal cord – the neural folds remain unfused. Thus the posterior aspect of the placode is what would have been the internal aspect of the spinal cord with an ependymal lining. The anterior aspect of the placode is the outer surface of a normally developed spinal cord with pia mater.
- A tethered cord is usually due to congenital abnormality but can be acquired. Acquired causes of a tethered cord include infection, scarring and tumours.
- Spinal lipomas are collections of fat and connective tissue that is connected to the leptomeninges or the spinal cord. Spinal lipomas can be further subclassified into intradural lipomas, lipomyeloceles/lipomyelomeningoceles and lipomas derived from caudal cell masses.

Further reading

Barkovich AJ. *Pediatric Neuroimaging*, 4th edn. Philadelphia, PA: Lippincott Williams & Wilkins, 2005; 710–31.

Raghavan N, Barkovich AJ, Edwards M, Norman D. MR imaging in the tethered spinal cord syndrome. *AJR Am J Roentgenol* 1989; **152**: 843–52.

Neuroradiology Case 35

JESSIE AW

Clinical history
Fire-cracker into eye.

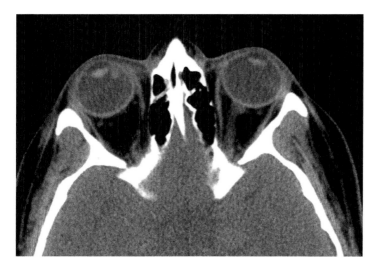

Figure 4.35a

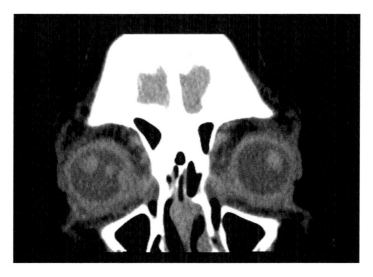

Figure 4.35b

Model answer
These are selected images from a non-contrast CT orbit examination (Figures 4.35a, 4.35b) showing abnormality in the right orbital globe and right medial epicanthus

region. There is soft tissue swelling in the right medial epicanthus region, and two foci of high attenuation in the vitreous chamber just posterior to the lens. The findings are consistent with an acute right intravitreous chamber haemorrhage. The anterior chamber appears clear and intact. No radio-opaque foreign body or air identified in either of the globes. The right lens does not appear dislocated or subluxed.

Questions

1. **What is the term for haemorrhage into the anterior chamber?**
   It is called a hyphaema.
2. **How do you tell if the lens is subluxed on imaging?**
   The lens will change its normal shape and will be biconcave.
3. **Which is more common: subluxation or dislocation?**
   Subluxation of the lens is more common than complete dislocation and needs to be assessed. Lens dislocation is seen in more severe cases of trauma.

Key points

- Vitreous haemorrhage is caused by a closed globe injury and has to be followed up very closely. Surgical treatment may be necessary if there is delayed clearing or if glaucoma develops.
- It is important to assess for intraocular foreign bodies preoperatively, especially when clinical evaluation is limited because of intraocular haemorrhage or cataracts.
- CT can detect metal, glass and stone.
- Wood is difficult to see on CT. If there is intraocular air, this may be a useful secondary sign in the appropriate clinical setting.

Further reading

Go JL, Vu VN, Lee KJ, Becker TS. Orbital trauma. *Neuroimaging Clin N Am* 2002; **12**: 311–24.

Reppucci VS, Movshovich A. Current concepts in the treatment of traumatic injury to the posterior segment. *Ophthalmol Clin N Am* 1999; **12**: 465–74.

Neuroradiology Case 36

JESSIE AW

Clinical history

Post motor vehicle accident.

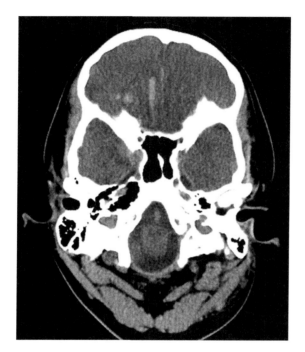

Figure 4.36a

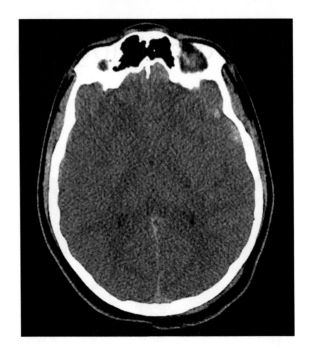

Figure 4.36b

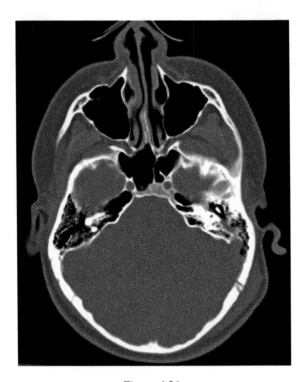

Figure 4.36c

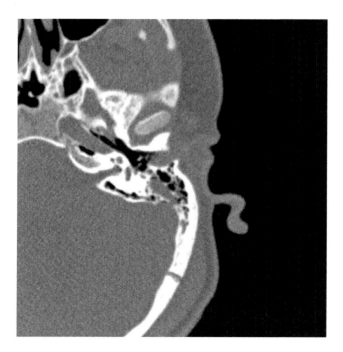

Figure 4.36d

Model answer

These are selected brain soft tissue and bone window images from a CT scan of the head. The axial soft tissue window image (Figure 4.36a) shows foci of intra-axial high density in the right inferobasal frontal region. Figure 4.36b shows more foci of high density in the subcortical region at the grey–white matter junction of the left frontal lobe.

Figures 4.36c and 4.36d show the temporal bony regions. There is pneumocephalus adjacent to the left sigmoid plate. The focused image of the left mastoid region shows a subtle disruption of the bony cortex of the left sigmoid plate with adjacent non-specific soft tissue opacification in the mastoid air cells. The left lambdoid suture is widened.

The constellation of findings and clinical history is consistent with bifrontal contusion with left lambdoid suture diastasis, left sigmoid plate fracture and pneumocephalus. The opacification in the left mastoid air cells may represent CSF, blood or serous fluid.

Questions

1. **What would be your next imaging modality, and why?**
   The next imaging modality of choice would be MRI, to assess sequelae of this post-traumatic head injury case. MRI is more sensitive than CT in detecting diffuse axonal injury, oedema and subtle subarachnoid blood.
2. **Which sequence is more sensitive for detecting blood products?**
   $T2^*$ gradient echo imaging is the technique of choice, as it is sensitive in detecting blood products. The $T2^*$ effect is the imaging technique used as a basis for susceptibility-weighted imaging (SWI).
3. **Is there any limitation of gradient echo imaging that you should be aware of?**
   The bone–air interface at the floor of the frontal and temporal bones can cause susceptibility artefact.
4. **What do you think about the opacification of the mastoid air cells?**
   Mastoid air cell opacification in conjunction with a bony cortical break of the sigmoid plate represents an open fracture that may result in a CSF leak and is associated with a risk of meningitis and venous sinus thrombosis.

Key points

- Diffuse axonal injury (DAI) is a severe brain injury resulting from a combination of severe deceleration, acceleration and rotational forces. Shearing occurs at the grey–white matter interface.
- Infants are more susceptible to this type of injury than older children and adults because of their relative larger head size, weaker neck muscles, softer skull bones and increased CSF spaces.
- More severe injury can result in lesions in the centrum semiovale, the body and splenium of the corpus callosum, the brainstem, the dorsolateral midbrain, pons and cerebellar peduncles.
- Corpus callosal lesions can result in intraventricular haemorrhage, thought to be due to rupture of the subependymal veins.

Further reading

Chavhan GB, Babyn PS, Thomas B, Shroff MM, Haacke EM. Principles, techniques, and applications of T2*-based MR imaging and its special applications. *Radiographics* 2009; **29**: 1433–49.

Hammound DA, Wasserman BA. Diffuse axonal injury: pathophysiology and imaging. *Neuroimaging Clin N Am* 2002; **12**: 205–16.

Poussaint TY, Moeller KK. Imaging of pediatric head trauma. *Neuroimaging Clin N Am* 2002; **12**: 271–94.

Neuroradiology Case 37

JESSIE AW

Clinical history

Post motor vehicle accident.

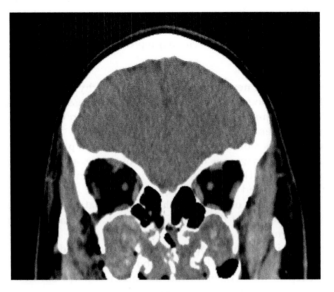

Figure 4.37a

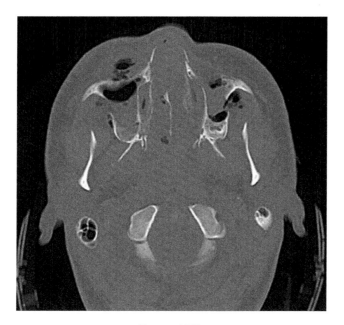

Figure 4.37b

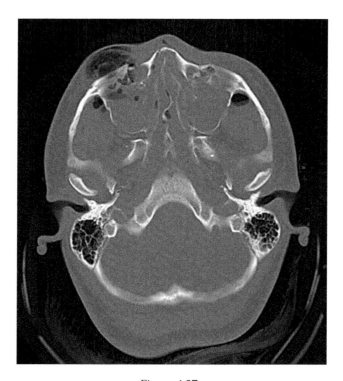

Figure 4.37c

Model answer

These are two axial bone window images and a coronal soft tissue window image from a CT scan of the head (Figures 4.37a–4.37c). The coronal image shows heterogeneous high-density opacification within the maxillary antra and nasal cavity. There are fractures of the lateral maxillary walls. The limited view of the brain shows no abnormality.

The axial images show subcutaneous emphysema in the soft tissues of the mid face and infratemporal fossae bilaterally. There are air–fluid levels in the maxillary antra. There are extensive comminuted and displaced craniofacial fractures. The naso-ethmoid-orbital complex may also be fractured. I would like to review the rest of the imaging to further characterize the fractures, as well as to look for associated injuries.

Questions

1. **What associated intracranial injuries would you assess for?**

I would assess for diffuse axonal and contra-coup injuries, intra- or extra-axial haemorrhage/collections, midline shift, oedema, skull base or calvarial fractures, and sutural diastasis.

2. **Which bone is at risk in naso-ethmoid-orbital fractures?**

The cribriform plate. Fracture of the cribriform plate would provide an open communication into the anterior cranial fossa, resulting in CSF leaks.

3. **Would you be concerned about the globes?**

Yes, I would assess for any associated ocular injuries such as ocular haemorrhage, lens displacement/subluxation and radio-opaque foreign bodies.

4. **What ducts are associated with naso-ethmoid-orbital fractures?**

The nasolacrimal and nasofrontal ducts.

Key points

- There are several classifications for facial fractures. They can be classified according to anatomy or by the amount of energy in the trauma/impact (low-, medium- and high-energy trauma).
- Anatomical classification is based on the location of the bony injuries, and they are classified as limited, transfacial and smash fractures.
  - Limited fractures can be either simple (e.g. a nasal fracture) or complex (e.g. a malar fracture).
  - Transfacial fractures are those that follow the fracture lines described by Le Fort (in their various combinations). A pure classic Le Fort fracture is rare.
  - Smash fractures are severely comminuted fractures, which do not follow the classic transfacial fracture lines described by Le Fort. They are fractures involving the naso-ethmoid-orbital, midface or craniofacial structures.
- A simplified scheme to work out the different types of Le Fort fractures (Rhea and Novelline 2005):
  - The pterygoid process is involved in almost every Le Fort fracture
  - Le Fort 1 – fracture of the lateral margin of the nasal fossa
  - Le Fort 2 – fracture of the inferior orbital rim
  - Le Fort 3 – fracture of the zygomatic arch
- More than one Le Fort fracture can be present (e.g. Le Fort 2 and 3 can occur together). Also, Le Fort fractures do not have to be bilateral and symmetric.

Further reading

Rhea JT, Novelline RA. How to simplify the CT diagnosis of Le Fort fractures. *AJR Am J Roentgenol* 2005; **184**: 1700–5.

Sun JK, LeMay DR. Imaging of facial trauma. *Neuroimaging Clin N Am* 2002; **12**: 295–309.

Neuroradiology Case 38

JESSIE AW

Clinical history
Patient presents with continuous ear discharge.

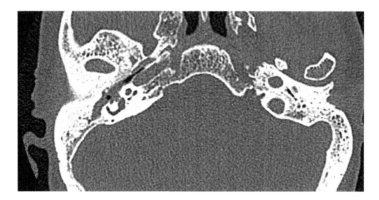

Figure 4.38a

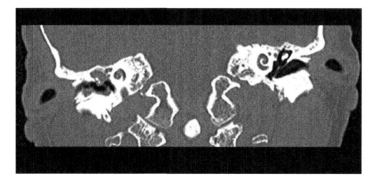

Figure 4.38b

Model answer
These are selected images from a high-resolution CT temporal bone series (Figures 4.38a, 4.38b). The right external auditory canal (EAC) and middle ear cavity are abnormal. There is soft tissue along the floor of the right EAC. The floor itself appears irregular. The ipsilateral tympanic membrane is retracted.

There is further soft tissue opacification seen in the right epitympanum and meso-tympanum. The soft tissue is extending into the aditus ad antrum. I would also like to assess the sinus tympanum, which is not seen on these two selected images.

The bony margin over the right vestibule is highly attenuated and may be eroded with fistula formation. The soft tissue is abutting the tympanic segment of the right facial nerve and dehiscence cannot be excluded. The tegmen tympani is intact. The majority of the ossicular chain is eroded and the margin of the scutum is irregular. All these features are consistent with a cholesteatoma with a possible vestibular fistula.

The mastoid air cells are under-pneumatized bilaterally; there may have been chronic otitis externa in childhood.

The left middle ear cavity appears normal on these selected images.

Questions

1. What is a cholesteatoma?

Cholesteatoma is a cystic lesion with keratin debris formed by keratinized squamous epithelium, which is thought to have migrated into the middle ear from the external canal.

2. What are the differential diagnoses for the case?

Granulation tissue, debris, cholesterol granuloma, fibrous tissue and mucoid secretions.

3. What are the possible complications of a cholesteatoma?

Cholesteatomas can block the aditus ad antrum, which is the route into and out of the mastoid air cells. The presence of infected material within the mastoid air cells can be associated with spread of infection through the mastoid cortex, resulting in a subperiosteal abscess.

Erosion of the tegmen tympani can also occur, resulting in the transgression of the cholesteatoma into the middle cranial fossa.

4. How are cholesteatomas treated?

They are treated surgically, but there is a high risk of recurrence.

Key points

- Cholesteatomas invade soft tissue structures and bone due to a combination of pressure effects and osteoclastic enzyme activity.
- Cholesteatomas can be either congenital or acquired. Acquired cholesteatomas can either be primary or secondary. Primary acquired cholesteatomas (also known as attic cholesteatomas) present without evidence of tympanic membrane perforation or infection. Secondary acquired cholesteatoma is associated with tympanic membrane perforation (e.g. due to trauma or infection).
- High-resolution CT of the temporal bone is the imaging modality of choice. The absence of abnormal soft tissue or bony destruction on temporal bone HRCT has a high negative predictive value.

Further reading

Aikele P, Kittner T, Offergeld C, *et al*. Diffusion-weighted MR imaging of cholesteatoma in pediatric and adult patients who have undergone middle ear surgery. *AJR Am J Roentgenol* 2003; **181**: 261–5.

Semaan MT, Megerian CA. The pathophysiology of cholesteatoma. *Otolaryngol Clin N Am* 2006: **39**; 1143–59.

Shohet JA, de Jong AL. The management of pediatric cholesteatoma. *Otolaryngol Clin N Am* 2002; **35**: 841–51.

Smith JA, Danner CJ. Complications of chronic otitis media and cholesteatoma. *Otolaryngol Clin N Am* 2006; **39**: 1237–55.

Neuroradiology Case 39

JESSIE AW

Clinical history

A 68-year-old presents with tiredness, memory problems and worsening visual problems.

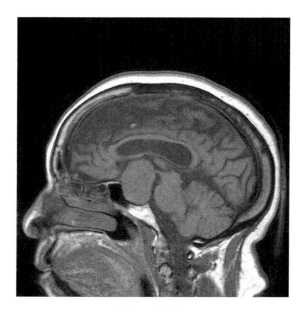

Figure 4.39a

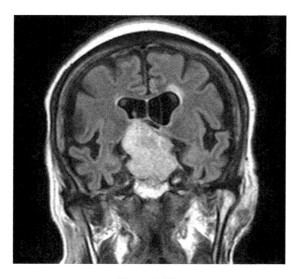

Figure 4.39b

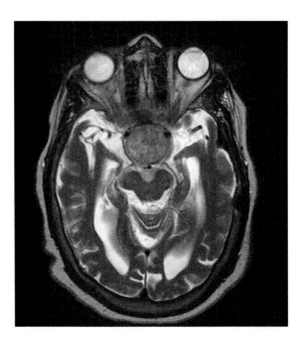

Figure 4.39c

Model answer

These are selected sagittal non-contrast T1, coronal FLAIR and axial T2 images from an MRI of the brain (Figures 4.39a–4.39c).

There is a large mass arising from the expanded pituitary fossa. The mass extends superiorly into the suprasellar cistern, effaces the third ventricle and compresses the floor of the lateral ventricles. It also exerts a mass effect on the fornices, predominantly on the right. The lesion is of homogeneously low T1 signal, has a heterogeneous high signal on FLAIR, and has a mixed signal on the T2-weighted sequence. The small foci of intratumoral high signal on T2 suggests small intratumoral cysts. The mass displaces the cavernous segments of the internal carotid arteries laterally. The optic chiasm is not visualized but is almost certainly compressed. The features are consistent with a large pituitary macroadenoma.

There are background changes of generalized sulcal prominence and ventriculomegaly consistent with atrophy.

Questions

1. **What are the differential diagnoses for a sellar tumour?**

   The differential diagnosis for a sellar lesion includes a pituituary adenoma, Rathke's cleft cysts, craniopharyngiomas, meningioma of the tuberculum sellae, metastases, hamartoma and optic glioma.

2. **What is the most common sellar lesion?**

   A pituitary adenoma.

3. **What is the treatment for symptomatic non-hormone-producing pituitary macroadenomas?**

   Surgical decompression is the treatment of choice, in order to debulk and decompress the tumour. Indications for surgery include size of the tumour, change in size and mass effect.

4. **How useful is the postoperative post-contrast MRI?**

   The postoperative MRI is useful to predict recurrence of tumour. If there is residual tumour present, then up to a third of patients will have recurrent growth.

Key points
- The transsphenoidal approach is the favoured surgical method to decompress most sellar and suprasellar lesions (except craniopharyngioma).
- Tumours that are enlarging or causing significant mass effect should be considered for surgery. Hypopituitarism and visual defects are also indications for surgery. Sellar or suprasellar lesions that are difficult to approach using the transsphenoidal route can be accessed by subfrontal, anterior interhemispheric and transcallosal approaches.
- 10% of pituitary microadenomas grow significantly. Follow-up imaging is usually indicated annually or every two years. Shorter follow-up imaging is only indicated if significant growth occurs.

Further reading
Jagannathan J, Kanter AS, Sheehan JP, Jane JA, Laws ER. Benign brain tumors: sellar / parasellar tumors. *Neurol Clin* 2007; **25**: 1231–49.
Molitch ME. Nonfunctioning pituitary tumors and pituitary incidentalomas. *Endocrinol Metab Clin N Am* 2008; **37**: 151–71.

Neuroradiology Case 40

JESSIE AW

Clinical history
A young female with a history of asthma presents with persistent stuffiness and post-nasal drip.

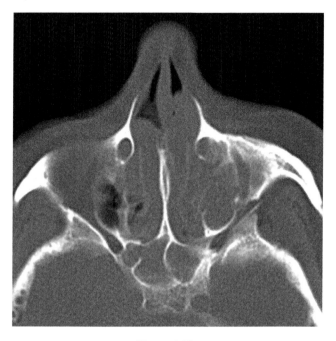

Figure 4.40a

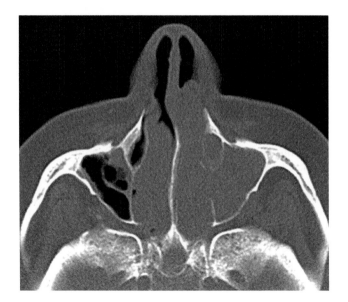

Figure 4.40b

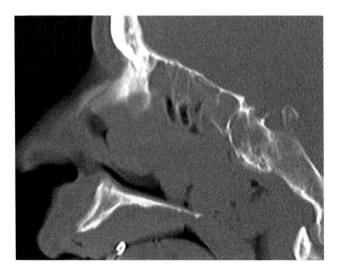

Figure 4.40c

Model answer

These are two axial and one sagittal bone window images from a CT scan of the sinuses (Figures 4.40a–4.40c). The axial images show virtually complete soft tissue opacification of the anterior and posterior ethmoid air cells, the left maxillary antrum and sphenoid sinuses. There is some mucosal thickening in the right maxillary antrum in association with a few air bubbles. These soft tissue opacifications have polypoid morphology on the sagittal image. Some are entering into the nasopharynx. The bones appear normal, with no evidence of hyperostosis, destruction or severe thinning due to chronic pressure effects. The findings are compatible with severe nasal polyposis.

Questions

1. **Who has a predisposition for nasal polyps?**
   Asthmatics, aspirin-sensitive people and cystic fibrosis patients.
2. **What are the surgical options available for patients with polyposis?**
   Polypectomy and functional endoscopic sinus surgery (FESS).
3. **What CT features could suggest neoplasm?**
   Unilateral opacification of the sinuses with positive mass effect and bony destruction would suggest a more aggressive disease process.
4. **How would you evaluate this further?**
   MRI of the sinuses with contrast can be performed to differentiate benign paranasal sinus disease from other aggressive paranasal entities.

Key points

- The aetiology of nasal polyps is unknown. It is a separate form of chronic rhinosinusitis.
- Nasal polyps tend to occur in narrow areas of mucosal contact such as the middle meatus.
- Polyps can be treated either medically or surgically. The mainstay of medical management is steroid therapy – with intranasal being first-line treatment and systemic steroids as a medical form of polypectomy.
- Surgery is reserved for patients who are refractory to medical treatment. The surgical technique used is known as FESS: functional endoscopic sinus surgery.
- CT is the imaging modality of choice and best depicts the bony architecture of the paranasal sinuses. MRI is reserved for the evaluation of soft tissue masses and intercompartmental spread, as it is better at defining the soft tissue planes and assessing possible tumour versus secretions.

Further reading

Aygun N, Zinreich SJ. Imaging for functional endoscopic sinus surgery. *Otolaryngol Clin N Am* 2006; **39**: 403–16.

Becker SS. Surgical management of polyps in the treatment of nasal airway obstruction. *Otolaryngol Clin N Am* 2009; **42**: 377–85.

Bikhazi NB. Contemporary management of nasal polyps. *Otolaryngol Clin N Am* 2004; **37**: 327–37.

Neuroradiology Case 41

JESSIE AW

Clinical history
A 64-year-old male presents with a several-month history of bleeding and painful gums.

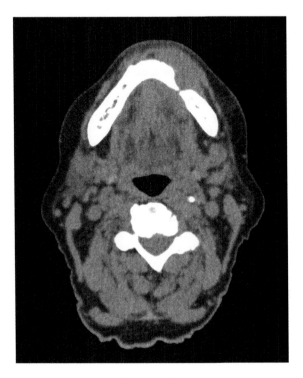

Figure 4.41a

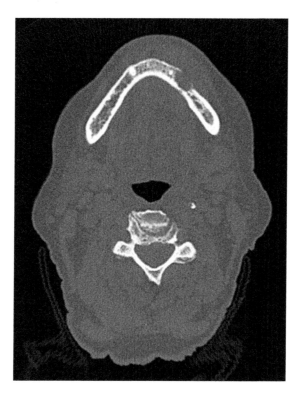

Figure 4.41b

Model answer

These are selected images from a non-contrast-enhanced CT examination of the cervical soft tissue (Figures 4.41a, 4.41b). The two axial images show an area of abnormality in the left hemimandible. There is a focal area of bony destruction. The bony lesion has ill-defined irregular margins and is associated with a large soft tissue mass, which extends anteriorly. The surrounding fat planes appear clean. The limited view of the mandible shows that the patient is nearly edentulous. No cervical lymphadenopathy is seen on these selected images.

The differential diagnoses include squamous cell carcinoma of the buccal mucosa and periodontal abscess. A biopsy of the lesion is required. The patient will require a staging CT scan of the chest and abdomen if malignancy is diagnosed.

Questions

1. **What would you do next, if the patient were still on the scanner?**
   Repeat the CT with intravenous contrast.
2. **If this were a tumour, where would you define the anatomical subsite for the lesion?**
   The subsite would be in the oral cavity.
3. **What is the posterior margin of the oral cavity?**
   The posterior margin is the anterior tonsillar pillars.
4. **Is the tongue base included in the oral cavity?**
   No, the tongue base is part of the oropharynx.

Key points

- The anatomical boundaries of the oral cavity are from the lips to the junction of the hard and soft palate. Its inferior extent is the circumvallate papillae, which separates the oral tongue from the base of the tongue. The posterior margin of the oral cavity is the anterior tonsillar pillars.

- The mucosa of the oral cavity and oropharynx are different, and thus tumours in these subsites behave differently.
- Smoking and alcohol are risk factors in head and neck cancer. Both these factors potentiate each other to increase the risk further.
- CT is excellent for assessing bone invasion.
- Squamous cell carcinoma on MRI is isointense to muscle on T1- and iso- to hyper-intense on T2-weighted sequences, with homogeneous moderate enhancement.

Notes
The diagnosis in this case was squamous carcinoma.

Further reading
Crozier E, Sumer BD. Head and neck cancer. *Med Clin North Am* 2010; **94**: 1031–46.
Stambuk HE, Karimi S, Lee N, Patel SG. Oral cavity and oropharynx tumors. *Radiol Clin North Am* 2007; **45**: 1–20.

Neuroradiology Case 42

JESSIE AW

Clinical history
Routine eye test finds abnormality in a 2½-year-old boy.

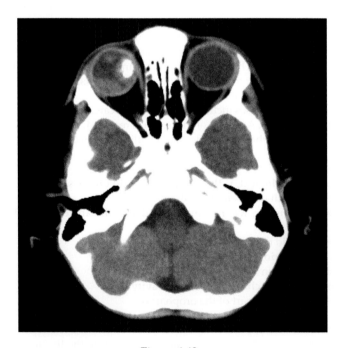

Figure 4.42a

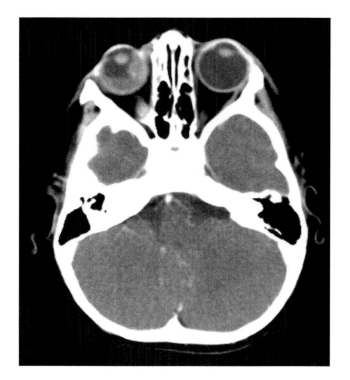

Figure 4.42b

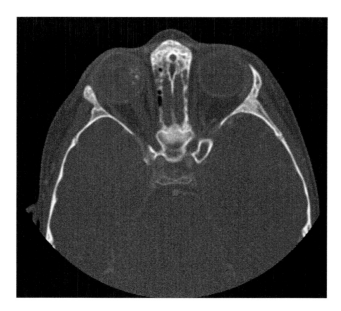

Figure 4.42c

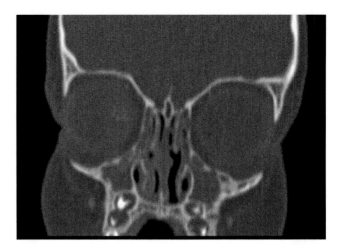

Figure 4.42d

Model answer

These are selected images from a CT head with and without contrast (Figures 4.42a–4.42d). There is a large lobulated mass in the posterior part of the right globe that contains areas of calcification and enhances homogeneously with intravenous contrast. The lesion does not extend beyond the globe. The retro-orbital fat remains normal. The optic nerve appears normal.

The left globe appears normal. The visualized brain and CSF spaces appear unremarkable. The appearances suggest retinoblastoma of the right eye.

Questions

1. **What is the inheritance pattern in familial retinoblastoma?**
   Autosomal dominant. Some cases may be sporadic.
2. **Does the presence of calcification help with the imaging diagnosis?**
   The presence of calcification is very characteristic for retinoblastoma, and CT is the imaging modality of choice to detect foci of calcification. (*NB: calcification occurs in over 70% of retinoblastomas.*)

Key points

- It is the commonest childhood ocular tumour. The tumour occurs either sporadically (60%) or is inherited in an autosomal dominant fashion (40%).
- There is no racial or gender predilection.
- MRI is complementary in the management. A baseline MRI is helpful to detect retrobulbar spread, and to determine intracranial spread and the presence of concurrent tumours.
- Trilateral retinoblastoma means bilateral retinoblastomas and an intracranial tumour, commonly in the pineal gland, suprasellar or parasellar region.

Further reading

Apushkin MA, Apushkin MA, Shapiro MJ, Mafee MF. Retinoblastoma and simulating lesions: role of imaging. *Neuroimaging Clin N Am* 2005; **15**: 49–67.

Neuroradiology Case 43

JESSIE AW

Clinical history
Visual disturbance.

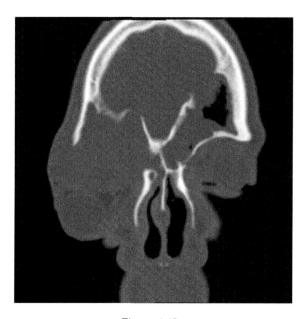

Figure 4.43a

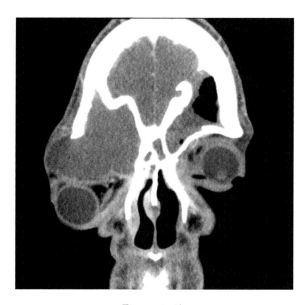

Figure 4.43b

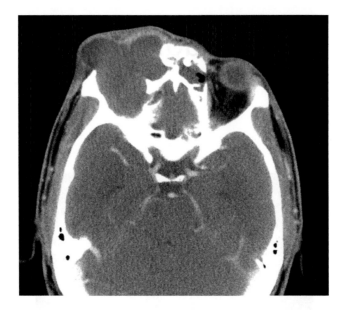

Figure 4.43c

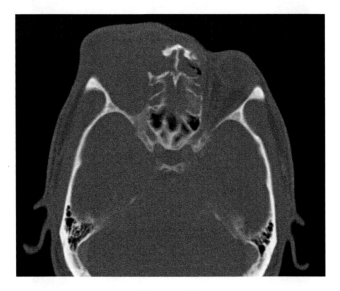

Figure 4.43d

Model answer

These are selected coronal and axial bone and soft tissue window images of the frontal sinuses and orbits (Figures 4.43a–4.43d).

The coronal images show soft tissue opacification within the right frontal sinus. The anterior wall of the right frontal sinus and the roof of the right orbit are eroded, and the soft tissue mass is causing mass effect and inferior displacement and deformity of the right globe. There is incomplete opacification of the left frontal sinus. The right nasal bone also appears eroded, with complete opacification with soft tissue density. The ethmoid air cells are opacified bilaterally.

This appearance is suggestive of an aggressive paranasal sinus tumour.

Questions

1. How would you take this case further?

I would contact the referring clinician with the results. Further imaging with a contrast-enhanced MRI would be required in order to characterize the non-specific soft tissue opacification and to determine if there is any underlying soft tissue mass.

2. What is a mucocele?

A mucocele is an abnormal epithelial-lined mucus-filled cavity.

3. How do paranasal mucoceles develop?

They usually develop because of obstruction of the outflow drainage pathway of the paranasal sinuses.

Key points

- The frontal sinus outflow is surgically less accessible and narrowed compared to the other sinuses.
- The most common paranasal sinus to develop a mucocele is the frontal sinus.
- There are two surgical options: open or endoscopic treatment. There is a trend towards a transnasal endoscopic approach for the surgical treatment of frontal mucoceles.
- Surgery is preferred when the sinonasal region is not infected.

Notes

This was an extreme case of frontal mucocele. In the FRCR examination, one would not be expected to provide a definitive diagnosis, and this would be a case used for further discussion about management.

Further reading

Aygun N, Zinreich SJ. Imaging for functional endoscopic sinus surgery. *Otolaryngol Clin N Am* 2006; **39**: 403–16.

Har-El G. Transnasal endoscopic management of frontal mucoceles. *Otolaryngol Clin N Am* 2001; **34**: 243–51.

McMains KC, Kountakis SE. Fronto-orbital-ethmoid mucoceles. *Oper Tech Otolaryngol* 2006; **17**: 19–23.

Neuroradiology Case 44

JESSIE AW

Clinical history
A 50-year-old male presents with nasal stuffiness, nasal swelling and right eye pain.

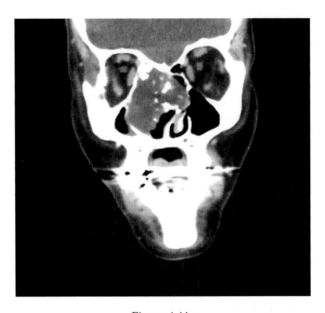

Figure 4.44a

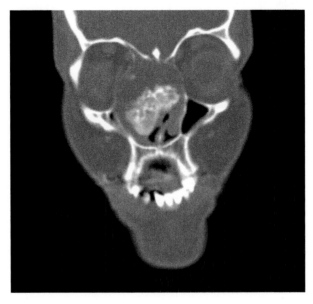

Figure 4.44b

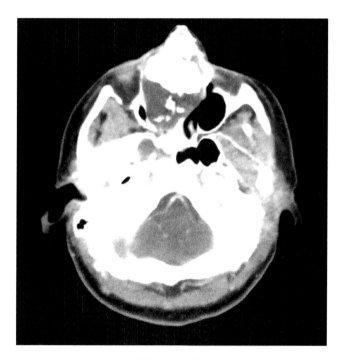

Figure 4.44c

Model answer

One soft tissue window axial image, and selected coronal soft tissue and bone window images from a CT sinus examination are presented (Figures 4.44a–4.44c). There is a large expansile mass in the right nasal cavity, causing mass effect on the nasal septum, which is deviated to the left. The lesion is indenting the medial wall of the right maxillary antrum and the medial walls of both orbits. These bony margins appear highly attenuated. The cribriform plate is not well demonstrated. However, there is a high probability of cribriform plate involvement. The mass is centred on the ethmoid air cells. There are foci of heterogeneous calcification within the inferior part of the mass. The extraconal fat appears clean bilaterally, and the lesion is indenting the right medial rectus muscle.

The findings are consistent with a sinonasal tumour. The differential diagnoses for a calcified mass in this region include chondroma, chondrosarcoma and osteosarcoma. Squamous cell carcinoma, adenocarcinoma and adenoid cystic carcinoma are less likely differential diagnoses. (NB: The latter three are the major differential diagnoses for non-calcified sinonasal masses.)

I would like to review the rest of the imaging on a workstation to look for the extent of disease. The findings need to be urgently communicated to the referring clinician, and the lesion should be biopsied. A contrast-enhanced MRI scan would be helpful to assess the extent of soft tissue spread and to assess for any intracranial extension.

Questions

1. **What imaging features would suggest a benign lesion versus an aggressive lesion?**

   Benign lesions cause bony remodelling, while aggressive lesions cause bony destruction and soft tissue infiltration. Benign lesions can also cause hyperostosis of the underlying bone and, unlike with aggressive lesions, there is an absence of soft tissue infiltration. Size is also an important indicator of malignancy, which is particularly important in this case. The major differential diagnosis lies between chondroma and chondrosarcoma.

2. **What are the other sinonasal tumours?**

Squamous cell carcinoma is the commonest tumour in the paranasal sinuses and are generally non-calcified. Other tumours include adenocarcinomas, juvenile angiofibromas and inverted papillomas. Olfactory neuroblastomas may be calcified.

Key points

- Sarcomas are rare in the sinonasal region. The most common of sarcomas to occur in the sinuses is a chondrosarcoma.
- CT is useful to show the calcified chondroid matrix.
- 50% of head and neck chondrosarcomas occur in the sinonasal region, with the remainder in the mandible and larynx.
- Chondrosarcomas usually occur in the third and fourth decade of life, with no gender predominance.
- Surgical resection is the curative treatment of choice for chondrosarcoma.

Further reading

Hamilton BE, Weissman JL. Imaging of chemosensory loss. *Otolaryngol Clin N Am* 2004; **37**: 1255–80.

Potter BO, Sturgis EM. Sarcomas of the head and neck. *Surg Oncol Clin N Am* 2003; **12**: 379–417.

Neuroradiology Case 45

JESSIE AW

Clinical history

Recurrent ear infections.

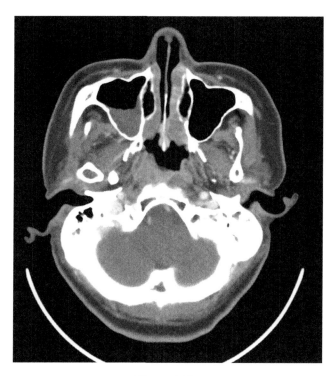

Figure 4.45a

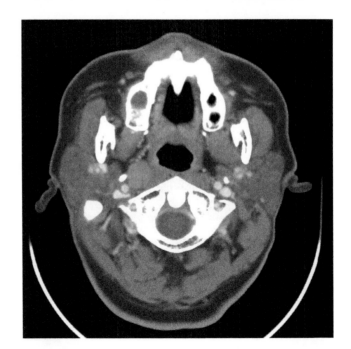

Figure 4.45b

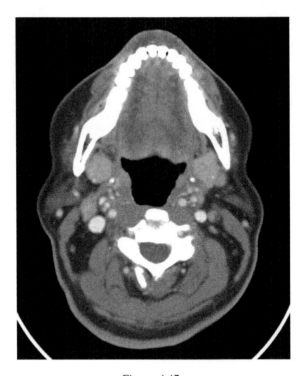

Figure 4.45c

Model answer

These are selected images from a CT soft tissue of the neck with IV contrast. Figure 4.45a shows asymmetry of the nasopharynx with soft tissue thickening with enhancement on the right. There is abnormal enhancing soft tissue obliterating the right fossa of Rosenmuller and more soft tissue anteriorly at the opening of the Eustachian tube. The right torus tubarius muscle is not well visualized and is most likely involved.

Figure 4.45b shows an enlarged separate soft tissue mass in the right retropharyngeal region consistent with a retropharyngeal node. Figure 4.45c shows an enlarged right level 2b lymph node and a small left level 2b node. The mastoid air cells appear clear bilaterally.

The findings are highly suspicious for a right nasopharyngeal tumour with a right retropharyngeal enlarged node and most likely an involved right level 2b node. The left level 2b node seen is indeterminate.

I would like to check the bony windows for any evidence of skull base bony erosion.

Questions

1. **Why is the patient getting recurrent ear infections?**
   The right Eustachian tube is blocked by the tumour mass, leading to secondary otitis media.
2. **Where is a frequent site for nasopharyngeal carcinomas (NPCs) to originate in?**
   The fossa of Rosenmuller and its surrounding areas are a frequent site.
3. **Is there an increased risk for NPC in any particular racial group?**
   Chinese, particularly southern Chinese.
4. **Is there a gender predilection?**
   There is a higher incidence in men than in women.
5. **Is there a relationship between NPC and smoking or alcohol?**
   No. Unlike squamous cell carcinoma in the head and neck region, there is no relationship to smoking or alcohol.

Key points

- NPC has a bimodal incidence peak. One peak is in the 30- to 40-year-olds and the second peak occurs in the fifth and sixth decades of life.
- The parapharyngeal space is the most common site for NPC invasion.
- Common nodal sites for NPC are retropharyngeal (as in this case), levels 2, 3 and 5.
- The primary treatment for NPC is radiotherapy.
- In advanced T3 or T4 lesions, additional chemotherapy can be added to the treatment regimen.

Further reading

Weber AL, Arayedh SA, Rashid A. Nasopharynx: clinical, pathologic, and radiologic assessment. *Neuroimaging Clin N Am* 2003; **13**: 465–83.

Neuroradiology Case 46

JESSIE AW

Clinical history
Previously healthy 55-year-old female presents with right hand and finger weakness.

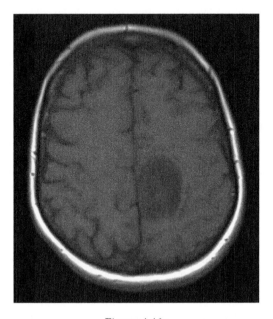

Figure 4.46a

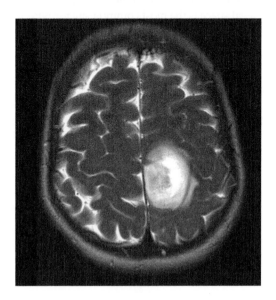

Figure 4.46b

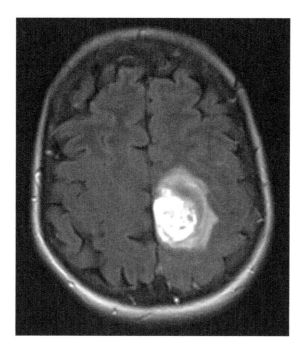

Figure 4.46c

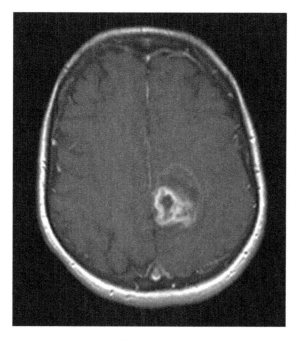

Figure 4.46d

Model answer

These are selected images from a pre- and post-contrast MRI of the brain (Figures 4.46a–4.46d), showing an intra-axial lesion in the mesial left frontoparietal region. It appears to be straddling the pre- and postcentral gyri. The lesion returns a heterogeneous high signal on T2 and is of low signal on T1. Part of the T2 high signal within the lesion suppresses with FLAIR. The lesion demonstrates intense irregular rim enhancement with ill-defined borders. There is high T2-weighted signal in the white matter adjacent to the mass. The findings are consistent with a mass that contains central necrosis and with associated surrounding peritumoral oedema. There is local mass effect but no midline shift. I would further evaluate the remainder of the study to check for any other lesions or hydrocephalus.

If this were a solitary lesion, then I would favour a primary glial neoplasm over metastases. The enhancement and features that suggest necrosis would suggest that this is a high-grade rather than a low-grade primary lesion.

Questions

1. **What are the differential diagnoses for a ring-enhancing lesion?**
   Metastases, abscesses, an active multiple sclerosis plaque, haematoma, and atypical infective lesions such as neurocystercosis or tuberculosis.
2. **What is the commonest primary intra-axial tumour in adults?**
   Astrocytomas. They have varying degrees of malignancy, depending on histological grading.
3. **Where do primary glial tumours occur?**
   Primary glial tumours usually arise in the deep white matter of the brain and do not usually involve grey matter.
4. **Which compartment does glioblastoma multiforme nearly always occur in – supra- or infratentorial?**
   Glioblastomas almost always occur in the supratentorial compartment.

Key points

- Glioblastoma multiforme (GBM) is a World Health Organization grade 4 tumour. They are histologically similar to anaplastic astrocytomas except that there are more features of anaplasia and the presence of necrosis.
- Primary brain tumours infiltrate locally into the adjacent white matter. The peritumoral oedema seen may contain microscopic tumour cells.
- The disease is considered incurable. Treatment can prolong survival. Poor prognostic factors include older age at diagnosis, higher histological grade, a short duration of symptoms and low Karnofsky performance score.
- Current treatment is surgical resection and postoperative radiotherapy.

Further reading

Altman DA, Atkinson DS, Brat DJ. Best cases from the AFIP: glioblastoma multiforme. *Radiographics* 2007; **27**: 883–8.

Neuroradiology Case 47

JESSIE AW

Clinical history
A 40-year-old female presents with arm weakness and paraesthesia.

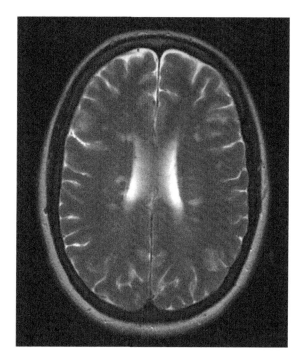

Figure 4.47a

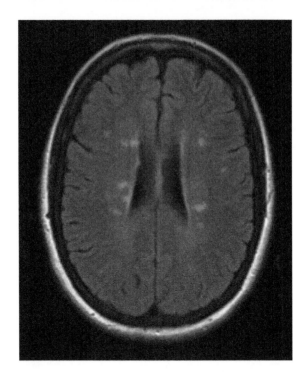

Figure 4.47b

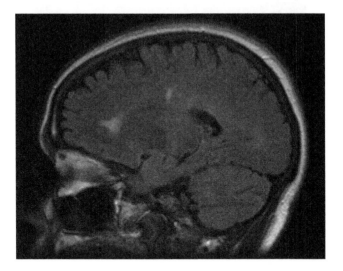

Figure 4.47c

Model answer

The images are from a non-contrast MRI brain study: axial T2-weighted, FLAIR and sagittal FLAIR (Figures 4.47a–4.47c). There are multiple high T2/FLAIR signal foci in the white matter of both cerebral hemispheres in a periventricular distribution. They are orientated perpendicular to the lateral ventricle, which is more apparent on the sagittal image, and at least one has a 'flame-shaped' appearance. The appearance is non-specific and the differential would include demyelination, ischaemic and inflammatory causes.

I would like to assess the remainder of the examination for any pericallosal, sub-cortical U-fibre or brainstem lesions. If there were such lesions present then multiple sclerosis is favoured.

An MRI of the spinal cord should be performed if multiple sclerosis is suspected.

Questions

1. **What are the subtypes of multiple sclerosis (MS)?**

   MS has several subtypes, based on the clinical course of the disease. The subtypes are relapsing and remitting, secondary progressive, primary progressive and progressive relapsing.

2. **What are the other less common forms of demyelinating diseases?**

   They are acute disseminated encephalomyelitis (ADEM), Devic's neuromyelitis optica, Balo's concentric sclerosis and Marburg.

   ADEM and Devic's are distinct diseases, while the latter two are rare variants of MS.

3. **Can MS affect men?**

   MS can affect men, and has a more aggressive course in men than in women.

4. **Which sequence is best to assess lesions in the posterior fossa and brainstem?**

   The T2-weighted sequence.

5. **Which sequence is best for assessing supratentorial lesions?**

   The FLAIR sequence in the axial and sagittal planes.

Key points

- Multiple sclerosis is thought to be a chronic immune-mediated disease.
- Oligoclonal bands are not specific for MS.
- In a patient with MS the spinal cord is commonly involved. Spinal cord lesions are not found in healthy individuals, unlike the non-specific high T2 white matter signal foci, which occur and increase with age.
- Contrast-enhancing lesions in the brain can occur, either the already identified high T2/FLAIR signal foci or other lesions, which may be inconspicuous on the non-contrast study but are active MS lesions.
- ADEM is another immune-mediated demyelinating disease. It is preceded by an infection (viral or bacterial) or vaccination and usually occurs in children, but it has been reported in adults.

Further reading

Bot JC, Barkhof F. Spinal-cord MRI in multiple sclerosis: conventional and nonconventional MR techniques. *Neuroimaging Clin N Am* 2009; **19**: 81–99.

Courtney AM, Treadaway K, Remington G, Frohman E. Multiple sclerosis. *Med Clin North Am* 2009; **93**: 451–76.

Lubin FD, Reingold SC. Defining the clinical course of multiple sclerosis: results of an international survey. *Neurology* 1996; **46**: 907–11.

Simon JH, Kleinschmidt-DeMasters BK. Variants of multiple sclerosis. *Neuroimaging Clin N Am* 2008; **18**: 703–16.

Neuroradiology Case 48

JESSIE AW

Clinical history
Post cardiac arrest, altered mental status and function.

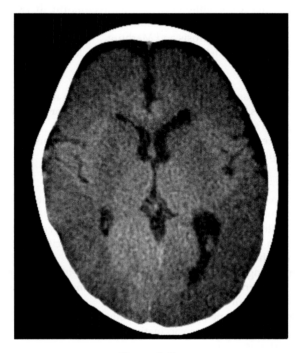

Figure 4.48a

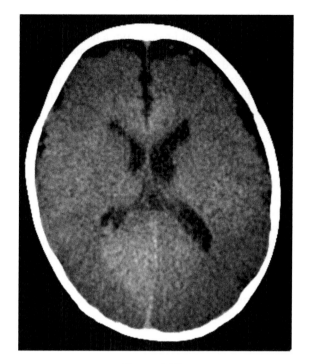

Figure 4.48b

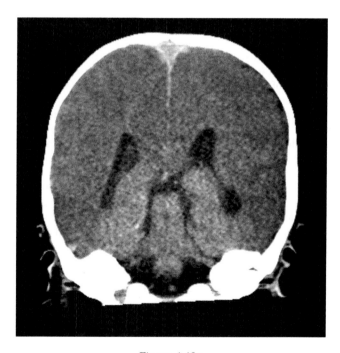

Figure 4.48c

Model answer

These are selected axial and coronal images from a non-contrast CT brain (Figures 4.48a–4.48c). The images show extensive bilateral abnormalities of the cerebral hemispheres. There is generalized sulcal effacement with reversal of the grey–white matter differentiation. The basal ganglia are also affected bilaterally, with symmetric low density. There is no midline shift, intra- or extra-axial haemorrhage or herniation on these selected images.

The findings are consistent with diffuse hypoxic–ischaemic injury. Reversal of grey and white matter differentiation is a poor prognostic sign. I would immediately contact the clinical team to relay the findings urgently.

Questions

1. **What is the imaging modality of choice for hypoxic–ischaemic injury?**
   MRI with diffusion-weighted imaging.
2. **What would you see on diffusion-weighted imaging?**
   Restricted diffusion will be seen in the affected areas, so ischaemia or acute infarct will be bright on diffusion and dark on the corresponding ADC map.

Key points

- Hypoxic–ischaemic injury (HII) could be due to reduced blood oxygenation, reduced cerebral perfusion or a combination of the two. Hypoxaemia, often aggravated by secondary hypoxic cardiac impairment, is the most common cause of HII in children. Hypoperfusion, with secondary tissue hypoxia, is the commonest underlying cause of HII in adults. The severity and duration of the insult, brain maturity and the timing of the imaging study can all influence the pattern of injury seen. In general, the most metabolically active brain cells and those containing the highest amounts of excitatory neurotransmitters, such as glutamate, are most vulnerable to HII. These are usually the neurones in the deep and superficial grey matter. In preterm neonates, less severe HII can result in intraventricular and cerebellar haemorrhage due to germinal matrix injury. More severe HII damages the deep grey matter (especially the thalami). Periventricular leukomalacia, where there is evidence of periventricular white matter changes, is another form of HII which affects premature infants.
- Severe HII in term infants tends to affect the deep grey matter nuclei with relative sparing of the cortex. More prolonged HII will affect cortical grey matter. Prolonged moderate HII in term infants can present with damage to the watershed areas due to shunting of blood from the cortical regions to the deep grey matter nuclei.
- Severe HII in infants aged 1–2 tends to affect the deep and cortical grey matter, with relative sparing of the thalami. Watershed changes are seen in moderate HII.
- Severe HII in older children and adults affects the deep and cortical grey matter. Cerebellar damage is commoner in this age group. Watershed changes are seen in moderate HII.

Further reading

Barkovich AJ. *Pediatric Neuroimaging*, 4th edn. Philadelphia, PA: Lippincott Williams & Wilkins, 2005; 205–6.
Yuang BY, Castillo M. Hypoxic–ischemic brain injury: imaging findings from birth to adulthood. *Radiographics* 2008; **28**: 417–39.

Neuroradiology Case 49

JESSIE AW

Clinical history
Known to have headaches and seizures. Increasing frequency of seizures.

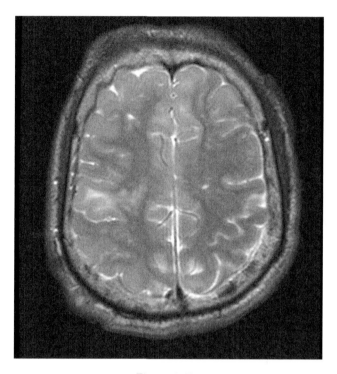

Figure 4.49a

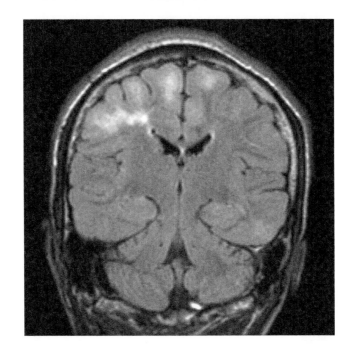

Figure 4.49b

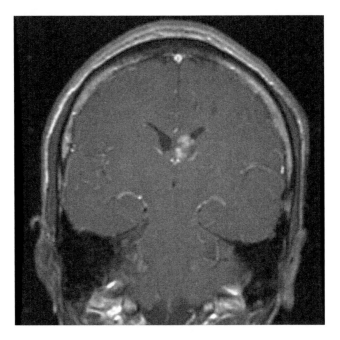

Figure 4.49c

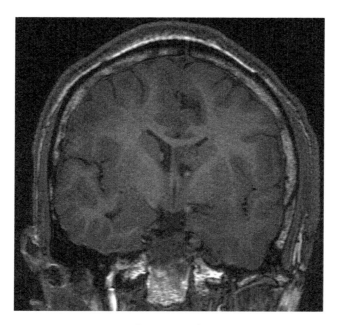

Figure 4.49d

Model answer

These are selected axial T2, coronal FLAIR, T1 pre- and post-contrast images from an MRI brain (Figures 4.49a–4.49d). The axial T2-weighted image shows high T2 signal in the subcortical and deep white matter affecting the right frontal lobe in the precentral gyrus. The coronal FLAIR sequence shows multiple areas of high signal in the subcortical and deep white matter of both cerebral hemispheres. The coronal precontrast shows subependymal nodules lining the lateral ventricles bilaterally and there is a lesion at the left foramen of Monro, which enhances with contrast.

The enhancing lesion in the left foramen of Monro is a subependymal giant-cell astrocytoma, and the high subcortical lesions represent cortical tubers. The features are diagnostic of tuberous sclerosis. I will inform the clinicians of the findings and will compare the findings with previous imaging, if available. The patient will require yearly MRI to follow up the subependymal giant-cell astrocytoma.

Questions

1. **What is the inheritance pattern for tuberous sclerosis (TS)?**
   TS is an autosomal dominant disorder with variable clinical expression.
2. **What are cortical tubers?**
   Cortical tubers are benign hamartomas.
3. **Which other organs does TS affect?**
   - Heart – cardiac rhabdomyomas
   - Eyes
   - Skin – hypomelanotic macules, facial angiofibromas, ungula fibromas
   - Kidneys – cysts, angiomyolipomas and rarely renal cell carcinoma
   - Lungs – lymphangioleiomyomatosis
4. **What should you be concerned about in a patient with giant-cell astrocytoma who develops a headache?**
   An enlarging giant-cell astrocytoma and the development of obstructive hydrocephalus. The latter can occur relatively quickly. Any symptom of raised intracranial pressure is an indication for urgent neuroimaging.

Key points

- The diagnosis of tuberous sclerosis is based on well-defined clinical and imaging criteria. These are listed by Umeoka *et al.* (2008).
- Tuberous sclerosis is inherited in an autosomal dominant pattern, although a significant proportion of cases can be attributed to new mutations.
- Tubers are usually seen at the grey–white junction, and they are detected by T2-weighted or FLAIR sequences.
- Subependymal nodules can calcify and are best seen on CT. They will demonstrate low T2 signal.
- Non-calcified subependymal nodules will be isointense to white matter on T1- and T2-weighted sequences. They are usually found along the walls of the lateral ventricles.
- Giant-cell astrocytomas do not usually grow after 20 years of age.

Further reading

Umeoka S, Koyama T, Miki Y, *et al.* Pictorial review of tuberous sclerosis in various organs. *Radiographics* 2008; **28**: e32.

Genitourinary Case 1

KIAT T. TAN AND RICHARD HOPKINS

Clinical history
Patient involved in road traffic accident.

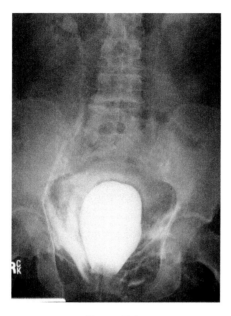

Figure 5.1a

Model answer
This is a selected image from a cystogram (Figure 5.1a). A catheter is in the well-distended bladder. Contrast has refluxed into both ureters and pelvicalyceal systems. There is leakage of contrast from the urinary bladder that is contained within the pelvis. The contrast has not outlined any intraperitoneal structures such as bowel loops. There are bilateral pubic rami fractures. The sacroiliac joints are normal.

The findings are consistent with extraperitoneal rupture of the bladder that is associated with fractures of the pubic rami. This patient will require a CT scan of the abdomen and pelvis for further characterization of the bladder injury as well as for the detection of occult injuries. The patient will need to be referred to the urologists and orthopaedic surgeons for management of the bladder injury and pubic rami fractures. The catheter should remain in position.

Questions
1. **What are the different types of bladder injury?**
   Bladder injuries are classified into five types:
   Type 1 refers to partial tears of the mucosa which are often undetectable by imaging. This is believed to be the commonest bladder injury, although its exact incidence is uncertain.
   Type 2 refers to intraperitoneal rupture of the bladder.
   Type 3 is used to describe intramural tear, with an intact serosa.
   Type 4 refers to extraperitoneal rupture.

Type 5 describes cases in which there is combined intraperitoneal and extraperitoneal rupture.

Intraperitoneal (type 2) accounts for 10–20% of major bladder injury detected on imaging, extraperitoneal (type 4) 80–90% and combined 5–10%. Intraperitoneal rupture is usually caused by blunt trauma to a distended bladder. Extraperitoneal injuries are associated with penetrating injury, and are often caused by pubic bone fractures. From a clinical point of view, it is important to differentiate between an extraperitoneal and an intraperitoneal rupture.

2. **How do you differentiate between extraperitoneal and intraperitoneal bladder ruptures?**

The presence of 'flame-shaped' contrast superior and lateral to the bladder is indicative of extraperitoneal rupture. Contrast in the paracolic gutters and/or outlining bowel wall is diagnostic of intraperitoneal bladder rupture.

3. **What are the main differences in the management of the different types of bladder rupture?**

Intraperitoneal rupture requires acute surgical repair. Extraperitoneal ruptures are treated conservatively with catheter drainage and antibiotics unless a cystogram at 7–10 days demonstrates persistent leakage.

4. **What precautions need to be taken before performing a cystogram in a trauma setting?**

A urethral injury needs to be excluded before the insertion of a Foley catheter, especially if there is bleeding per urethram. A *retrograde urethrogram* should be performed prior to undertaking the cystogram.

Key points

- It is clinically important to distinguish between extraperitoneal and intraperitoneal bladder rupture.
- Intraperitoneal rupture most often results from blunt trauma to a full bladder. Extraperitoneal rupture is caused by penetrating injury.

Notes

Figure 5.1b, which illustrates intraperitoneal bladder rupture, is provided for comparison.

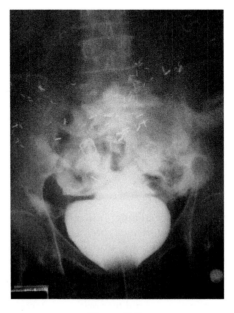

Figure 5.1b

Further reading

Ramchandani P, Buckler PM. Imaging of genitourinary trauma. *AJR Am J Roentgenol* 2009; **192**: 1514–23.

Vaccaro JP, Brody JM. CT cystography in the evaluation of major bladder trauma. *Radiographics* 2000; **20**: 1373–81.

Genitourinary Case 2

KIAT T. TAN AND RICHARD HOPKINS

Clinical history

12-year-old boy with a two-day history of scrotal pain.

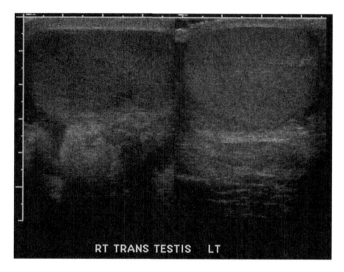

RT TRANS TESTIS   LT

Figure 5.2a

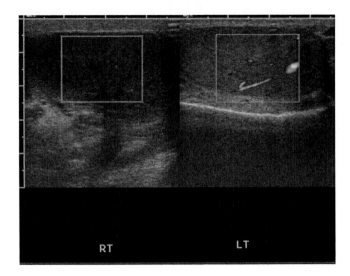

Figure 5.2b

Model answer

These are selected images from a scrotal ultrasound scan, including a power Doppler study (Figures 5.2a, 5.2b). There is a normal power Doppler flow pattern in the left testicle but no flow in the right. The right testicle has an inhomogeneous appearance and contains echo-poor regions. The findings are in keeping with right testicular infarction, which is most likely caused by testicular torsion. I would like to review the remaining images to look for a contralateral bell-clapper testicle. Although the affected testicle is unsalvageable, the patient will require urgent urological opinion with a view to orchidectomy to prevent gangrene and/or subfertility. Surgical fixation of a contralateral bell-clapper testicle (if present) should be performed prior to discharge.

Questions

1. **What is the pathophysiology of testicular torsion, and what do you mean by a bell-clapper deformity?**

   Testicular torsion occurs when the spermatic cord twists around itself as a result of testicular rotation. Normally, the testicle is fixed to the posterior part of the scrotum. Inadequate testicular fixation allows torsion to develop. The 'bell-clapper testicle' is a sign of poor testicular fixation and refers to a testicle that is lying with its long axis in a transverse plane, as opposed to the longitudinal orientation of a normal testicle.

2. **What are the risk factors for testicular torsion?**

   Age 10–15, bell-clapper deformity and previous torsion on the contralateral side.

3. **What is the differential diagnosis of acute scrotal pain and scrotal swelling in children?**

   Testicular torsion, torsion of testicular appendage, epididymo-orchitis, testicular tumour including lymphoma and scrotal hydrocele.

4. **What are the determinants of viability in a torted testicle?**

   The duration of torsion is an important indicator of testicular viability. There is an 80% chance of testicular recovery if the surgery is performed within six hours of symptom onset. This drops to 20% in 24 hours. Ultrasonically, hypoechogenicity is an indicator of non-viability.

Key points

- Testicular torsion is a medical emergency.
- Clinical examination can be non-specific in a significant proportion of patients.
- Viability is determined by duration of ischaemia and ultrasound findings.

Further reading

Berman L. The male reproductive system. In Adam A, Dixon AK, eds., *Grainger and Allison's Diagnostic Radiology*, 5th edn. London: Churchill Livingstone, 2008 (ebook).

Genitourinary Case 3

KIAT T. TAN AND RICHARD HOPKINS

Clinical history

No history.

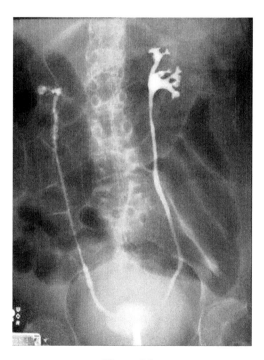

Figure 5.3a

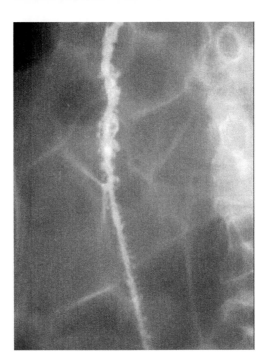

Figure 5.3b

Model answer

These are two images from a retrograde study of both ureters, with a magnified view of the right ureter (Figures 5.3a, 5.3b). The cystoscope is visualized in the bladder. The right ureter is abnormal, with multiple tiny flask-shaped outpouchings seen along its entire length. The left pelvicalyceal system and the left ureter are normal. The ureteric findings are typical of ureteral pseudodiverticulosis. The full-length image shows an abnormal right calyceal branching pattern, with only a small bulbous area just above the proximal ureter filling with contrast. Possible causes would include extensive renal infiltration by tumour such as transitional cell carcinoma and advanced renal atrophy/scarring. As there is an association between ureteral pseudodiverticulosis and urological cancers, a CT scan should be obtained for further characterization of the urinary tract. The patient will need to have urine cytology. Follow-up imaging by either IVU or CT is advised.

Questions

1. **What is ureteral pseudodiverticulosis, and what is its clinical significance?**
   Ureteral pseudodiverticulosis occurs when there are multiple small (less than 5 mm) outpouchings of hyperplastic epithelial cells into the submucosa, resulting in the formation of 'crypts'. The lesions do not extend past the lamina propria. The condition is often bilateral and most often affects the upper to middle parts of the ureter. The exact aetiology of the condition is uncertain, although it appears to be associated with chronic inflammation and epithelial proliferation. It is therefore not surprising that 25–50% of patients with ureteral pseudodiverticulosis have or will develop transitional cell carcinomas.

Key points

- Ureteral pseudodiverticulosis is rare.
- It is not a true diverticulum, as the outpouchings do not extend through the external muscular layer of the ureter.

- It is associated with chronic inflammatory stimuli and regarded as generalized urothelial disease.
- It is associated with urothelial malignancy.

Further reading

Wasserman NF, Zhang G, Posalaky IP, Reddy PK. Ureteral pseudodiverticula: frequent association with uroepithelial malignancy. *AJR Am J Roentgenol* 1991; **157**: 69–72.

Genitourinary Case 4

KIAT T. TAN AND RICHARD HOPKINS

Clinical history

No history. Report the control radiograph from the IVU series first.

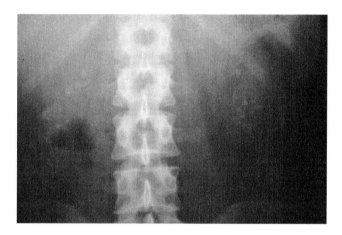

Figure 5.4a

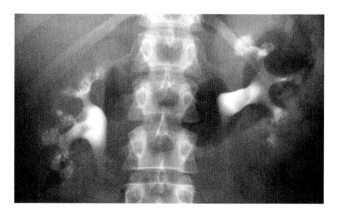

Figure 5.4b

Model answer

I am presented with the control image from an IVU series (Figure 5.4a). There are punctate and nodular opacities in the medullary regions of both kidneys. The findings are consistent with medullary nephrocalcinosis. Bones are normal. The most common cause of medullary nephrocalcinosis is medullary sponge kidney. Medullary nephrocalcinosis can also be due to hypercalciuria, which may or may not be related to hypercalcaemia. Causes of hypercalciuria include hyperparathyroidism, renal tubular acidosis, prolonged immobilization and sarcoidosis. I would like to review the other images from the IVU, as medullary sponge kidney has a characteristic appearance on this examination.

The excretion phase of the study (Figure 5.4b) confirms the medullary site of calcification. The papillae demonstrate streaky linear hyperdense areas, consistent with the diagnosis of medullary sponge kidney. No further investigation is required, unless the patient has coexisting problems or complications of medullary sponge kidney.

Questions

1. What are the different types of nephrocalcinosis and what are their causes?

Nephrocalcinosis can be classified into medullary, cortical and 'miscellaneous' forms, depending on the site and pattern of calcium deposition. Cortical nephrocalcinosis can be due to acute cortical necrosis, chronic glomerulonephritis and transplant rejection. 'Miscellaneous' causes include tuberculosis, carcinoma and renal cyst calcification

2. What causes the linear contrast densities in medullary sponge kidney on an IVU?

Contrast filling of the dilated collecting tubes found in the condition.

Key points

- Medullary sponge kidney (MSK) is a poorly understood congenital dilatation of kidney collecting ducts.
- The condition is most often asymptomatic, although there is a predisposition to stone formation.
- IVU/CTU findings are characteristic. Plain radiographic features are indistinguishable from other causes of medullary nephrocalcinosis. Medullary sponge kidney tends to be associated with normal-sized or enlarged kidneys, unlike other causes of nephrocalcinosis.

Further reading

Dyer RB, Chen MY, Zagoria RJ. Abnormal calcifications in the urinary tract. *Radiographics* 1998; **18**: 1405–24.

Rottenberg G, Sandhu C. Radiology of the upper urinary tract. In Adam A, Dixon AK, eds., *Grainger and Allison's Diagnostic Radiology*, 5th edn. London: Churchill Livingstone, 2008 (ebook).

Images courtesy of Dr John Curtis, University Hospital Aintree, Liverpool.

Genitourinary Case 5

KIAT T. TAN AND RICHARD HOPKINS

Clinical history

36-year-old man. Palpable lump in right testis.

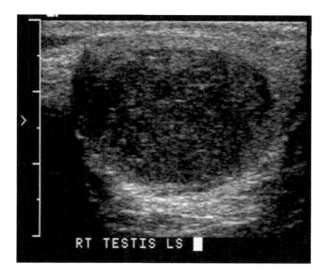

Figure 5.5a

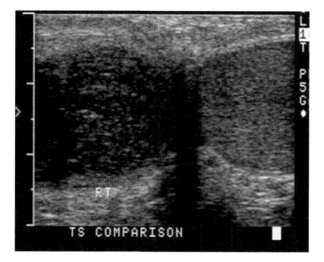

Figure 5.5b

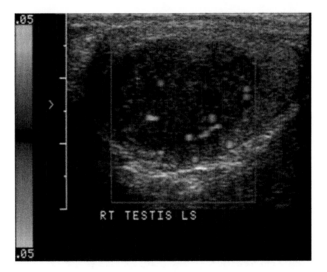

Figure 5.5c

Model answer

These are three images from a scrotal ultrasound series, including an image of a colour Doppler examination (Figures 5.5a–5.5c). There is an oval, well-defined hypoechoic mass measuring about 2 cm by 1.5 cm in the right testicle. Normal testicular parenchyma can be seen peripheral to the oval mass. The colour Doppler image shows scattered areas of vascularity. The findings are consistent with testicular cancer, most likely a seminoma. The patient will need an urgent urological opinion as well as a staging CT scan of the chest, abdomen and pelvis.

Questions

1. **What are the risk factors for testicular carcinoma?**
   Undescended testis, infertility, previous contralateral testicular cancer, positive family history.
2. **What other conditions can cause intratesticular masses or mass-like lesions? Are there any features which help to distinguish them?**
   - Testicular stromal tumours. These are less common than germ-cell tumours. They may be small at presentation with clinical symptoms arising from hormone production, e.g. testosterone (virilization in children) or oestrogen (gynaecomastia, impotence).
   - Epidermoid. Classical echo-poor 'onion-skin' appearance on ultrasound.
   - Lymphoma. This occurs in the older age group, and is frequently bilateral.
   - Testicular torsion and infarction. Diffuse hypoechoic changes throughout the testicle can mimic a seminoma.
   - Haematoma. Generally this is associated with a history of trauma or contact sports. A history of anticoagulation may be present.
   - Focal infection. Increased lesional vascularity, often associated with changes of epididymitis. Systemic symptoms of fever, night sweats may be present. Inflammatory markers and white blood cell count may be raised.
   - Testicular metastasis. This is more common in the middle-aged and elderly population. Metastases may be multiple, multifocal and bilateral. Review of other imaging studies may help. Tumour markers PSA (prostate), CEA (colorectal) may confirm the diagnosis.

Key points

- Seminoma is the commonest testicular carcinoma. The lesion is classically round and uniformly echo-poor on ultrasound.
- There is significant overlap between the radiological appearances of the various testicular tumours, and ultrasound is *not* a replacement for histology.
- hCG, αFP and LDH are testicular tumour markers.
- Testicular microlithiasis (i.e. a testicle with multiple echogenic foci on ultrasound) may be associated with carcinoma, although the relationship is poorly understood.

Further reading

Woodward PJ, Sohaey R, O'Donoghue MJ, Green DJ. From the archives of the AFIP. Tumors and tumorlike lesions of the testis: radiologic–pathologic correlation. *Radiographics* 2002; **22**: 189–216.

Genitourinary Case 6

KIAT T. TAN AND RICHARD HOPKINS

Clinical history

40-year-old male with a history of blunt abdominal trauma.

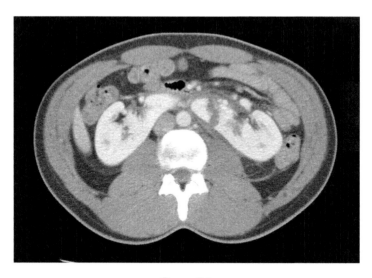

Figure 5.6

Model answer

The image is taken from an intravenous contrast-enhanced CT scan of the abdomen (Figure 5.6). There is a horseshoe kidney. There is a laceration in the part of the horseshoe kidney that is overlying the spine. This is associated with a small perirenal haematoma. I would like to review the CT scan on a workstation to assess the extent of renal injury and the size of the haemorrhage as well as to look for other injuries. The patient will need to be referred to a urologist for inpatient management.

1. What are the complications of horseshoe kidney?

Horseshoe kidney is an isolated finding in most patients. The remaining patients may have associated congenital anomalies in the cardiovascular, central nervous and musculoskeletal systems. Urinary tract complications of horseshoe kidney include collecting system dilatation (which may or may not be associated with pelviureteric junction obstruction), increased susceptibility to stone formation, recurrent urinary tract infections and an increased risk of developing Wilms' tumour. The low-lying position of the kidney anterior to the spine predisposes it to injury in blunt trauma.

2. Is there a classification system that would help you assess the degree of renal damage and prognosis in trauma patients?

Yes. The American Association for the Surgery of Trauma has classed renal injury into five categories:

Grade I – haematuria with one of the following: no imaging findings, contusion or a subcapsular haematoma with an intact capsule

Grade II – superficial cortical laceration (< 1 cm) with no evidence of medullary/ collecting system injury *or* non-expanding perinephric haematoma

Grade III – deep lacerations (> 1 cm) with no collecting system injury

Grade IV – laceration with collecting system involvement, laceration with vascular involvement (which does not qualify for grade V: see below)

Grade V – completely shattered kidney, complete disruption of main renal artery or vein

Higher-grade injuries are associated with greater degrees of renal impairment.

Key points

- Post-traumatic haematuria, whether macro- or microscopic, should always be investigated.
- Absence of haematuria does *not* exclude significant renal injury.
- Always check the integrity of the normal kidney.
- Percutaneous angiographic embolization can be a useful method to control bleeding in renal trauma and may result in preservation of a kidney that would formerly have been removed.
- Conservative management (including percutaneous embolization) is now the mainstay of treatment for grades I–III (and certain forms of grade IV) renal trauma.

Further reading

Alonso RC, Nacenta SB, Martinez PD, Guerrero AS, Fuentes CG. Kidney in danger: CT findings of blunt and penetrating renal trauma. *Radiographics* 2009; **29**: 2033–53.

De Bruyn R, Gordon I, McHugh K. Imaging of the kidneys, urinary tract and pelvis in children. In Adam A, Dixon AK, eds., *Grainger and Allison's Diagnostic Radiology*, 5th edn. London: Churchill Livingstone, 2008 (ebook).

Genitourinary Case 7

KIAT T. TAN AND RICHARD HOPKINS

Clinical history
Palpable abdominal mass.

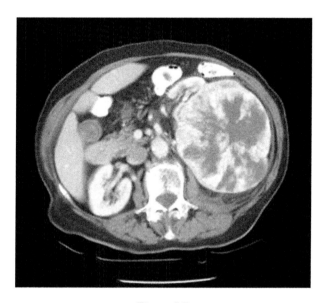

Figure 5.7

Model answer
This is an axial image from an intravenous and oral contrast-enhanced CT scan of the upper abdomen (Figure 5.7).

A large exophytic well-circumscribed mass is seen arising posteriorly from the left kidney. The lesion displaces the kidney anteromedially and is of mixed attenuation, with peripheral hyperattenuation and central hypoattenuation. There is no evidence of local invasion, with preserved perinephric fat planes. The left renal vein is not identified on this image. There is no lymphadenopathy. The visualized liver, IVC and right kidney are normal. A stone is noted in the gallbladder.

The differential diagnoses include renal cell carcinoma (RCC) and oncocytoma. I would like to review the rest of the imaging to look for any evidence of invasion of adjacent structures, with particular attention to the IVC, and distant metastasis. The patient is likely to require nephrectomy, and should be referred to the urologists.

Questions
1. **What is an oncocytoma?**
   A benign well-vascularized tumour arising from the collecting ducts. It is impossible to differentiate an oncocytoma from a renal cell carcinoma on imaging.
2. **What is your recommended treatment plan?**
   The patient will require either partial or complete nephrectomy. Radiofrequency ablation is an unsuitable option for lesions of this size. Conservative management with radiological follow-up is an option for those who are unfit or unwilling to undergo surgery.

Key points
- Oncocytomas are benign renal tumours.
- They are indistinguishable from renal cell carcinomas and are treated identically.
- Cryotherapy/radiofrequency ablation (hopefully by the interventional radiologist) of suspected oncocytomas/RCCs are promising minimally invasive treatment options.

Further reading
Rottenberg G, Rankin S. Renal masses. In Adam A, Dixon AK, eds., *Grainger and Allison's Diagnostic Radiology*, 5th edn. London: Churchill Livingstone, 2008 (ebook).

Genitourinary Case 8

KIAT T. TAN AND RICHARD HOPKINS

Clinical history
No history.

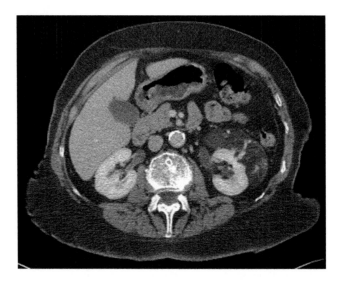

Figure 5.8

Model answer
This is a single image from a contrast-enhanced CT scan of the abdomen (Figure 5.8). There is a fat-containing mass arising from the left kidney. The mass is connected to the kidney by large feeding vessels. The radiological findings are consistent with those of an angiomyolipoma. I would like to review the rest of the CT scan to evaluate if this is an isolated lesion or whether there are multiple angiomyolipomas. Angiomyolipomas are associated with tuberous sclerosis, and it would be of value to ascertain if this patient has this condition.

Questions

1. **What is a possible radiological treatment for angiomyolipoma (AML)?**
   Angiomyolipoma can be treated by arterial embolization. Lesions over 4 cm in diameter are likely to bleed and should be considered for embolization.
2. **What is the association between angiomyolipoma and tuberous sclerosis?**
   Between 50% and 80% of patients with tuberous sclerosis will have at least one angiomyolipoma.
3. **What are the other imaging findings of tuberous sclerosis?**
   Tuberous sclerosis is typically manifested radiologically by the presence of calcified cortical and/or subependymal periventricular nodules. In addition, central nervous system gliomas (astrocytomas) and retinal tumours may be present. On the chest radiograph, 5% of cases will demonstrate cystic lung disease – lymphangioleiomyomatosis, with relative preservation of lung volume.

Key points

- Angiomyolipomas characteristically contain fat.
- Lesions containing minimal amounts of fat can be difficult to differentiate from renal cell carcinoma. Multiphase CT may be useful in this situation.
- Angiomyolipomas are associated with tuberous sclerosis and lymphangioleiomyomatosis.
- The blood vessels in angiomyolipomas are friable and liable to rupture.

Further reading

Evans JC, Curtis J. The radiological appearances of tuberous sclerosis. *Br J Radiol* 2000; **73**: 91–8.

Halpenny D, Snow A, McNeill G, Torreggiani WC. The radiological diagnosis and treatment of renal angiomyolipoma: current status. *Clin Radiol* 2010; **65**: 99–108.

Israel GM, Bosniak MA. Pitfalls in renal mass evaluation and how to avoid them. *Radiographics* 2008; **28**: 1325–38.

Umeoka S, Koyama T, Miki Y, *et al.* Pictorial review of tuberous sclerosis in various organs. *Radiographics* 2008; **28**: e32.

Genitourinary Case 9

KIAT T. TAN AND RICHARD HOPKINS

Clinical history
No history.

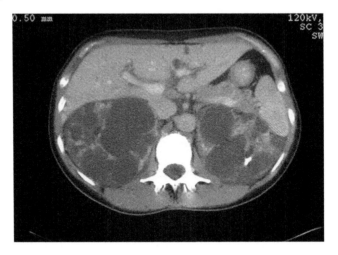

Figure 5.9

Model answer
This is a single image of a contrast-enhanced CT scan of the abdomen (Figure 5.9). It demonstrates bilateral renal enlargement. The kidneys are virtually replaced by multiple large cysts. Some of these cysts contain dense calcification. The appearances are those of adult polycystic kidney disease. Intravenous contrast has been used, and it is important to monitor the patient's renal function post scan, although this may not be relevant if he or she is undergoing dialysis. I would also like to review the rest of the CT examination (along with previous imaging), as there is an association between polycystic kidney disease and renal cell carcinoma. The patient may benefit from either CT or MR cerebral angiography, as there is also an association with cerebral aneurysms. However, both CT and MR contrast administration may be an issue in this patient. The patient should be followed up by nephrology. Genetic testing of family members should be considered.

Questions
1. **What are the appearances of adult polycystic kidney disease on IVU?**
   The IVU typically demonstrates a 'spider-leg appearance' due to contrast filling of calyces that are elongated and deformed by the cysts. There may also be filling defects within the renal pelvis. Occasionally the cyst walls may calcify.
2. **You mentioned that both CT and MR contrast could be an issue. Please explain why.**
   CT contrast can cause or aggravate renal failure, particularly in those with pre-existing renal disease. Gadolinium contrast agents can cause nephrogenic systemic fibrosis in patients with renal impairment.
3. **What other organs are involved in adult polycystic kidney disease?**
   Approximately 30% of patients with adult polycystic kidney disease also have polycystic changes to the liver. Splenic and pancreatic cysts are also seen. Approximately 10% of patients have intracranial aneurysms.

4. How do adult polycystic kidney (APCK) patients present, and what is the mode of inheritance?

APCK is inherited as an autosomal dominant condition. The patient with APCK can present with hypertension and/or renal impairment. Family members of patients with known APCK should be screened.

Key points

- Adult polycystic kidney disease is different from childhood polycystic kidney disease. Both can cause bilateral gross renal enlargement. Clinical differentiation can be difficult in adolescent patients, and radiology is crucial in this age group.
  - Adult polycystic kidney disease: large cysts, adult onset, autosomal dominant.
  - Childhood polycystic kidney disease: small cysts, onset in infancy (most common) to adolescence, autosomal recessive.

Further reading

Rottenberg G, Rankin S. Renal masses. In Adam A, Dixon AK, eds., *Grainger and Allison's Diagnostic Radiology*, 5th edn. London: Churchill Livingstone, 2008 (ebook).

Genitourinary Case 10

KIAT T. TAN AND RICHARD HOPKINS

Clinical history

Symptoms of pneumaturia for several weeks, now passing urine per rectum. Raised CEA level.

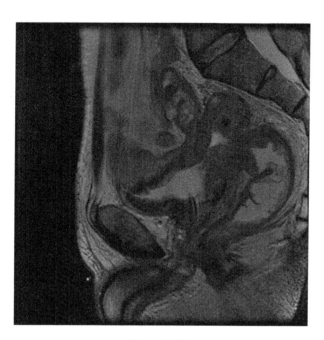

Figure 5.10a

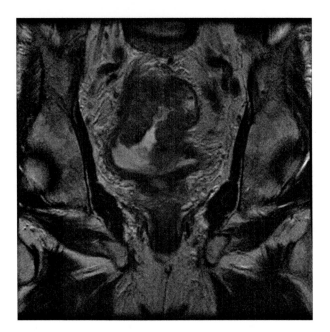

Figure 5.10b

Model answer

I am presented with one sagittal and one coronal T2-weighted image from a pelvic MRI scan (Figures 5.10a, 5.10b). The bladder is catheterized. There is a large irregular mass invading the anterior part of the upper rectum and the posterior part of the bladder. A well-defined track is present between rectum and bladder, and there is fluid in the rectum.

When combined with the finding of a raised carcinoembryonic antigen (CEA), the features are consistent with a malignant rectovesical fistula due to a primary colonic tumour. I would like to review the rest of the MR images on a workstation to assess the degree of local disease spread and lymphadenopathy. The patient will require a CT scan of the chest and abdomen to look for distant metastasis and peritoneal spread. I will discuss the case at the local cancer multidisciplinary team meeting as part of the treatment planning process.

Questions

1. **What other imaging modalities can be used to image a rectovesical fistula?**
   If MRI is unavailable, either a CT or fluoroscopic cystogram may be considered. MRI remains the gold standard in the evaluation of local disease in most pelvic pathology.
2. **What are the common causes of rectovesical fistulas?**
   Infective or inflammatory causes such as diverticulitis and Crohn's disease; pelvic malignancy such as colorectal, bladder or uterine cancers; trauma from surgery; and congenital anomalies.

Key points

- MRI is the most useful modality in imaging pelvic fistulas.
- Gas within a non-catheterized bladder is a sign of bladder fistulas. The presence of this finding should always prompt a careful search for its cause.

Further reading

Avritscher R, Madoff DC, Ramirez PT, *et al*. Fistulas of the lower urinary tract: percutaneous approaches for the management of a difficult clinical entity. *Radiographics* 2004; **24**: S217–36.

Genitourinary Case 11

KIAT T. TAN AND RICHARD HOPKINS

Clinical history
Chronic urological condition.

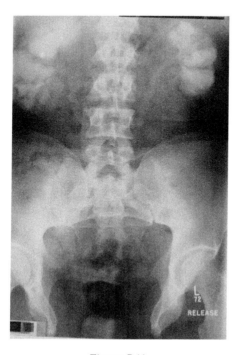

Figure 5.11

Model answer
The image is a single 'release' film from an IVU series (Figure 5.11). The calyces appear to be filled with contrast and are markedly dilated bilaterally. I would like to confirm this as well as to exclude the presence of radio-opaque stones by referring to the control radiograph. The left ureter is dilated. The right ureter is not clearly visualized. There is a prominent loop of small bowel in the right lower quadrant that appears to be filled with contrast agent, which I would again confirm by referring to the control radiograph. The pubic bones are widely separated. The findings are consistent with bladder exstrophy, with a possible ileal conduit. The marked hydronephrosis bilaterally could be due to associated long-standing vesicoureteric reflux or pelviureteric junction obstruction. The former is more likely in this patient in the presence of a hydroureter.

Questions
1. **What is bladder exstrophy?**
   Bladder exstrophy is part of the exstrophy–epispadias complex affecting the genitourinary system. In bladder exstrophy, there is a midline defect in the abdominal wall with exposure of the bladder mucosa. This is almost always associated with gross widening of the pubic symphysis and divergence of the recti. The condition is also associated with a wide range of other urogenital, gastrointestinal and musculoskeletal abnormalities.

2. **What are the other causes of pubic symphysis widening?**

Apart from the exstrophy–epispadias complex, pubic symphysis widening could be due to trauma (especially during childbirth) and infection.

Key points

- Incidence of the exstrophy–epispadias complex is around 1 in 10 000, with a male predominance of 1.5–6 : 1.
- The spectrum of disease ranges from mild distal epispadia, where there is a gaping meatus, to severe bladder exstrophy.
- It is a congenital problem, resulting from abnormal cloacal development.

Further reading

De Bruyn R, Gordon I, McHugh K. Imaging of the kidneys, urinary tract and pelvis in children. In Adam A, Dixon AK, eds., *Grainger and Allison's Diagnostic Radiology*, 5th edn. London: Churchill Livingstone, 2008 (ebook).

Ebert A, Reutter H, Ludwig M, Rosch WH. The exstrophy–epispadias complex. *Orphanet J Rare Dis* 2009; **4**: 23.

Genitourinary Case 12

KIAT T. TAN AND RICHARD HOPKINS

Clinical history

No history. Report the control film first.

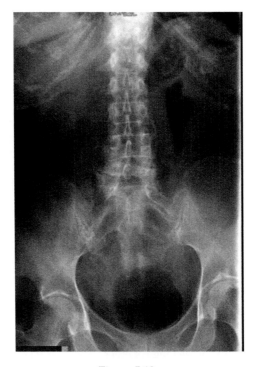

Figure 5.12a

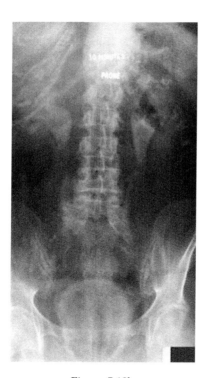

Figure 5.12b

Model answer

This is the control film from an IVU series (Figure 5.12a). The images show lucencies within the renal collecting systems, ureters and bladder, consistent with intraluminal gas. There is a curvilinear shadow that delineates the bladder wall consistent with gas within the bladder wall. The radiological findings are due to emphysematous cystitis. I would like to review the other images from the IVU series to assess the anatomy of the urinary tract as well as to look for fistulas between the urinary tract and gas-containing structures.

The prone 30-minute film (Figure 5.12b) confirms the presence of gas within the urinary tract. There is good contrast opacification of the bladder, which has a mottled appearance. No fistulous tract evident on this study. A clinical history, either from the referring clinician or from the patient, would be invaluable. Emphysematous cystitis most often affects patients with diabetes, although those who are generally debilitated or have underlying urinary tract abnormalities are also at risk. Urine cultures should be obtained prior to starting antibiotics.

Questions

1. **What are the causes of intraluminal gas within the urinary tract?**

   Infection by gas-forming organisms, urinary tract fistulas, trauma (including surgery and instrumentation).

2. **How is emphysematous cystitis treated?**

   The treatment of emphysematous cystitis depends on the clinical picture. Conservative management with antibiotics is successful in the vast majority of patients. Surgical management is reserved for severe cases or those not responding to conservative treatments.

Further reading

Rankin S. Renal parenchymal disease, including renal failure, renovascular disease and transplantation. In Adam A, Dixon AK, eds., *Grainger and Allison's Diagnostic Radiology*, 5th edn. London: Churchill Livingstone, 2008 (ebook).

Thomas AA, Lane BR, Thomas AZ, *et al.* Emphysematous cystitis: a review of 135 cases. *BJU Int* 2007; **100**: 17–20.

Genitourinary Case 13

KIAT T. TAN AND RICHARD HOPKINS

Clinical history

Young female with lower abdominal pain.

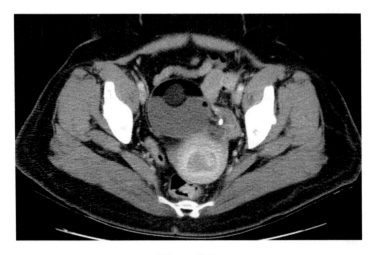

Figure 5.13

Model answer

This is a selected image from an intravenous and oral enhanced CT scan of the abdomen and pelvis (Figure 5.13). There is a large uniformly thin-walled lesion in the right adnexal region. The lesion is sharply demarcated into two halves, with an anterior hypoattenuating region and a more hyperattenuating part posteriorly. A heterogeneous nodule can be seen in the centre of this lesion. There is no associated calcification. I think this lesion is a dermoid cyst. I would like to confirm my diagnosis by measuring the Hounsfield unit of the anterior hypoattenuating region, which should be of fat attenuation in a dermoid cyst. The central heterogeneous region may be free-floating hair or a Rokitansky nodule. I will confirm the presence of a Rokitansky nodule by examining the MPR images. I would also like to look for features of malignant degeneration such as invasion of adjacent structures, although this is rare, especially in a young patient.

Questions
1. **What is a dermoid cyst?**
   A mature cystic teratoma, also known as a dermoid cyst, is a germ-cell tumour that contains at least two derivative components out of the three germ-cell layers. Any tissue subtype could therefore be present in the cyst. Common contents include skin, hair, fat, mucosal epithelium and teeth. A Rokitansky nodule is a focal prominence in the cyst wall that is found in most dermoid cysts.
2. **What are the complications of a dermoid cyst?**
   Dermoid cysts can rupture, undergo torsion, become infected or undergo malignant degeneration. Malignant degeneration is rare and tends to occur in the older patient. It occurs when cancerous cells arise from differentiated tissues. The risk of malignant degeneration is estimated to be 1–2%. There is a rare association between autoimmune haemolytic anaemia and dermoid cysts. Removal of the cyst may result in a cure.
3. **What are the radiological features of a dermoid cyst that has undergone malignant transformation?**
   As expected, there is considerable overlap between the imaging features of benign dermoid cysts and those that have undergone malignant change. Typical malignant dermoid cysts demonstrate invasion of adjacent structures and have irregular soft tissue outlines that enhance with contrast. Malignant tissue tends to form an obtuse angle with the inner wall of the cyst. Other risk factors for malignancy include age (> 45 years) and a tumour that is larger than 9.9 cm in diameter.

Key points
- Mature cystic teratomas do not usually cause symptoms.
- Mature cystic teratomas should be differentiated from immature cystic teratomas, which are aggressive lesions containing embryonic tissues. Indeed, malignant degeneration of mature cystic teratomas results in the formation of cancerous cells that are often indistinguishable from their non-germ-cell counterparts (e.g. squamous cell carcinoma, adenocarcinoma, thyroid carcinoma).
- The presence of one teratoma (whether mature or immature) is a risk factor for the coexistence of another. The radiologist should always look for the presence of synchronous tumours.

Further reading
Outwater EK, Siegelman ES, Hunt JL. Ovarian teratomas: tumor types and imaging characteristics. *Radiographics* 2001; **21**: 475–90.
Park SB, Kim JK, Kim KR, Cho KS. Imaging findings of complications and unusual manifestations of ovarian teratomas. *Radiographics* 2008; **28**: 969–83.

Genitourinary Case 14

KIAT T. TAN AND RICHARD HOPKINS

Clinical history

18-year-old female patient. Normal secondary sexual characteristics. Irregular but otherwise normal periods. Increasing abdominal pain and bloating for several weeks. Enlarged uterus on ultrasound scan.

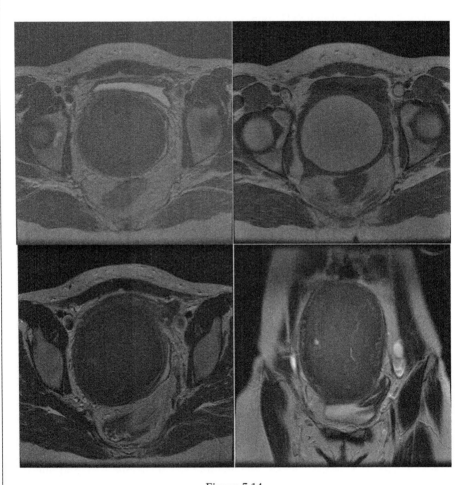

Figure 5.14

Model answer

These are selected T1 axial, T2 axial and T2 coronal MRI images from the lower abdomen and pelvis (Figure 5.14). There is a very dilated uterus that extends out of the pelvis and into the lower abdomen. The uterine cavity is distended and filled with material which is of high signal on T1 and intermediate signal on T2, consistent with altered blood products. There is a slit-like cavity to the left of the distended uterine body that contains a central area of high signal on T2. The findings are consistent with uterus didelphys with right unilateral haematometra, which would be in keeping with the clinical history and ultrasound findings.

Questions

1. **What is the difference between haematometra and haematocolpos?**
   Haematometra is due to retained secretions and products of menstruation within the uterine cavity, where the level of obstruction is at the cervix. Haematocolpos refers to retained menstrual products within the vagina, in which the level of obstruction is lower, for example in cases of imperforate hymen.

2. **Describe the anatomy of a didelphic uterus.**
   Uterus didelphys is one of the Müllerian duct abnormalities. It results from complete failure of fusion of the separate Müllerian ducts. The individual horns are fully developed and there are two cervices present. The condition is usually (but not always) associated with a longitudinal septum in the vagina.

Key points

- Unicornuate uterus – one horn is atrophic or hypoplastic.
- Didelphic uterus – two distinct uterine horns, two cervices and usually two vaginas.
- Bicornuate uterus – large fundal cleft.
- Septate uterus – large fibrous or muscular septum dividing the uterine cavity.
- Arcuate uterus – minor contour abnormality of the endometrial cavity at the fundus.

Further reading

Sala E, Allison S, Ascher SM, Hricak H. Imaging in gynecology. In Adam A, Dixon AK, eds., *Grainger and Allison's Diagnostic Radiology*, 5th edn. London: Churchill Livingstone, 2008 (ebook).

Genitourinary Case 15

KIAT T. TAN AND RICHARD HOPKINS

Clinical history
Chronic pelvic pain.

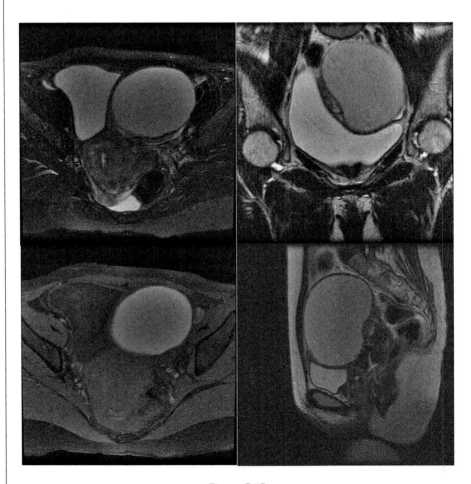

Figure 5.15

Model answer
These are selected axial fat-saturated T2, coronal T2, axial fat-saturated T1 and sagittal T2 images from an MRI scan (Figure 5.15). There is a large oval collection arising from the left adnexa which is of high signal on T1- and T2-weighted sequences and does not suppress with fat saturation. It appears to be arising from the left ovary, which is draped around the medial aspect of the lesion. Imaging characteristics suggest that the lesion contains blood products. In this clinical context, the radiological features are consistent with a large endometrioma. The patient will need to be seen by a gynaecologist for further management.

Questions

1. **What are the common symptoms of endometriosis?**
   Chronic pelvic pain, reduced fertility, dyspareunia, dysmenorrhoea.
2. **What is adenomyosis, and what are its imaging signs?**
   Adenomyosis refers to ectopic endometrial glandular tissue within the myometrium. On ultrasound the uterus is bulky and has a heterogeneous reflectivity without discrete masses being identified. The imaging hallmark on ultrasound is the presence of single or multiple small cystic lesions of a few millimetres in diameter. MRI features of adenomyosis include diffuse enlargement of the uterus, patchy areas of reduced signal intensity on T1 and T2 sequences and thickening of the junctional zone.

Key points

- Endometriomas are hyperintense on T1 and usually hypointense on T2, although they may be iso- or hyperintense on T2.
- On barium enema, endometriosis is typically seen along the anterior wall of the upper rectum or at the rectosigmoid junction. Endometriosis most often shows up as a serrated/notched, corrugated irregularity of the mucosal surface with a mass of variable size associated with the serosal surface and bowel wall. A variable fibrotic reaction may be present. The appearance is almost impossible to distinguish from serosal malignancy.
- On ultrasound, endometriomas are hypoechoic with diffuse low-level internal echoes. The wall is generally thin and unilocular.

Further reading

Bis KG, Vrachliotis TG, Agrawal R, *et al*. Pelvic endometriosis: MR imaging spectrum with laparoscopic correlation and diagnostic pitfalls. *Radiographics* 1997; **17**: 639–55.

Kuligowska E, Deeds L, Lu K. Pelvic pain: overlooked and underdiagnosed gynecologic conditions. *Radiographics* 2005; **25**: 3–20.

Genitourinary Case 16

KIAT T. TAN AND RICHARD HOPKINS

Clinical history
Female, 68 years old. Symptoms of abdominal pain and bloating.

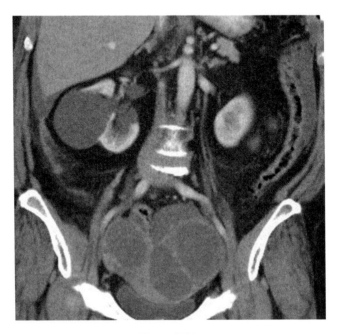

Figure 5.16a

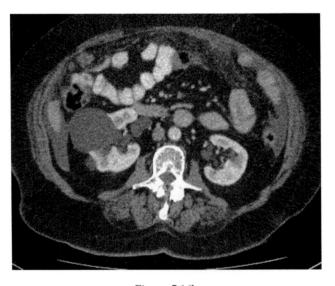

Figure 5.16b

Model answer

I am presented with a coronal and an axial image from a CT examination (Figures 5.16a, 5.16b). There is a mass arising from the central pelvis that contains both cystic and solid components. Multiple thick irregular septations are present. The bladder is displaced inferiorly. On both the images, there is a small amount of free fluid in the left paracolic gutter and inferior to the liver. There is nodularity and fat stranding in the greater omentum. Simple cysts are noted in the right kidney.

The radiological findings are consistent with a primary ovarian tumour that has spread to the peritoneum and omentum. The diagnosis could be confirmed by measuring tumour markers such as the CA125 level. The CT result should be communicated to the referring clinical team to expedite patient management.

Questions

1. **Which tumours can involve the peritoneum?**
   Secondary tumour deposits are the commonest form of peritoneal malignancy. These include tumours from the ovary, gastrointestinal tract, breast and endometrium. Primary malignant mesothelioma of the peritoneum is rare and is usually related to previous asbestos exposure.
2. **Which non-malignant process can give rise to peritoneal thickening, nodularity and ascites?**
   Peritoneal tuberculosis.
3. **What investigations would you recommend in cases where the peritoneal pathology is uncertain?**
   Clinical history, review imaging for evidence of primary, measure tumour markers (e.g. CA125, CEA), ascitic fluid cytology and omental biopsy.

Key points

- Tumour spread to the peritoneum is by direct invasion, lymphatics, intraperitoneal seeding and via the blood.
- Barium studies are non-specific. Signs include tethering, speculation, mass effect and pseudosacculation.
- Peritoneal seeding can occur by inadvertent/inappropriate puncture of a malignant ovarian cyst. These lesions are best removed en bloc at surgery.
- Peritoneal deposits in children are mostly secondary to adenocarcinoma and germ-cell tumours.

Further reading

Shaw MS, Healy JC, Reznek RH. Imaging the peritoneum for malignant processes. *Imaging* 2000; **12**: 21–33.

Genitourinary Case 17

KIAT T. TAN AND RICHARD HOPKINS

Clinical history
Please review this single image from an IVU study. The control film is normal.

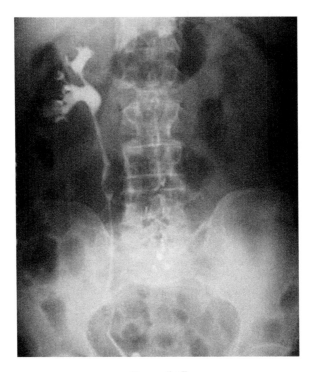

Figure 5.17

Model answer
This is the post-release radiograph from an IVU series (Figure 5.17). The left kidney and ureter are missing. The right pelvicalyceal system is normal. There is an irregular expansile filling defect within the right ureter with associated luminal narrowing at the level of L4 to L5. However, this is not causing significant obstruction as the proximal pelviureteric system is not dilated and there is good contrast opacification of the distal ureter and bladder. The appearance is strongly suspicious of urothelial tumour. Presumably, the left kidney and ureter have been removed for previous contralateral tumour. Less likely differential diagnoses would include a blood clot and fungus ball, although one would expect a blood clot of this size to cause significant obstruction. The shape, radiolucency and lack of obstructive features make urolithiasis unlikely. As part of good clinical practice, I would like to review the rest of the IVU series. In particular, I would like to look for synchronous tumours in the bladder and renal pelvis. I would like to obtain a clinical history to confirm a history of previous urothelial malignancy. The patient will need to have a staging CT scan of the chest, abdomen and pelvis. The patient should have urine cytology and culture. He or she should be referred to the urologists for cystoureteroscopy and definitive treatment.

Questions

1. What are the risk factors for urothelial malignancy?

Exposure to carcinogens (smoking, cyclophosphamide, aniline dyes), previous urinary malignancy, chronic urinary tract infection, urolithiasis and hereditary non-polyposis colorectal cancer. Horseshoe kidneys increase the risk of urothelial malignancy.

2. What are the forms of urothelial malignancy that you know of?

Transitional cell (> 90%) and squamous cell carcinomas.

3. You mentioned you would expect a stone or blood clot of this size to cause obstruction. Why are there no features of urinary tract obstruction in this case?

The tumour grows slowly, allowing time for the ureter to dilate.

Key points

- The risk of synchronous or metachronous urothelial carcinoma is high. Up to 50% of patients with upper tract tumours develop bladder cancer.
- Haematuria and pain are the commonest presenting symptoms. Acute renal colic is uncommon unless associated with blood clots.
- CT urography is the ideal method for imaging the disease, although IVU is still frequently used.

Further reading

Rottenberg G, Caron S. Radiology of the upper urinary tract. In Adam A, Dixon AK, eds., *Grainger and Allison's Diagnostic Radiology*, 5th edn. London: Churchill Livingstone, 2008 (ebook).

Wong-You-Cheong JJ, Wagner BJ, Davis CJ. Transitional cell carcinoma of the urinary tract: radiologic–pathologic correlation. *Radiographics* 1998; **18**: 123–42.

Breast Case 18

IAIN D. LYBURN

Clinical history

52-year-old woman. Routine screening mammograms.

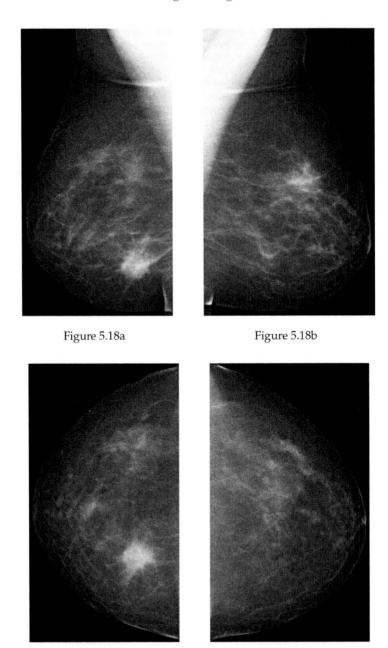

Figure 5.18a

Figure 5.18b

Figure 5.18c

Figure 5.18d

Model answer

These are bilateral mediolateral oblique and craniocaudal mammograms (Figures 5.18a–5.18d). After making a global inspection of both breasts, I would examine all the films under magnification, using workstation tools in the case of digital images or a magnifying glass with conventional analogue films, to assess for microcalcifications.

There is a spiculated ill-defined dense mass associated with fine pleomorphic microcalcification in the lower inner quadrant of the right breast. The remainder of the right breast is normal. The left breast is normal.

The mass in the lower inner right breast has an appearance suspicious for malignancy.

I would suggest recall for assessment with clinical examination, ultrasound and possible further mammographic views, with the intention to proceed to image-guided core biopsy.

Questions

1. **How are such masses evaluated in the assessment clinic?**
   A clinical examination should be performed to look for a palpable lesion in the breast, and also of the axilla to assess for lymphadenopathy. Further mammography, including focal paddle compression and lateral views, may confirm the presence, morphology and site of the mass. Ultrasound could be used to establish the nature of the mass. It is likely to have features suspicious for malignancy – heterogeneous and solid, with ill-defined margins. The lesion should undergo needle core biopsy. If the mass is not visible on ultrasound, stereotactic core biopsy of the mammographic abnormality should be performed. Ultrasound of the ipsilateral axilla should also be performed: any lymph nodes of configuration suspicious for malignancy should undergo needle core biopsy or fine needle aspiration (FNA).

2. **In the NHS Breast Screening Programme, what is the age range of the women invited, what is the screening interval, and what mammographic views are taken?**
   At present women are invited for bilateral two-view mammography – mediolateral oblique (MLO) and craniocaudal (CC) or superioinferior (SI) projections every three years between the ages of 50 and 70 years. The screening programme in the UK is currently being extended to incorporate women in the age range 47–73 years.

Key points

- Breast cancer is the most common cancer in women. Risk factors include:
  - history of breast or ovarian cancer in a first-degree relative
  - previous history of breast/ovarian cancer
  - obesity
  - HRT
  - early menarche, nulliparity
  - radiation exposure (especially in the under-30s)
  - late menopause
  - oral contraceptive usage
- Breast cancer is associated with the following genetic disorders: mutations in BRCA1 and 2; Li–Fraumeni syndrome; Cowden's disease.
- MRI is more sensitive than mammography at detecting breast cancer, although it has low specificity. Tumours usually enhance avidly with contrast.

Further reading

Liston J, Wilson R. *Clinical Guidelines for Breast Cancer*, 3rd edn. NHSBSP Publication 49. Sheffield: NHS Breast Screening Programme, 2010.
Breast Screening: a Pocket Guide. Sheffield: NHS Breast Screening Programme, 2008.

Breast Case 19

IAIN D. LYBURN

Clinical history

A 72-year-old woman. Swollen, painful left breast with peau d'orange getting rapidly progressively worse for two months.

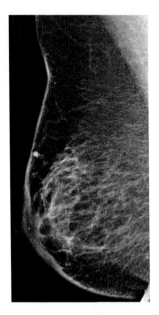 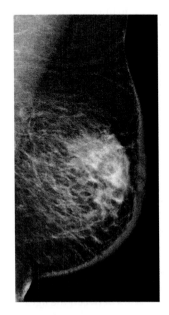

Figure 5.19a   Figure 5.19b

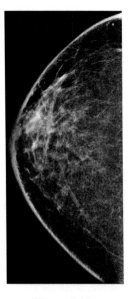 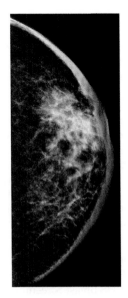

Figure 5.19c   Figure 5.19d

Model answer

These are bilateral mediolateral oblique and craniocaudal mammograms (Figures 5.19a–5.19d). After making a global inspection of both breasts, I would examine all the films under magnification, using workstation tools in the case of digital images or a magnifying glass with conventional analogue films, to assess for microcalcifications.

The left breast is of generalized increased density relative to the contralateral one. There is trabecular prominence and skin thickening, with inversion of the nipple. No obvious calcification. The right breast is normal. The appearances of the left breast are very suggestive of an inflammatory carcinoma. The patient will need to have a biopsy of the lesion for definitive diagnosis.

Questions

1. What are the differential diagnoses of such an appearance?
- Inflammatory breast carcinoma
- Infection: mastitis with possible associated abscess
- Post-radiotherapy inflammation
- Non-breast malignancy: leukaemia, lymphoma or adenocarcinoma (of the lung)
- Post trauma

2. What proportion of breast cancers is inflammatory?
Inflammatory carcinoma of the breast accounts for 1% of breast cancers.

Key points

- Inflammatory carcinoma of the breast is due to spread of malignant ductal cells into the epidermis.
- A negative mammogram does not exclude malignancy. MRI may be helpful in these cases. Biopsy should be performed in all cases where malignancy is clinically suspected.

Further reading

Kushwaha AC, Whitman GJ, Stelling CB, Cristofanilli M, Buzdar AU. Primary inflammatory carcinoma of the breast: retrospective review of mammographic findings. *AJR Am J Roentgenol* 2000; **174**: 535–8.

Breast Case 20

IAIN D. LYBURN

Clinical history
A 52-year-old woman. Screening mammograms.

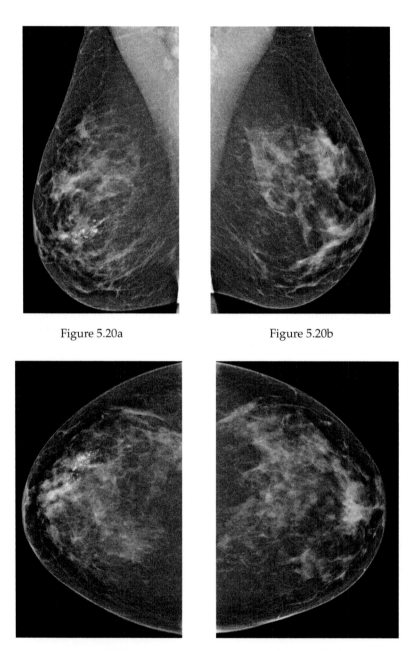

Figure 5.20a

Figure 5.20b

Figure 5.20c

Figure 5.20d

Model answer

These are bilateral mediolateral oblique and craniocaudal mammograms (Figures 5.20a–5.20d). After making a global inspection of both breasts, I would examine all the films under magnification, using workstation tools in the case of digital images or a magnifying glass with conventional analogue films, to assess for microcalcifications.

There is extensive pleomorphic microcalcification distributed in a clustered linear distribution in the retroareolar and lateral aspects of the right breast. The linear distribution of the calcification would be consistent with intraductal calcification. The features are suspicious for ductal carcinoma in situ (DCIS). I would suggest magnification views to further characterize the nature of the microcalcification and ultrasound to assess for the presence of a mass in the right breast. If a mass is identified, ultrasound-guided biopsy should be performed; if not, the patient should have stereotactic biopsy of the microcalcifications.

Questions

1. **How would you define mammographic microcalcification?**
   The individual components of microcalcification measure < 0.5 mm in diameter. (The components of macrocalcification are ≥ 0.5 mm in diameter.)
2. **What are some of the features of calcification suspicious for malignancy?**
   - Pleomorphic microcalcification – the components are of varying size and shape; branching linear forms are particularly suspicious.
   - Microcalcification of segmental or clustered distribution (as opposed to being scattered throughout the breast).
   - Associated localized soft tissue opacity.
   - Macrocalcification may be seen in malignancy.
   - Very often the appearances are not definitive – if there is any doubt from the imaging or clinical perspective there should be a low threshold to proceed to image-guided biopsy.

Key points

- Ductal carcinoma in situ (DCIS) refers to neoplastic cells that are restricted to the mammary ducts, and it is a risk factor for invasive breast cancer. The proportion of DCIS that will become invasive breast cancer is uncertain.
- Ratio of DCIS to invasive breast cancer is 1 : 4.
- When assessing microcalcifications in the breast, describe the site, distribution (widespread versus localized), shape, heterogeneity (are the calcifications of the same size and shape?) and density.

Further reading

Allegra CJ, Aberle DR, Ganschow P, *et al*. NIH state-of-the-science conference statement: diagnosis and management of ductal carcinoma in situ. *NIH Consens State Sci Statements* 2009; **26**: 1–27.

Bassett LW. Mammographic analysis of calcifications. *Radiol Clin North Am* 1992; **30**: 93–105.

Sickles EA. Breast calcification: mammographic evaluation. *Radiology* 1986; **160**: 289–93.

Breast Case 21

IAIN D. LYBURN

Clinical history

36-year-old man. Tender soft lump behind the left nipple.

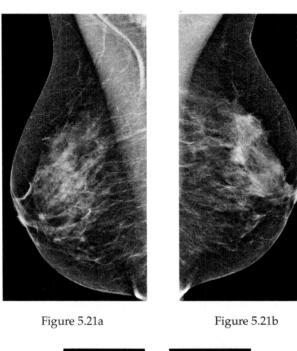

Figure 5.21a   Figure 5.21b

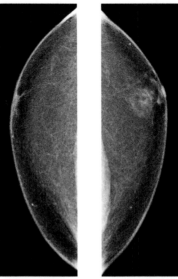

Figure 5.21c   Figure 5.21d

Model answer

These are bilateral mediolateral oblique and craniocaudal mammograms (Figures 5.21a–5.21d). After making a global inspection of both breasts, I would examine all the films under magnification, using workstation tools in the case of digital images or a magnifying glass with conventional analogue films, to assess for microcalcifications.

There is a flame-shaped density which merges into surrounding fatty tissue in the retroareolar aspect of the left breast. The right breast is normal.

The density in the left breast has features consistent with gynaecomastia. I will discuss the case with the referring clinician, as further investigation, if required, is guided by the clinical presentation. The patient's testicles should be examined for tumour.

Questions

1. **What are some of the causes of gynaecomastia?**
   Gynaecomastia is due to a hormonal imbalance: a relative excess of serum level of oestradiol and a decreased serum level of testosterone. There are a number of categories of causes:
   - physiological changes at puberty and senescence
   - endocrine disorders: hypo- and hyperthyroidism
   - systemic diseases: chronic renal failure and cirrhosis
   - testicular tumours: germ cell, Leydig and Sertoli
   - non-testicular neoplasms: liver, lung and renal cell
   - pharmacological: anabolic steroids, digoxin, cimetidine, spironolactone and marijuana
2. **How common is male breast cancer?**
   Male breast cancer accounts for less than 1% of male cancers and less than 1% of breast cancers in the Western world. The mean age of presentation is 70 years. Predisposing factors include Klinefelter's syndrome and previous breast irradiation.

Key points

- Gynaecomastia can occur at any age but is most commonly found in infancy (due to maternal oestrogen), puberty and old age.
- Many cases of gynaecomastia require no treatment and resolve spontaneously. The mainstay of treatment is medical, and involves pharmacological hormonal manipulation. Surgery is reserved for those in whom medical management has failed.

Further reading

Braunstein GD. Clinical practice: gynecomastia. *N Engl J Med* 2007; **357**: 1229–37.
Chantra PK, So GJ, Wollman JS, Bassett LW. Mammography of the male breast. *AJR Am J Roentgenol* 1995; **164**: 853–8.

Breast Case 22

IAIN D. LYBURN

Clinical history
A 53-year-old woman. Screening mammograms. Report the mammograms first.

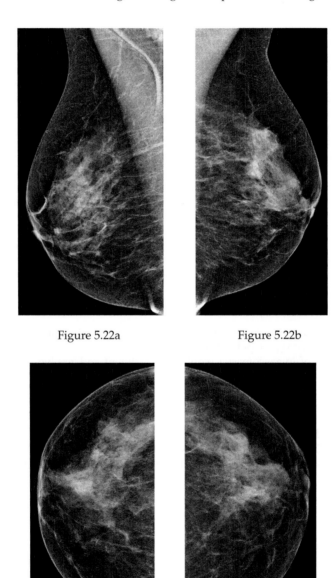

Figure 5.22a

Figure 5.22b

Figure 5.22c

Figure 5.22d

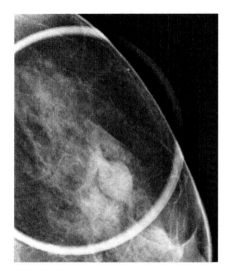

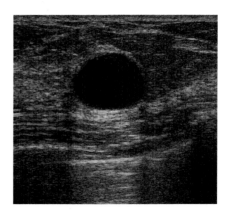

Figure 5.22e   Figure 5.22f

Model answer

These are bilateral mediolateral oblique and craniocaudal mammograms, along with a spot compression view (Figures 5.22a–5.22e). There is an ovoid mass in the upper outer quadrant of the left breast. The spot compression view confirms the presence of a smooth ovoid opacity with well-defined margins. There is no associated spiculation or calcification. The differential diagnoses include a cyst, papilloma, fibroadenoma, fat necrosis and a well-circumscribed carcinoma. I would like to arrange an ultrasound for further characterization.

The ultrasound (Figure 5.22f) demonstrates an ovoid homogeneously anechoic mass with through transmission and posterior acoustic enhancement. No associated nodularity. The appearances are consistent with a simple cyst.

Questions

1. **How could you further manage this lesion?**

   The cyst could be aspirated to dryness under ultrasound guidance if it was painful or if the patient wished to have an aspiration. There is a high probability of recurrence post aspiration. If the cyst is not causing any distress, no intervention is necessary.

Key points

- Ultrasound is the imaging examination of choice in women under the age of 35.
  - useful for further characterization of lesions found on mammography or palpable lumps not visualized on mammography
  - is usually the image-guided modality of choice for biopsy of breast lesions (if visible)
  - allows differentiation of cystic versus solid lesions
- Ultrasound features associated with benign lesions include oval shape, uniform echotexture, posterior enhancement, smooth echogenic pseudocapsule, 'wider than deep'.

Further reading

Berg WA, Campassi CI, Ioffe OB. Cystic lesions of the breast: sonographic–pathologic correlation. *Radiology* 2003; **227**: 183–91.

Feig SA. Breast masses: mammographic and sonographic evaluation. *Radiol Clin North Am* 1992; **30**: 67–92.

Breast Case 23

IAIN D. LYBURN

Clinical history
64-year-old woman. Screening mammograms.

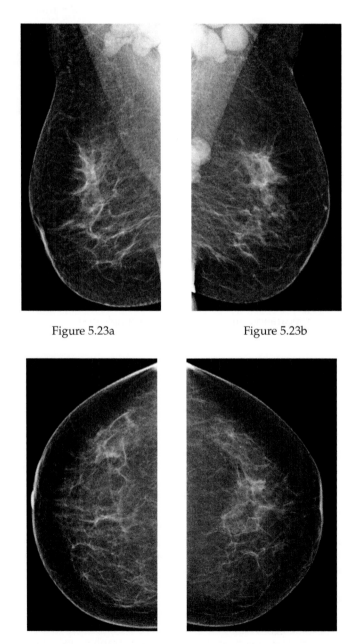

Figure 5.23a

Figure 5.23b

Figure 5.23c

Figure 5.23d

Model answer

These are bilateral mammograms. I am presented with mediolateral oblique and craniocaudal views (Figures 5.23a–5.23d). After making a global inspection of both breasts, I would examine all the films under magnification, using workstation tools for digital images or a magnifying glass for analogue films, to look for microcalcifications.

There are enlarged nodes in both axillae. The parenchyma in both breasts is normal. Differential diagnoses of bilateral axillary lymphadenopathy include: lymphoproliferative diseases (lymphoma and leukaemia); granulomatous diseases (sarcoidosis and tuberculosis); collagen vascular diseases (e.g. rheumatoid arthritis); and HIV.

Questions

1. **What are the commonest causes of unilateral axillary adenopathy?**
   - Reactive – infection or inflammation.
   - Breast carcinoma metastases – the primary may be mammography-occult.
   - Metastases from melanoma or lung carcinoma.
   - Silicone granulomatous infiltration from current or prior rupture or leak of a breast prosthesis.

Key points

- Axillary lymph nodes are classified as follows:
  - level 1 nodes lie inferior and lateral to pectoralis minor muscle
  - level 2 nodes lie beneath pectoralis minor muscle (Rotter nodes)
  - level 3 nodes lie superior to pectoralis minor muscle

Further reading

Walsh R, Kornguth PJ, Soo MS, Bentley R, DeLong DM. Axillary lymph nodes: mammographic, pathologic and clinical correlation. *AJR Am J Roentgenol* 1997; **168**: 33–8.

Breast Case 24

IAIN D. LYBURN

Clinical history

A 62-year-old woman. Screening mammograms.

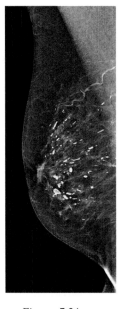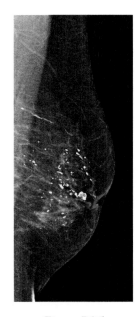

Figure 5.24a   Figure 5.24b

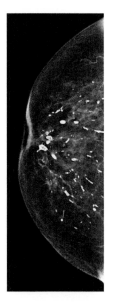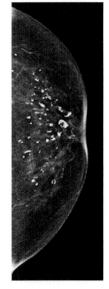

Figure 5.24c   Figure 5.24d

Model answer

These are bilateral mediolateral oblique and craniocaudal mammograms (Figures 5.24a–5.24d). After making a global inspection of both breasts, I would examine all the films under magnification, using workstation tools in the case of digital images or a magnifying glass with conventional analogue films, to assess for microcalcifications.

There is diffuse scattered well-defined microcalcification in both breasts. The components are linear and rod-like with radiolucent centres. Both nipples are inverted. There are no associated soft tissue masses. The features are benign and are most likely due to duct ectasia.

Questions

1. **What are some of the differential diagnoses for diffuse benign micro-calcification?**
   - Plasma cell mastitis and duct ectasia.
   - Vascular – usually secondary to medial atherosclerosis. These often have a characteristic 'train-track' configuration.
   - 'Milk of calcium'. This can be diagnosed as benign with orthogonal magnification mammograms. The CC view demonstrates calcifications as poorly defined and smudgy; the ML view demonstrates calcifications as sharply defined and linear or crescent-shaped.

2. **What proportion of malignant lesions have microcalcification identifiable on mammography?**
   About a third of malignancies contain microcalcification demonstrable on mammography.

Key points

- Duct ectasia is due to inspissated secretions that calcify.
- Nipple retraction refers to when a slit like area of the nipple is pulled inward; nipple inversion refers to when the entire nipple is pulled inward. Both retraction and inversion may be either congenital or acquired. When it is a normal variant, nipple inversion may be reversible by applying manual pressure at the margins of the nipple. Acquired causes include:
  - malignancy – invasive or in situ carcinoma, which may be associated with Paget's disease of the nipple (carcinoma in situ involving the nipple epidermis)
  - duct ectasia (dilatation)
  - fat necrosis
  - abscess
  - mastitis
  - post-surgical change
- Bilateral slowly progressive or long-standing nipple retraction is more likely benign. Women with acquired unilateral nipple inversion should undergo clinical and imaging evaluation.

Further reading

Bassett LW. Mammographic analysis of calcifications. *Radiol Clin North Am* 1992; **30**: 93–105.

Sickles EA. Breast calcification: mammographic evaluation. *Radiology* 1986; **160**: 289–93.

Breast Case 25

IAIN D. LYBURN

Clinical history
62-year-old woman in the symptomatic breast clinic. Firm mass central left breast. Report the mammograms first.

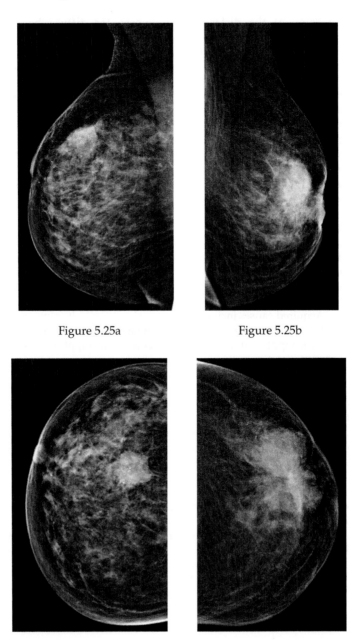

Figure 5.25a

Figure 5.25b

Figure 5.25c

Figure 5.25d

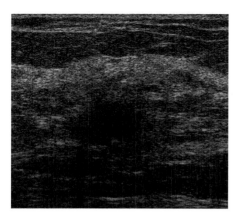

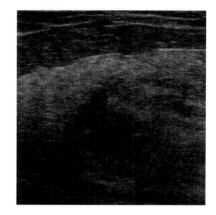

| Figure 5.25e | Figure 5.25f |

Model answer

These are bilateral mediolateral oblique and craniocaudal mammograms (Figures 5.25a–5.25d). After making a global inspection of both breasts, I would examine all the films under magnification, using workstation tools in the case of digital images or a magnifying glass with analogue films, to assess for microcalcifications.

There is a large area of ill-defined opacification associated with distortion in the central left breast. This is associated with nipple retraction. There is an ill-defined semi-spiculate mass associated with clustered pleomorphic microcalcification in the superior central right breast. The patient will require ultrasound and biopsy of these lesions.

I am presented with ultrasound images of both lesions (Figures 5.25e, 5.25f). The ultrasound features of both masses are similar. The masses are hypoechoic, with irregular poorly defined margins and obscuration of the posterior margins. The imaging features are highly suggestive of bilateral breast carcinomas. Biopsy of these lesions and ultrasound of both axillae to assess for nodal involvement is suggested.

Questions

1. **What is the incidence of bilateral breast carcinoma?**
   About 2%.
2. **What is the lifetime probability of a woman with no known risk factors developing breast carcinoma?**
   About 12%.

Key points

- Ultrasound features that could suggest malignancy include: irregular shape, echogenic halo, hypoechogenicity, obscuration of the posterior margins, calcification, gross vascularity on Doppler, extension across tissue planes, 'deeper than wide'.

Further reading

Breast Screening: a Pocket Guide. Sheffield: NHS Breast Screening Programme, 2008.
National Institute for Health and Clinical Excellence. NICE guidelines. Familial breast cancer: the classification and care of women at risk of familial breast cancer in primary, secondary and tertiary care (partial update of CG14). www.nice.org.uk/cg41.

Breast Case 26

IAIN D. LYBURN

Clinical history
73-year-old woman. Previous breast surgery.

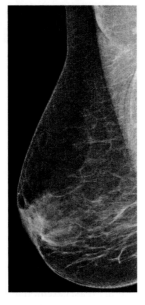 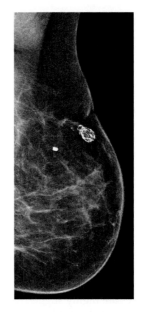

Figure 5.26a   Figure 5.26b

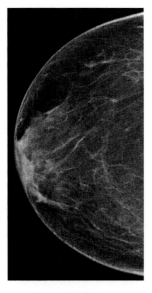 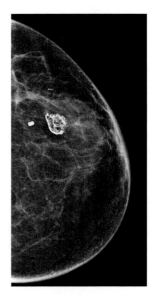

Figure 5.26c   Figure 5.26d

Model answer

These are bilateral mediolateral oblique and craniocaudal mammograms (Figures 5.26a–5.26d). After making a global inspection of both breasts, I would examine all the films under magnification, using workstation tools in the case of digital images or a magnifying glass with conventional analogue films, to assess for microcalcifications.

The left breast is smaller than the right. There is trabecular distortion. In the upper outer quadrant there is focal coarse calcification with a lucent centre. Appearances are suggestive of fat necrosis within a surgical excision bed.

Questions

1. What are some of the differential diagnoses for fat necrosis?
- Blunt trauma, including seat-belt injury.
- Post surgery – lumpectomy, reduction, implantation, reconstruction.
- Spontaneous – in patients with diabetes and collagen vascular disease.
- No history of prior trauma or surgery in up to 50% of cases.

2. What are some of the mammographic appearances post breast conservation therapy?
Post-treatment findings include:
- architectural distortion
- scarring
- oedema
- skin thickening
- calcifications

Key points

- Post-surgical changes may mimic or mask local recurrent malignancy. Recurrent malignancy and post-treatment change can usually be distinguished by comparing findings on follow-up studies.
- Postoperative masses and oedema usually resolve. Post-treatment calcification is usually elongated, lucent-centred and coarse. Pleomorphic and granular microcalcifications are suggestive of recurrent cancer.

Further reading

Chala LF, de Barros N, de Camargo Moraes P, *et al*. Fat necrosis of the breast: mammographic, sonographic, computed tomography and magnetic resonance imaging findings. *Curr Probl Diagn Radiol* 2004; **33**: 106–26.

Krishnamurthy R, Whitman GJ, Stelling CB, Kushwaha AC. Mammographic findings after breast conservation therapy. *Radiographics* 1999; **19**: S53–62.

Acknowledgements

Richard Hopkins would like to acknowledge the help of the following individuals in the preparation of the genitourinary part of this chapter: Dr C. Cook, Dr S. Gandhi, Dr R. Singh, Dr J. Rowlands, Dr A. Isaac.

Paediatric Case 1

RACHANA SHUKLA

Clinical history
None given.

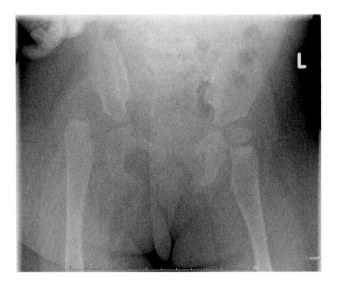

Figure 6.1

Model answer
This is an AP view of the pelvis in an infant who is less than six months old (Figure 6.1). There is a shallow right acetabulum consistent with developmental dysplasia of the right hip. There is superolateral subluxation of the right femoral head secondary to this. The right femoral head ossification centre is smaller than that on the contralateral side, which is due to delayed ossification often observed in the unstable hip. The left hip is normal, with a correctly located femoral head. I would like to discuss the findings with the relevant paediatrician/surgeon, as this disorder needs to be treated to prevent long-term disability.

Questions
1. **Is this the best method for diagnosing developmental dysplasia of the hip (DDH) in an infant?**

   A screening programme is in place in the UK whereby all infants at risk of DDH – namely, breech presentations, infants with a family history of DDH or abnormal hip examinations – should have an ultrasound of the hips at six weeks of age. Ultrasound is 99% sensitive for the diagnosis of DDH and is the modality of choice in an infant less than 4–5 months of age. X-ray diagnosis is preferred in older infants who may have been missed or lost on follow-up, and for late presentation of DDH. X-ray is preferred because there is poor resolution of ultrasound in this age group.

2. **What is likely to happen to this patient if he/she is not treated?**
   The displaced femoral head can cause the formation of a neoacetabulum in the innominate bone, with which it articulates. This can lead to secondary degenerative changes and long-term disability, with pain and reduced function. There is distorted anatomy of the hip joint and correcting this is a demanding surgical procedure.
3. **What are Hilgenreiner's and Perkin's line? What is their clinical significance?**
   The line of Hilgenreiner is the line through the centre of the triradiate cartilage. Perkin's line is perpendicular to Hilgenreiner's line and is drawn in the sagittal plane through the outer border of the acetabulum. These lines divide the hip into quadrants. The femoral head should lie in the inferomedial quadrant in the normal hip. DDH is suspected if this is not the case.

Key points

- DDH is a neonatal condition in which there is hip instability. This affects femoral and acetabular development.
- Risk factors: breech presentation, females, positive family history, first child.
- Hip ultrasound is the initial imaging investigation in the majority of cases. The alpha angle, which is the angle between the line through the acetabular roof and the innominate bone in the coronal plane, should be more than 60 degrees in normal individuals. The beta angle (the angle between the long axis of the innominate bone and the inclination line) is used to assess the degree of acetabular coverage of the femoral head. This should be more than 55 degrees.
- Stress manoeuvres can be performed to assess hip joint stability during ultrasonography. The Barlow manoeuvre, where the femur is held in adduction and the knee at 90 degrees while applying backward pressure on the knee, is used in most centres.
- Other modalities such as CT or MRI can also be used in patients who present late or have persistent dysplasia. However, CT has considerable radiation risk and both modalities most probably require anaesthesia, which is an additional risk in itself.

Further reading

DiPietro MA, Harcke T. Developmental dysplasia of the hip. In Slovis TL, ed., *Caffey's Pediatric Diagnostic Imaging*, 11th edn. Philadelphia, PA: Elsevier, 2007.

Grissom L, Harcke HT, Thacker M. Imaging in the surgical management of developmental dislocation of the hip. *Clin Orthop Relat Res* 2008; **466**: 791–801.

Luther AZ, Clarke NM. Developmental dysplasia of the hip and occult neurologic disorder. *Clin Orthop Relat Res* 2008; **466**: 871–7.

Paediatric Case 2

RACHANA SHUKLA

Clinical history
Right iliac fossa pain and redcurrant-jelly stools.

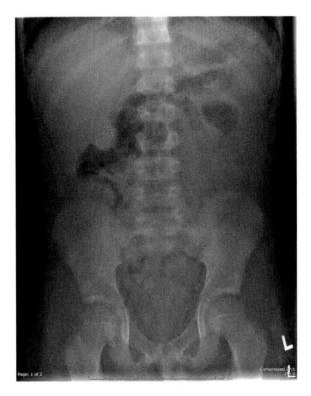

Figure 6.2a

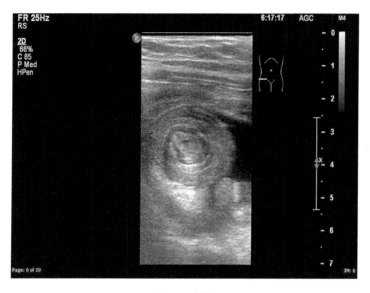

Figure 6.2b

Model answer

The frontal radiograph of the abdomen (Figure 6.2a) shows a filling defect within the caecum with a 'claw-sign' configuration that would be suspicious for a filling defect due to an intussusception. No pneumoperitoneum or bowel wall pneumatosis is visible. An ultrasound would be advisable for confirmation.

The ultrasound of the right iliac fossa (Figure 6.2b) reveals a rounded lesion with multiple alternating echo-dense and echo-lucent layers. Appearances would be consistent with ileo-colic intussusception. There is fluid and fat within the intussusceptum along with a long segment of small bowel. The case will need to be urgently discussed with the relevant surgeon. A cautious reduction with an air enema may be attempted under fluoroscopy if the patient is clinically suitable.

Questions

1. **How is an intussusception treated?**
   First-line treatment for uncomplicated intussusception is an air enema with a fluoroscopy-assisted reduction of intussusception. The child needs to be fluid-resuscitated, with IV access and the appropriate surgeon on standby to operate/intervene on an emergent basis if the reduction is unsuccessful or if bowel perforation occurs. Surgery is the first-line treatment if there are complications such as bowel perforation or if the intussusception is long-standing.
2. **What are the complications of untreated intussusception?**
   Bowel perforation and bowel necrosis.

Key points

- Intussuception occurs when part of a hollow organ prolapses into another segment, analogous to the way in which a retractable antenna or telescope can be shortened.
- The intussusceptum is the part of the organ that prolapses, and the intussuscipiens is the segment that contains the intussusceptum.
- It is a paediatric abdominal emergency, presenting usually at an age between five months and three years. Delay in diagnosis may lead to bowel obstruction, ischaemia, perforation and peritonitis.

- The condition is most commonly idiopathic in children. Non-idiopathic intussusception is due to the presence of a lead point in the bowel, which could be secondary to lymph nodes, diverticulum, scarring, neoplasm or focal haemorrhage. In adults, intussusception is usually due to the presence of a lead point.
- Ultrasound is used as the initial imaging diagnostic modality of choice, in order to confirm the diagnosis prior to attempts at hydrostatic enema reduction.
- A high-frequency (5–10 MHz) linear probe is recommended.
- The appearance of alternating hypo- and hyperechogenic layers seen on ultrasound is due to the different layers of bowel. If there is oedema resulting from venous congestion and obstruction, the alternating layers become more difficult to visualize.

Further reading
Parker BR. Small intestine. In Kuhn JP, Slovis TL, Haller JO, eds., *Caffey's Pediatric Diagnostic Imaging*, 10th edn. Philadelphia, PA: Mosby, 2003; 1616–48.

Paediatric Case 3

RACHANA SHUKLA

Clinical history
A 4-year-old girl presents with a limp.

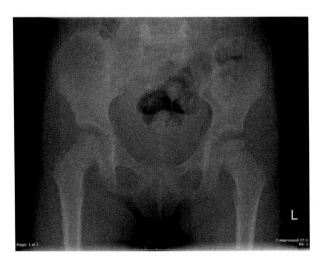

Figure 6.3

Model answer
This is an AP radiograph of the pelvis (Figure 6.3). There is increased density and mild flattening of the left femoral head consistent with Perthes' disease, which is avascular necrosis of the femoral head. The right hip is normal.

Questions

1. **What are the other diagnostic modalities available for diagnosis?**
   Technetium bone scans are useful to diagnose Perthes' disease before it is evident on plain radiographs. MRI would also be helpful in delineating the extent of avascular change prior to x-ray diagnosis.
2. **What is the typical age range of the affected child?**
   Perthes' disease commonly affects 4- to 12-year-old children.
3. **What determines prognosis in idiopathic Perthes' disease?**
   Patients younger than eight years of age tend to do well. Patients with less than 50% involvement of the femoral head fare much better than those with more severe involvement.
4. **What are the causes of avascular necrosis?**
   Most cases of Perthes' disease are idiopathic. However, avascular necrosis of the femoral head can be secondary to trauma, steroid use and sickle cell disease.

Key points

- Perthes' disease (or Legg–Calvé–Perthes) is idiopathic ischaemic necrosis of the femoral head, subchondral fracture, bone necrosis and subsequent bone resorption and repair.
- Early diagnosis and surgery before the appearance of subluxation, and femoral head flattening on radiography, can help prognosis. Bone-scan imaging is the modality of choice for early diagnosis.
- Once Perthes' disease has been diagnosed, MRI is excellent and useful for the evaluation of the extent of epiphyseal necrosis.
- Complications of untreated Perthes' disease are arthritis and severe osseous destruction.

Further reading

Dwek JR. The hip: MR imaging of uniquely pediatric disorders. *Radiol Clin North Am* 2009; **47**: 997–1008.

Kaniklides C. Diagnostic radiology in Legg–Calvé–Perthes disease. *Acta Radiol Suppl* 1996; **406**: 1–28.

Kaniklides C, Lonnerholm T, Moberg A. Legg–Calvé–Perthes disease. Comparison of conventional radiography, MR imaging, bone scintigraphy and arthrography. *Acta Radiol* 1995; **36**: 434–9.

Paediatric Case 4

RACHANA SHUKLA

Clinical history
A 17-month-old infant with drooling and very distressed.

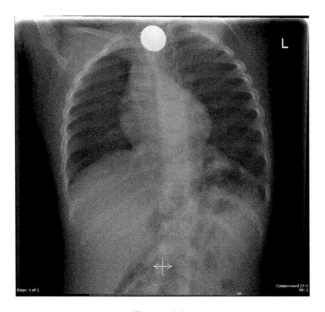

Figure 6.4a

Model answer
This is an AP view of the neck and upper chest in a small child (Figure 6.4a). There is a metallic radiodensity suggestive of a coin projected in the coronal plane at the level of the thoracic inlet on this view. The presence of a large foreign body below the level of the larynx and a coronal orientation of the coin would indicate that the foreign body is located in the oesophagus. If the coin were in the trachea, it would have a sagittal orientation because of the incomplete tracheal rings posteriorly.

Questions
1. **What will you do next?**
   A lateral view of the neck and chest would be advisable for confirmation (Figure 6.4b).

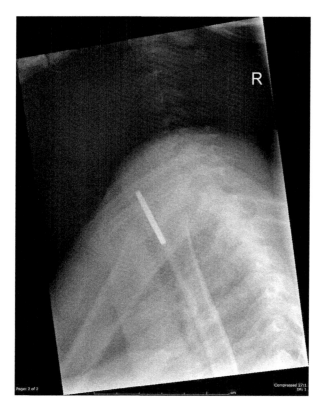

Figure 6.4b

2. How would you investigate a radiolucent oesophageal foreign body?
Direct endoscopy would be the preferred method in case of a witnessed ingestion. You might consider a contrast swallow if the diagnosis is uncertain.

Key points
- Foreign bodies (FBs) have different effects depending on site of impact and time duration. Their effects can range from complete upper airway obstruction with hypoxia to partial obstruction with cough, drooling, stridor and respiratory distress.
- FBs impacted in the upper airways, the larynx or trachea have a higher mortality rate than FBs lodged more distally.
- The peak age for FB impaction is two years.
- A child's airway differs from an adult's until about age eight years. These differences make the paediatric airway more prone to airway obstruction. Differences include:
  - large occiput, resulting in neck flexion in the supine position
  - increased soft tissue, flexible trachea and large tongue
  - more horizontal ribs, flatter diaphragm
  - smaller airway diameter
  - high and anterior airway, with a more acute angle between the tracheal opening and the epiglottis

Further reading
Castellote A, Vazquez E, Vera J. Cervicothoracic lesions in infants and children. *Radiographics* 1999; **19**: 583–600.
Wu IS, Ho TL, Chang CC, Lee HS, Chen MK. Value of lateral neck radiography for ingested foreign bodies using the likelihood ratio. *J Otolaryngol Head Neck Surg* 2008; **37**: 292–6.

Paediatric Case 5

RACHANA SHUKLA

Clinical history
Monoamniotic twin with an antenatal diagnosis of dextrocardia. Clinically stable with no respiratory distress.

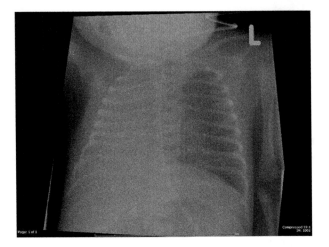

Figure 6.5

Model answer
This is a frontal chest radiograph of a neonate (Figure 6.5). There is complete opacification of the right lung with mediastinal shift to the right. There is decreased intercostal distance in the right hemithorax, indicating a loss of volume. The cardiac outline is not visible because of the significant mediastinal shift to the right. The gastric air bubble is present correctly on the left side. The nasogastric tube passes into the stomach. In the absence of acute respiratory symptoms, appearances would indicate a congenital hypoplasia or agenesis of the right lung.

I would like to look at previous imaging. I notice that this x-ray has been taken three days after birth. I would also like to have an echocardiogram to evaluate the dextrocardia, since there is a high association with congenital heart disease. A specialist referral to a paediatric respiratory physician would also be indicated, with a view to a CT chest/bronchoscopy for adequate delineation of the right chest.

Questions

1. You mentioned hypoplasia and agenesis of the lung. What is the difference?

Lung agenesis refers to complete non-development of the lung. In lung hypoplasia there is some pulmonary development, although the distal lung tissues are incompletely formed (to a varying degree).

2. What is lung aplasia?

This is complete absence of the lung with presence of rudimentary main bronchus.

3. What are the associated anomalies?

Renal disease, heart anomalies and congenital diaphragmatic hernias. There is also an association with the VACTERL syndrome (vertebral, anorectal, cardiac, tracheo-oesophageal, renal, limb).

4. What is the role of ultrasound in a child with a completely opaque hemithorax?

Ultrasound is portable, easy and relatively quick. Ultrasound can distinguish fluid from solid lung/mass and the diaphragm can be assessed in real time. Ultrasound is also useful in the workup of other associated anomalies, including ultrasound of the renal tract.

Key points

- Unilateral lung agenesis or lung aplasia can affect either side, with no predilection for one side or the other.
- There is no sex predilection with unilateral lung agenesis or lung aplasia.
- There is compensatory hyperinflation of the contralateral lung.
- Lung hypoplasia can be unilateral or bilateral. It can be primary, or it may be secondary to causes such as congenital diaphragmatic hernia, agenesis of diaphragm, large intrathoracic mass, excessive pleural fluid secondary to non-immune fetal hydrops, and oligohydraminos.

Further reading

Berrocal T, Madrid C, Novo S, *et al*. Congenital anomalies of the tracheobronchial tree, lung, and mediastinum: embryology, radiology, and pathology. *Radiographics* 2004; **24**(1): e17.

Effmann EL. Anomalies of the lung. In Kuhn JP, Slovis TL, Haller JO, eds., *Caffey's Pediatric Diagnostic Imaging*, 10th edn. Philadelphia, PA: Mosby, 2003; 899–902.

Paterson A. Imaging evaluation of congenital lung abnormalities in infants and children. *Radiol Clin North Am* 2005; **43**: 303–23.

Paediatric Case 6

RACHANA SHUKLA

Clinical history
A 10-year-old girl presents with left hip pain.

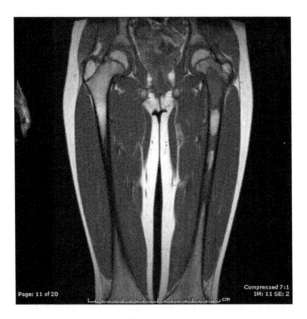

Figure 6.6a

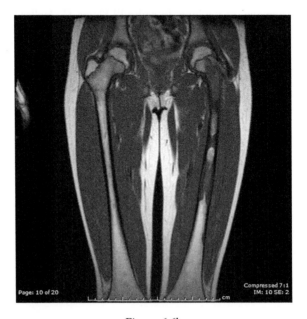

Figure 6.6b

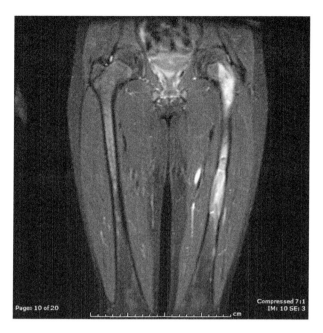

Figure 6.6c

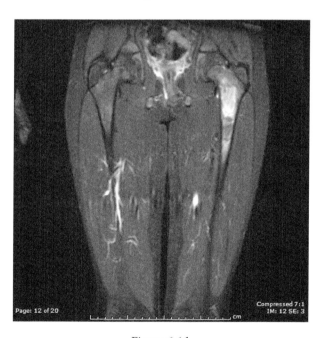

Figure 6.6d

Model answer

These are T1-weighted and STIR (fat-suppressed) coronal sequences through the hips and legs (Figures 6.6a–6.6d). There are multiple intramedullary expansile cystic areas involving the left femoral neck and shaft with sharp margins and a narrow zone of transition. The lesions have a homogeneous low signal on T1-weighted sequences and high signal on T2-weighted sequences. There is no evidence of an associated soft tissue mass or cortical destruction. However, there is a subtle transverse line through the medial femoral cortex at the level of the left femoral neck, which would be highly suspicious for an incomplete fracture. Appearances are suggestive of fibrous dysplasia of the left femur with a pathological fracture of the left femoral neck. I would like to compare the current imaging with previous plain radiographs of the pelvis to look at the bony detail. The patient should be referred to the orthopaedic surgeons for management of the left femoral fracture.

Questions

1. **What would be the initial radiology imaging modality for patients with bone lesions?**

   Plain radiographs are still essential for fibro-osseous lesions in both the adult and paediatric population. Then further characterization with MRI is warranted, as MRI is superior in assessing the tumour extent, extent of intramedullary involvement, joint assessment/involvement and soft tissue abnormalities. In particular, MRI is excellent in determining involvement of the neurovascular bundle and muscle.

2. **Are there associated abnormalities or syndromes associated with fibrous dysplasia?**

   Endocrine disturbances such as hyperparathyroidism, acromegaly and Cushing's syndrome may occur in a subset of patients. The disease forms part of the triad of McCune–Albright syndrome (the other two being precocious puberty and café-au-lait spots).

Key points

- Most cases of fibrous dysplasia are monostotic, and approximately one-fifth of cases are polyostotic.
- Can occur in any bone. Four main disease patterns: (1) monostotic, (2) polyostotic, (3) craniofacial, (4) cherubism.
- On plain radiography and CT, fibrous dysplasia is classically described as well-defined, sclerotic margins, expanded lesion with a ground-glass appearance.
- On MRI it is seen as an intramedullary lesion, iso to low T1-weighted signal, on T2-weighting heterogeneous and high signal. There is no cortical destruction. There is a hypointense rim (dark) on all sequences due to the sclerotic margin.

Further reading

Kaste SC, Strouse PJ, Fletcher BD, Neel MD. Benign and malignant bone tumors. In Slovis TL, ed., *Caffey's Pediatric Diagnostic Imaging*, 11th edn. Philadelphia, PA: Elsevier, 2007.

Wootton-Gorges SL. MR imaging of primary bone tumors and tumor-like conditions in children. *Magn Reson Imaging Clin N Am* 2009; **17**: 469–87.

Paediatric Case 7

RACHANA SHUKLA

Clinical history
An 8-year-old child presents with cough and chest pain.

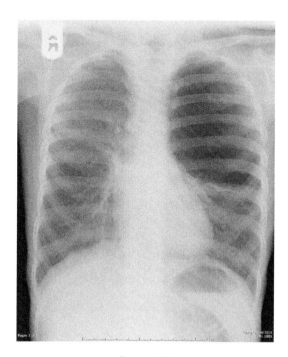

Figure 6.7

Model answer
This frontal chest radiograph (Figure 6.7) shows an expanded hyperlucent left upper lobe with paucity of lung markings. This is associated with some compressive atelectasis of the left lower lobe. The right lung is clear. The heart is normal. Appearances would be consistent with congenital lobar emphysema involving the left upper lobe. Specialist chest physician referral would be indicated, with a view to further imaging with a CT scan to characterize lung morphology.

Questions
1. **What is congenital lobar emphysema (CLE)?**
   Congenital lobar emphysema is a hyperinflation of a pulmonary lobe due to air trapping.
2. **What are the causes of congenital lobar emphysema?**
   Lobar emphysema can be congenital or acquired. Acquired lobar emphysema may be secondary to extrinsic or intrinsic compression and/or narrowing. There may be extrinsic compression by vascular lesions, vascular rings, the pulmonary artery, or enlarged lymph nodes. Intrinsic causes include bronchomalacia, bronchial stenosis, bronchotorsion, aspirated meconium and foreign bodies.

3. **Which pulmonary lobes can be involved?**
   The left upper lobe is the commonest site (40%), followed by the middle lobe (30%), the right upper lobe (20%) and the lower lobes (< 10%).
4. **What is the treatment of choice?**
   Surgical resection.

Key points

- Male predilection.
- Approximately half the patients present in the neonatal period and within six months of birth.
- Chest radiograph is the initial imaging modality of choice and is diagnostic.
- Imaging pitfall – it is important *not* to mistake this for a pneumothorax. Attenuated lung markings will be present in CLE.
- CT chest is useful to assess for secondary causes: vascular lesions or mediastinal masses.

Further reading

Effmann EL. Anomalies of the lung. In Kuhn JP, Slovis TL, Haller JO, eds., *Caffey's Pediatric Diagnostic Imaging*, 10th edn. Philadelphia, PA: Mosby, 2003; 904.

Mendeloff EN. Sequestrations, congenital cystic adenomatoid malformations and congenital lobar emphysema. *Semin Thorac Cardiovasc Surg* 2004; **16**: 209–14.

Paterson A. Imaging evaluation of congenital lung abnormalities in infants and children. *Radiol Clin North Am* 2005; **43**: 303–23

Paediatric Case 8

RACHANA SHUKLA

Clinical history
A newborn infant presents with abdominal distension and scrotal oedema.

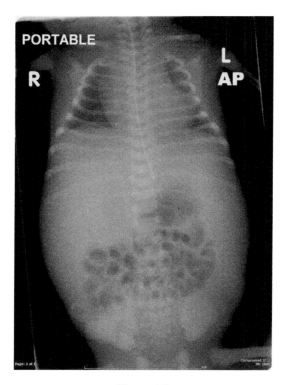

Figure 6.8

Model answer
Chest and abdominal radiograph in a neonate (Figure 6.8). There are flecks of calcification throughout the peritoneal cavity, relatively more marked in the right flank and right upper quadrant. There is an ovoid lucency in the right paramedian region of the central abdomen. Overall appearances are suggestive of meconium peritonitis with hollow viscus perforation. The small bowel loops are present centrally within the peritoneal cavity, indicating that there is probably some associated ascites. The nasogastric tube is correctly positioned in the stomach. Urgent referral to paediatric surgery would be indicated here.

Questions
1. **How will you confirm pneumoperitoneum in this infant?**
   I will do a lateral decubitus radiograph, right side up, to look for free gas against the hepatic edge.
2. **What is the condition associated with meconium peritonitis?**
   Distal intestinal obstruction syndrome (previously called meconium ileus) is almost always associated with cystic fibrosis. One would also need to exclude microcolon and bowel atresia.

3. Does the calcification persist into adulthood?

No. The calcification associated with meconium peritonitis virtually always resolves in childhood.

Key points

- Meconium peritonitis is an aseptic chemical peritonitis due to intestinal perforation.
- Meconium peritonitis seen in cystic fibrosis patients usually does not have intraperitoneal calcification.
- Meconium ileus should be differentiated from meconium plug syndrome, which is a transient disorder due to immaturity of the nerve cells in the intestine. Contrast enema classically shows a small empty colon with meconium in the ileum in meconium ileus, and long stringy meconium in meconium plug syndrome.
- Intraluminal meconium calcification can be misinterpreted as meconium peritonitis.

Further reading

Bloom DA, Slovis TL. Congenital anomalies of the gastrointestinal tract. In Slovis TL, ed., *Caffey's Pediatric Diagnostic Imaging*, 11th edn. Philadelphia, PA: Elsevier, 2007.

Chaudry G, Navarro OM, Levine DS, Oudjhane K. Abdominal manifestations of cystic fibrosis in children. *Pediatr Radiol* 2006; **36**: 233–40.

Finkel LI, Slovis TL. Meconium peritonitis, intraperitoneal calcifications and cystic fibrosis. *Pediatr Radiol* 1982; **12**: 92–3.

Paediatric Case 9

RACHANA SHUKLA

Clinical history

A 12-year-old girl referred by the GP with recurrent right hip pain and limited range of movement.

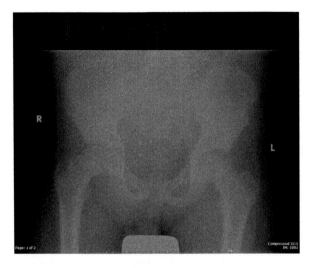

Figure 6.9a

Model answer

X-ray pelvis AP view (Figure 6.9a). There is an abnormal configuration to the right hip with widening of the epiphyseal growth plate. The Klein line (which is the line along the lateral edge of the femoral neck) does not transect the epiphysis. The left hip appears abnormal as well, with a similarly abnormal Klein line, although no epiphyseal widening is visible. Appearances are consistent with bilateral slipped capital femoral epiphyses.

Questions

1. **Is there any other investigation you will do to confirm your impression of the left hip?**
   A frog's-leg lateral view of both hips would be advisable to confirm the diagnosis. (At this point Figure 6.9b will probably be shown to you.)

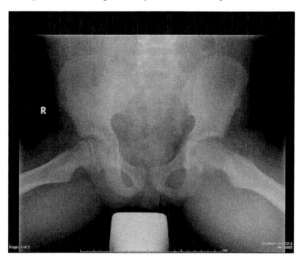

Figure 6.9b

2. **How is this condition treated, and what are the complications of treatment?**
   Pinning in situ is the treatment of choice at present. This may predispose the patient to avascular necrosis of the femoral heads.
3. **What is the age group affected?**
   The disorder typically occurs just after puberty, with a predilection for overweight boys.

Key points

- The aetiology of slipped capital femoral epiphysis (SCFE) is unknown.
- SCFE is the most common hip disorder in adolescents.
- Bilateral involvement occurs in 20–30% of cases.
- Early SCFE is easily missed. Radiographic signs include widening of the physis, a Klein line that does not intersect the femoral head, demineralization and the blanch sign (increased density in the metaphysis of the femur).
- Frog's-leg lateral views should be obtained only if absolutely necessary (or not at all), as they can result in further displacement of the femoral head.
- Lateral views may be useful.
- Stabilization and prevention of further slippage are the goals of surgical management, in order to prevent the complication of avascular necrosis and subsequent arthritis.
- There are several surgical options: pinning in situ, realignment with manipulation or osteotomy, and osteotomy alone.

Further reading

Carney BT, Weinstein SL, Noble J. Long-term follow-up of slipped capital femoral epiphysis. *J Bone Joint Surg Am* 1991; **73**: 667–74.

Crawford AH. Slipped capital femoral epiphysis. *J Bone Joint Surg Am* 1988; **70**: 1422–7.

Paediatric Case 10

RACHANA SHUKLA

Clinical history

A 6-week-old infant does not move the right leg.

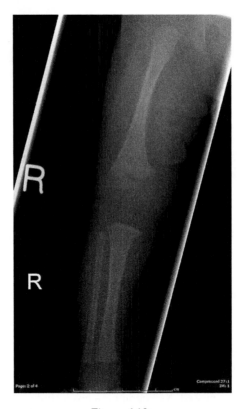

Figure 6.10a

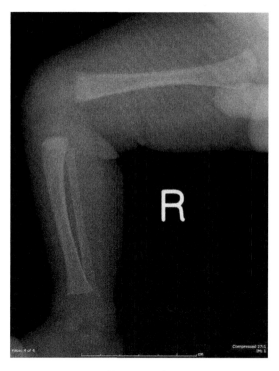

Figure 6.10b

Model answer

These are AP and lateral radiographs of the right leg (Figures 6.10a, 6.10b). There are corner fractures involving the distal femoral metaphysis with a diffuse periosteal reaction, indicating an injury at that site which is more than 7–10 days old. Appearances are suggestive of a non-accidental injury (NAI).

I will liaise with the consultant paediatrician. The patient needs to be recalled for a skeletal survey and CT head.

Questions

1. **What if the skeletal survey does not reveal any further fractures but the clinician is worried after this unexplained metaphyseal fracture?**
   A repeat skeletal survey has been recommended by the Royal College of Radiologists, 10–15 days after the initial presentation, to look for missed fractures. The follow-up skeletal survey two weeks after the initial skeletal survey increases the sensitivity in detection of NAI.
2. **What is the commonest sign of non-accidental injury?**
   Bruising and other soft tissue signs (contusions) are the commonest signs of NAI. Fractures are the second commonest sign.
3. **Why are fractures in a child of less than one year of age highly suspicious?**
   In children of that age group, bones have more plasticity and more force is required to fracture the bone. The bones usually deform before fracturing. Rib fractures, especially posterior rib fractures, have a high specificity for NAI.

Key points

- The classic metaphyseal fracture is commonly found in the distal femur, proximal tibia, proximal fibula, distal tibia, distal fibula and proximal humerus.

- Fractures in non-accidental injury are often due either to direct trauma or, more commonly, to shear force. Shear force results either from twisting injuries or when the child is shaken, resulting in flailing of the limbs.
- Corner fractures are due to the action of shear forces on growing bone adjacent to the growth plate.
- The classic metaphyseal fracture seen in a child older than one year of age is not specific to NAI. In a child less than one year, it is highly suspicious.
- There are other causes of metaphyseal fractures which should be borne in mind: birth trauma, iatrogenic (i.e. orthopaedic manipulation), metabolic bone disorders (rickets is one example) and bone dysplasias.
- Additional views should be used to evaluate equivocal fractures.
- Fractures which have a high specificity for NAI are classic metaphyseal fractures, posteromedial rib fractures, scapular fractures, spinous process fractures and sternal fractures.
- Head injury needs to be excluded in suspected NAI, as it accounts for the vast majority of deaths from the condition. Injuries that may be seen include subdural haematomas, subarachnoid bleeds, diffuse axonal injury, cerebral contusion, hypoxic injuries and skull fractures.

Further reading

Offiah A, van Rijn RR, Perez-Rossello JM, Kleinman PK. Skeletal imaging of child abuse (non-accidental injury). *Pediatr Radiol* 2009; **39**: 461–70.

Royal College of Radiologists, Royal College of Paediatrics and Child Health. *Standards for Radiological Investigations of Suspected Non-Accidental Injury.* London: RCR & RCPCH, 2008.

van Rijn RR. How should we image skeletal injuries in child abuse? *Pediatr Radiol* 2009; **39**: S226–9.

Paediatric Case 11

RACHANA SHUKLA

Clinical history

A 9-year-old with sudden-onset acute pain in the left leg and an antalgic gait.

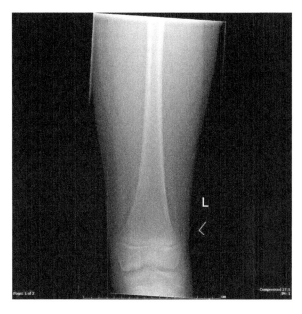

Figure 6.11a

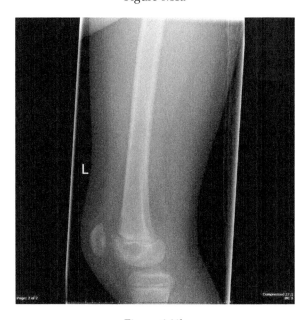

Figure 6.11b

Model answer

AP and lateral views of the left leg (Figures 6.11a, 6.11b). There is a plate-like defect involving the articular margin of the medial femoral condyle, best appreciated on the AP view. I cannot see a convincing ossific loose body on the given projections. Appearances are consistent with osteochondritis dissecans of the left knee.

Questions

1. **What would be the next investigative step?**

   An MRI of the knee is useful to look at the femoral bed at the site of bone avulsion and to grade the lesion. Clinical management of this condition depends on the grading of the lesion, with conservative management for stage I and II injuries and surgical management for stage III and IV injuries.

2. **Which are the other sites which may be affected by osteochondritis dissecans?**

   The humeral head, capitellum of elbow and talus. The knee is the commonest site affected.

Key points

- Staging of osteochondritis dissecans

Stage	Appearance on MRI	Stability of lesion
I	Thickening of articular cartilage and low signal changes	Stable
II	Articular cartilage interrupted, low-signal rim behind fragment showing that there is fibrous attachment	Stable
III	Articular cartilage interrupted, high-signal changes behind fragment and underlying subchondral bone	Unstable
IV	Loose body	Unstable

- Classically osteochondritis dissecans occurs at the medial femoral condyle of the knee, and the knee is the most commonly affected site.
- Other joints have been reported to be affected, including talus, patella, capitellum and the wrist.
- Unknown cause.
- Two distinct groups are affected:
  - juvenile form: aged 5–15 years
  - adult form: older than 15 years with closed physes
- The juvenile form has a better long-term prognosis than the adult form.

Further reading

Aurich M, Anders J, Trommer T, *et al*. Histological and cell biological characterization of dissected cartilage fragments in human osteochondritis dissecans of the femoral condyle. *Arch Orthop Trauma Surg* 2006; **126**: 606–14.

Strouse PJ, Harcke HT. Alignment disorders. In Slovis TL, ed., *Caffey's Pediatric Diagnostic Imaging*, 11th edn. Philadelphia, PA: Elsevier, 2007.

Paediatric Case 12

Clinical history

A 10-year-old girl presents with an eight-week history of headache and vomiting. She is found to have bilateral papilloedema on fundoscopy examination.

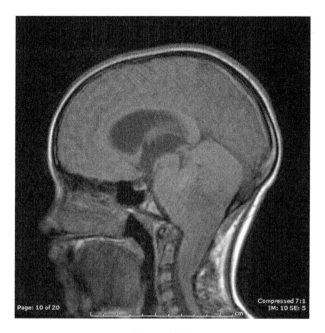

Figure 6.12a

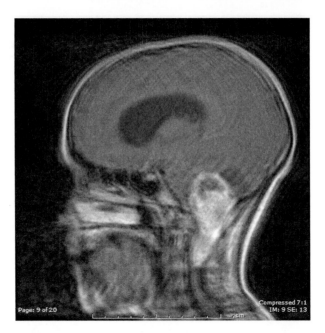

Figure 6.12b

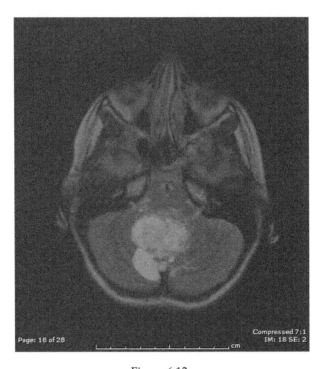

Figure 6.12c

Model answer

MRI of the brain: sagittal pre- and post-contrast T1-weighted and axial T2-weighted sequences (Figures 6.12a–6.12c). There is a heterogeneous lobulated posterior fossa mass, which appears to be arising from the fourth ventricle with secondary ventricular obstruction and hydrocephalus. The mass has solid and cystic components. The solid components are mildly hyperintense on T2-weighted sequence and hypointense on T1-weighted sequence with heterogeneous enhancement on post-contrast T1-weighted sequence. The mass extends inferiorly through the foramen magnum into the upper cord. The 'dripping candle wax' appearance and foraminal extension of this posterior fossa tumour would be consistent with an ependymoma. The differential diagnosis would include a medulloblastoma.

1. **What other investigation will you do to stage this tumour?**
   Ependymomas are prone to drop metastases. An MRI of the whole spine with contrast would therefore be essential.

2. **How do you differentiate a medulloblastoma from an ependymoma?**
   Differentiating between these two conditions can be difficult (or sometimes impossible) radiologically. However, the presence of calcification cysts and hyperdensity on CT would favour ependymoma. The 'dripping candle wax' appearance and foraminal extension with narrow tongues of tissue suggest ependymoma.

3. **What is the treatment for ependymomas?**
   Surgery is the main treatment. Histology confirms the diagnosis, the tumour is debulked or resected, and obstructive hydrocephalus is relieved. Postoperative radiotherapy is the standard adjuvant treatment.

Key points

- Ependymomas are commonly found in the posterior fossa. 90% of childhood ependymomas arise intracranially, while the majority of adult ependymomas occur in the spinal cord.
- Ependymomas arise from the ependymal cells lining the cerebral ventricles and the central canal of the cord.
- Their imaging signal is non-specific, but approximately 20% of these tumours are soft and pliable. They tend to grow through the foramens: Luschka (15%), Magendie (60%) and magnum.
- There are a few options for the treatment of hydrocephalus preoperatively: pre-operative steroids and then removal of tumour, preoperative ventricular drainage and shunt placement, and endoscopic third ventriculostomy.
- Ependymomas have an infiltrative growth pattern along the wall of the fourth ventricle, and therefore complete resection is difficult and the recurrence rate is high.
- Calcification is a feature of a significant number of ependymomas.

Further reading

Barkovich AJ. *Pediatric Neuroimaging*, 4th edn. Philadelphia, PA: Lippincott Williams & Wilkins, 2005; 525–7.

Helton KH, Steen RG. Intracranial neoplasms. In Slovis TL, ed., *Caffey's Pediatric Diagnostic Imaging*, 11th edn. Philadelphia, PA: Elsevier, 2007.

Schiffer D, Giordana MT. Prognosis of ependymoma. *Childs Nerv Syst* 1998; **14**: 357–61.

Shim KW, Kim DS, Choi JU. The history of ependymoma management. *Childs Nerv Syst* 2009; **25**: 1167–83.

Paediatric Case 13

RACHANA SHUKLA

Clinical history
A 12-year-old girl presents with frequent headaches, vomiting and ataxia.

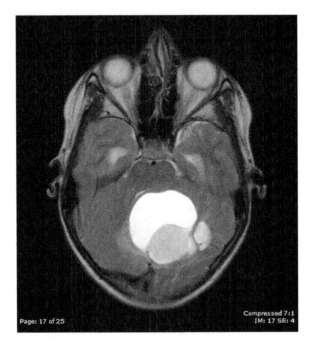

Figure 6.13a

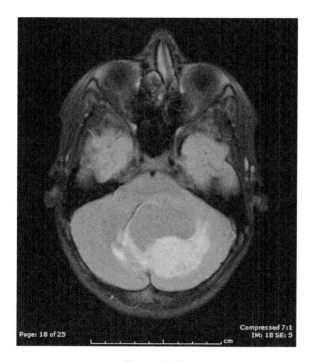

Figure 6.13b

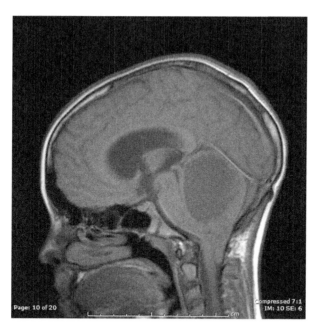

Figure 6.13c

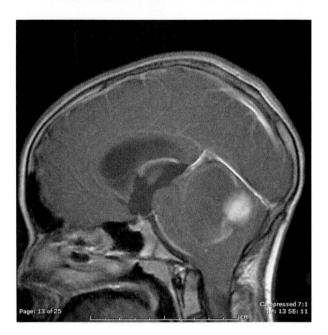

Figure 6.13d

Model answer

Axial T2-weighted and FLAIR sequences (Figures 6.13a, 6.13b). Sagittal T1-weighted pre- and post-contrast sequences (Figures 6.13c, 6.13d). There is a posterior fossa tumour located eccentrically in the left paramedian region of the cerebellum. This has a large cystic component, which is hyperintense on T2-weighted sequence and hypointense on T1-weighted sequences. There are peripheral solid nodules which are mildly hyperintense on T2-weighted and FLAIR sequence and isointense to grey matter on non-contrast T1-weighted sequence. There is intense enhancement of these solid nodules on post-contrast T1-weighted sequence. The mass causes anterior displacement of the fourth ventricle with secondary ventricular compression and hydrocephalus. There is inferior cerebellar tonsil herniation secondary to the raised intracranial pressure. Appearances would be consistent with a juvenile pilocytic astrocytoma in this age group.

Urgent referral to neurosurgery is advised.

Questions

1. **Which other tumours would you think of in an older individual?**
   The commonest posterior fossa tumour in an adult is a metastatic deposit. A haemangioblastoma would also give a similar MRI appearance of a predominantly cystic tumour with a solid nodule.
2. **What condition is juvenile pilocytic astrocytoma (JPA) associated with?**
   Juvenile pilocytic astrocytomas may be associated with neurofibromatosis type 1.
3. **What is the mainstay of treatment for JPAs?**
   Surgical resection. There is no role for radiotherapy as a standard primary treatment for JPAs.

Key points

- Juvenile pilocytic astrocytomas are generally intra-axial tumours, usually WHO grade 1.
- There is no gender predilection.

- Juvenile pilocytic astrocytomas on CT commonly appear as a cyst with a nodule of varying size. The nodule will enhance on post-contrast and there will be variable enhancement of the cyst wall. JPAs can be solid and they will mainly demonstrate homogeneous enhancement.
- Juvenile pilocytic astrocytomas on MRI will show hypo- to isointense nodule with homogeneous enhancement of the nodule on post-contrast. As with CT, there is variable enhancement of the cyst wall.

Further reading

Helton KH, Steen RG. Intracranial neoplasms. In Slovis TL, ed., *Caffey's Pediatric Diagnostic Imaging*, 11th edn. Philadelphia, PA: Elsevier, 2007.

Tonn JC, Westphal M, Rutka JT, eds. *Oncology of CNS Tumors*, 2nd edn. Berlin: Springer, 2010; 445–51.

Paediatric Case 14

RACHANA SHUKLA

Clinical history
A 14-year-old child with learning difficulties presents with ataxia and headache.

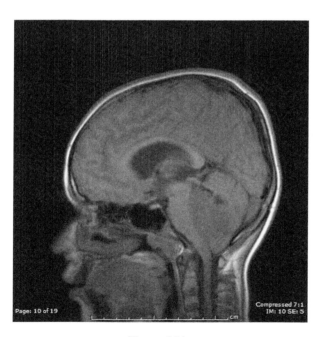

Figure 6.14a

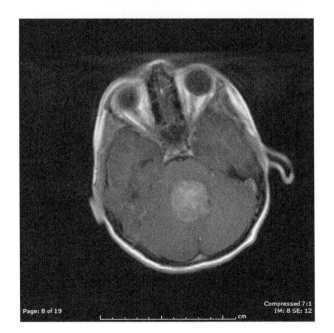

Figure 6.14b

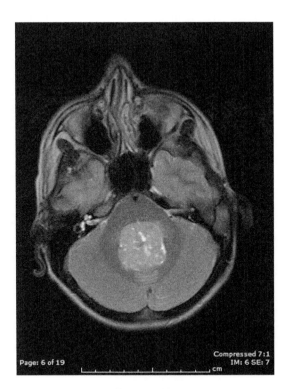

Figure 6.14c

Model answer

MRI of the brain: sagittal T1-weighted pre-contrast and axial post-contrast sequence (Figures 6.14a, 6.14b), axial T2-weighted MR sequence (Figure 6.14c). There is a lobulated midline solid mass probably arising from the cerebellar vermis with effacement of the fourth ventricle. The mass is heterogeneous with predominantly hyperintense signal characteristics on T2-weighted sequences and hypointense on T1-weighted sequences. Moderate enhancement is noted on intravenous contrast administration. There is secondary hydrocephalus. A non-contrast CT, if available, would be useful, as medulloblastomas are hyperdense on CT. The appearances would be suggestive of a medulloblastoma in this age group. The differential would include an ependymoma. As the mass is so large, it is difficult to tell if the lesion is truly arising from the cerebellar vermis or from within the fourth ventricle.

Questions

1. **What else would you like to do to complete the staging process?**
   I would like to do an MRI with contrast of the spine, since these lesions are prone to leptomeningeal spread and drop metastases.
2. **Do medulloblastomas have a particular gender predilection?**
   Males are affected more than females, up to 2–4 times more.

Key points

- Medulloblastoma is an aggressive primitive neuroectodermal tumour (PNET) that arises in the lining of the roof of the fourth ventricle.
- It is the most common tumour in 6- to 11-year-olds.
- Enhancement pattern of medulloblastomas on MR is variable: patchy or homogeneous.
- Histologically 80% are classic medulloblastomas. 15% are desmoplastic medulloblastomas, which is more prevalent in the adult population. Approximately 4% are a highly malignant variant (large-cell / anaplastic medulloblastoma), and the remainder are medulloblastomas with extensive nodularity.
- This tumour can spread via CSF pathways and metastasize via the bloodstream.
- Medulloblastomas are rarely calcified.

Further reading

Helton KH, Steen RG. Intracranial neoplasms. In Slovis TL, ed., *Caffey's Pediatric Diagnostic Imaging*, 11th edn. Philadelphia, PA: Elsevier, 2007.

Paediatric Case 15

RACHANA SHUKLA

Clinical history

A 2-month-old infant presents with poor growth of head circumference.

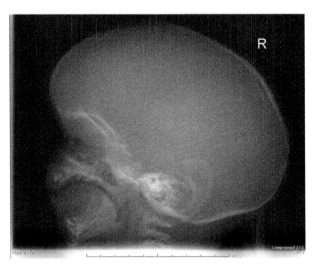

Figure 6.15a

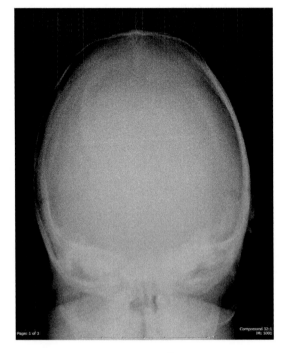

Figure 6.15b

Model answer

These radiographs of the skull are a lateral view and Towne's view (Figures 6.15a, 6.15b). There is an elongated boat-shaped head suggestive of scaphocephaly. The sagittal suture is not clearly visible on the Towne's view. Appearances are suggestive of craniosynostosis involving the sagittal suture. I will do a low-dose CT head for sutural delineation to confirm the diagnosis. A surgical referral is warranted, as the anomaly can be the case of significant cosmetic anomaly and has implications for the growing brain.

Questions

1. **Which is the commonest suture to be involved by craniosynostosis?**
   The sagittal suture is the commonest suture, involved in 50–58% of patients with craniosynostosis, followed by the coronal suture in 20–29%, the metopic suture in 4–10% and the lambdoid suture in 2–4%.
2. **What conditions are associated with craniosynostosis?**
   - Metabolic disorders: hyperthyroidism and rickets
   - Haematological disorders: thalassaemia, polycythaemia vera, sickle cell anaemia
   - Mucopolysaccharidoses
   - Iatrogenic: hydrocephalus with shunt
   - Chromosomal disorders: Apert's syndrome, Crouzon's syndrome
3. **What are the potential problems associated with craniosynostosis?**
   Early fusion of the skull suture lines can lead to significant craniofacial deformity. Raised intracranial pressure is a concern when more than one suture line is involved.
4. **What is the treatment for craniosynostosis?**
   Surgical management. The extent of surgery will depend on the severity of the anomaly. The goals of surgery are to restore normal anatomy and cosmesis, and to allow the brain to expand and develop normally.

Key points

- There are various types of craniosynostosis:
  - Scaphocephaly – fusion of the sagittal suture, producing a boat-shaped skull (Greek *skaphe*, boat).
  - Trigonocephaly – fusion of the metopic suture, producing a triangular shape of the forehead.
  - Plagiocephaly – unilateral synostosis of the coronal suture. On the affected side there is flattening of the forehead and the orbit is raised and triangular.
  - Brachycephaly – synostosis of the coronal sutures. The forehead is set back from normal position at the level of the supraobital rim. However, the forehead bulges over this ridge. The temporal fossa is also bulging.
  - Oxycephaly – late synostosis of the coronal sutures. The supraorbital ridge is set back and the forehead is tilted backwards.
  - Rare types – cloverleaf skull, plagiocephaly, faciocraniosynostosis.

Further reading

Silverman F. Congenital dysplasias. In Kuhn JP, Slovis TL, Haller JO, eds., *Caffey's Pediatric Diagnostic Imaging*, 10th edn. Philadelphia, PA: Mosby, 2003; 345–51.

Paediatric Case 16

RACHANA SHUKLA

Clinical history
A 15-year-old girl presents with neck swelling.

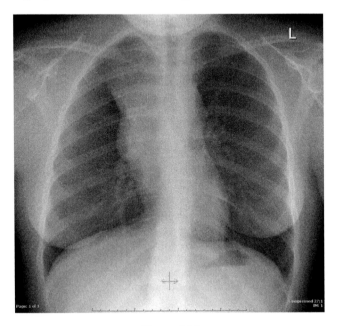

Figure 6.16

Model answer
This is a frontal radiograph of the chest (Figure 6.16). There is fairly extensive right paratracheal and right hilar bulky lymphadenopathy. Mild lobulation is also noted along the left margin of the superior mediastinum, suspicious for left paratracheal/anterior mediastinal lymphadenopathy. The lungs are clear. The heart is normal in size. In view of the cervical, hilar mediastinal and axillary lymphadenopathy, lymphoma or leukaemia are possible diagnoses.

Questions
1. **What would be your next investigative step?**
   A staging CT scan would be required, along with a lymph node biopsy for histopathological diagnosis.
2. **What would be the other causes for hilar and mediastinal lymphadenopathy in this age group?**
   - Infectious: infectious mononucleosis, tuberculosis
   - Reactive: Castleman's disease
   - Miscellaneous: sarcoidosis, Langerhans cell histiocytosis

Key points
- The majority of mediastinal lymphadenopathy in children is malignant rather than benign.

- Malignant mediastinal lymphadenopathy in children is most commonly due to lymphoma or leukaemia. The next commonest is neuroblastoma, and then rhabdomyosarcoma.
- In children Hodgkin's is more common than non-Hodgkin's lymphoma.
- Castleman's disease is also known as angiofollicular lymphoid hyperplasia. It is a disease of unknown aetiology and usually has a benign clinical course.
- Castleman's disease can be unicentric; it presents with single regional lymphadenopathy, usually in the hilum or mediastinum. It can also be multicentric, presenting with generalized lymphadenopathy and organomegaly.

Further reading

Binkovitz L, Binkovitz I, Kuhn J. Mediastinum. In Slovis TL, ed., *Caffey's Pediatric Diagnostic Imaging*, 11th edn. Philadelphia, PA: Elsevier, 2007.

Twist CJ, Link MP. Assessment of lymphadenopathy in children. *Pediatr Clin North Am* 2002; **49**: 1009–25.

Paediatric Case 17

RACHANA SHUKLA

Clinical history

A preterm infant is being started on oral feeds. Develops abdominal distension and bloody stools.

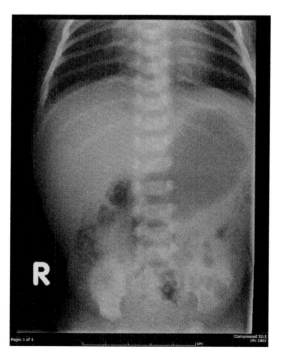

Figure 6.17

Model answer

Plain abdominal radiograph of a neonate (Figure 6.17). The nasogastric tube tip and side-hole are just within the stomach. For optimal positioning, the tube should be advanced slightly. There is mottled bowel shadowing in both flanks with curvilinear and 'bubbly' gas shadows on the right, suggestive of pneumatosis. There is no free gas, portal venous gas or bowel distension. Appearances are suggestive of necrotizing enterocolitis. I will speak to the relevant paediatrician immediately. The patient should have regular abdominal radiographs to check for disease progression as well as the development of perforation.

Questions

1. **Who is at risk of developing necrotizing enterocolitis (NEC)?**
   Premature infants have a relatively higher risk, with the incidence inversely related to birth weight and gestational age. Term infants with comorbidities such as birth asphyxia, metabolic abnormalities or a history of maternal placental insufficiency are also at higher risk of developing necrotizing enterocolitis.
2. **Which part of the intestine is most likely to be affected?**
   The caecum/ascending colon and terminal ileum.
3. **What are the complications?**
   Bowel perforation (can be multiple), strictures (single or multiple, and the colon is more frequently affected than the small intestine) and multiorgan failure.
4. **How do you treat necrotizing enterocolitis?**
   (a) stop enteral feeds
   (b) antibiotics
   (c) fluid resuscitation, ventilatory and inotropic support
   (d) surgical evaluation
   (e) surgery – there is no current consensus as to the best approach; peritoneal drainage or open laparotomy

Key points

- Incidence of necrotizing enterocolitis is increasing due to improved neonatal care, whereas in the past the preterm would have succumbed to a different aetiology.
- Clinical symptoms are often non-specific, and radiographic signs may precede and allow early diagnosis. Early radiographic signs may be non-specific: *dilated bowel loops*, either generalized or a bowel segment, and *intramural gas*, which can be difficult to distinguish from faecal material, and resolution of intramural gas does not necessarily mean a clinical improvement,
- Portal venous gas is not an early radiological sign. It was thought to be a premorbid sign but there are reported cases to the contrary. Portal venous gas can appear and disappear. This does not always indicate clinical improvement.
- Regular radiographic studies are justified and, depending on the severity, will help determine the frequency of radiographs. One institute recommends 4- to 6-hour intervals for severe cases, while mild cases can be imaged every 12–24 hours and continued daily until 7–10 days after clinical improvement to ensure there is no relapse/recurrence.

Further reading

Bloom DA, Slovis TL. Necrotizing enterocolitis. In Slovis TL, ed., *Caffey's Pediatric Diagnostic Imaging*, 11th edn. Philadelphia, PA: Elsevier, 2007.
Boston VE. Necrotising enterocolitis and localised intestinal perforation: different disease or ends of a spectrum of pathology. *Pediatr Surg Int* 2006; **22**: 477–84.
Daneman A, Woodward S, de Silva M. The radiology of neonatal necrotizing enterocolitis (NEC): a review of 47 cases and the literature. *Pediatr Radiol* 1978; **7**: 70–7.

Paediatric Case 18

RACHANA SHUKLA

Clinical history

A 13-month-old infant presents with recurrent urinary tract infections. He presents on this occasion with abdominal pain and distension. Urine culture grows *Proteus*.

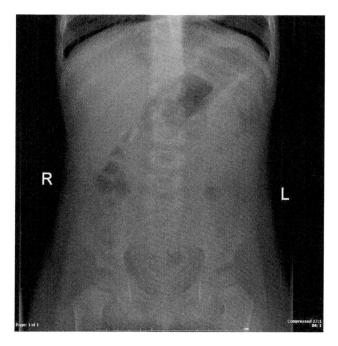

Figure 6.18

Model answer

This is a frontal radiograph of the abdomen (Figure 6.18). There is a lobulated calcific density overlying the renal shadow on the right side. This density follows the outline of the pelvicalyceal system. Appearances are consistent with a right-sided renal staghorn calculus. No radio-opaque stones seen in the left kidney. The bones are normal.

A urological opinion should be sought. The patient will require an ultrasound to search for congenital anomalies that could account for stone formation. A metabolic screen should also be performed to seek out an underlying stone-forming disorder.

Questions

1. **Is there a sex predilection of childhood urolithiasis?**
   No, there is equal occurence between the sexes.
2. **What are the metabolic causes of stone formation in childhood?**
   Any cause of hypercalciuria, such as hypercalcaemia of whatever cause (for example, primary hyperparathyroidism), chronic use of furosemide, immobility and idiopathic hypercalciuria. Other causes include hyperoxaluria and cystinuria.

Key points

- The clinical presentation of urolithiasis is different in the paediatric population. In preschool children urinary tract infection is a common presenation, while in adolescents abdominal, flank and pelvic pain is more common than infections.
- Stone analysis is helpful at directing the investigation for metabolic dysfunction.
- Normal urinary calcium excretion does not differ between the sexes, and racial differences have not been found.
- Performing a 24-hour urinary collection and assessing the urinary calcium excretion make the diagnosis of hypercalciuria.

Further reading

Sty JR. Urolithiasis, nephrocalcinosis, and trauma to the urinary tract. In Kuhn JP, Slovis TL, Haller JO, eds., *Caffey's Pediatric Diagnostic Imaging*, 10th edn. Philadelphia, PA: Mosby, 2003; 1796–9.

Paediatric Case 19

RACHANA SHUKLA

Clinical history

An 8-year-old girl presents with swelling of the left shoulder. There is no history of trauma.

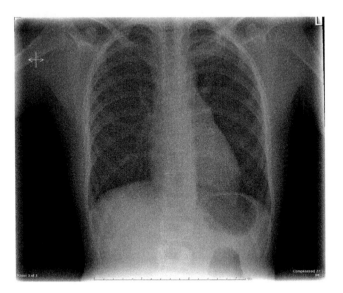

Figure 6.19

Model answer

The frontal chest radiograph (Figure 6.19) shows that there is diffuse expansion of the left clavicle with a permeative lytic lesion, along with extensive lamellar periosteal reaction. No other bony lesion is visible in the thoracic skeleton. The lungs are clear. Heart and mediastinal contours are normal.

The appearances are suggestive of an aggressive disease process, and the differential diagnosis would include an osteomyelitis or a neoplastic process such as Ewing's sarcoma or osteosarcoma. I will discuss the case with the referring clinician. In particular, I would like to know if the patient has any clinical features suggestive of an underlying infection.

Questions
1. **In which decade does osteosarcoma usually present?**
   They present in the second to third decade.
2. **Is there a gender predilection?**
   There is a male predilection.
3. **How will you make a definitive diagnosis?**
   An MRI would be useful to map the soft tissue and bone marrow involvement by the disease process. However, a definitive diagnosis is only possible on histopathology/microbiology.
4. **How would you stage the lesion?**
   A staging chest CT and a bone scan.

Key points
- Osteomyelitis is more common and should be considered in the differential diagnosis.
- The majority of osteosarcomas are located in the metaphyseal region.
- Osteosarcomas are seen on radiographs as destructive bony lesions with a soft tissue component and periosteal reactions: sunburst pattern, periosteal elevation with Codman's triangle.
- An important prognostic factor for osteosarcoma is the presence or absence of metastatic disease at presentation.
- Ewing's sarcoma is classically seen as a lytic permeative lesion in the long bones with soft tissue mass and an aggressive periosteal reaction.

Notes
This was a case of Ewing's sarcoma.

Further reading
Azouz EM. Infections in bone. In Slovis TL, ed., *Caffey's Pediatric Diagnostic Imaging*, 11th edn. Philadelphia, PA: Elsevier, 2007.

Kaste SC, Strouse PJ, Fletcher BD, Neel MD. Benign and malignant bone tumors. In Slovis TL, ed., *Caffey's Pediatric Diagnostic Imaging*, 11th edn. Philadelphia, PA: Elsevier, 2007.

Sforzo CR, Scarborough MT, Wright TW. Bone-forming tumors of the upper extremity and Ewing's sarcoma. *Hand Clin* 2004; **20**: 303–15.

Paediatric Case 20

RACHANA SHUKLA

Clinical history
A patient presents with pain and deformity of the right wrist.

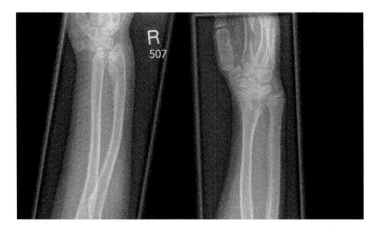

Figure 6.20

Model answer
AP and lateral radiographs of the right wrist (Figure 6.20). There is a growth disturbance of the distal radial epiphysis with radial deviation of the wrist. Dorsal subluxation of the ulna is noted on the lateral view. Appearances are consistent with Madelung's deformity.

Questions
1. **What is congenital or idiopathic Madelung's deformity?**
   It is a growth abnormality of distal radial development. There is triangular deformity and focal dysplasia of the physis and medial tilt of the distal radius.
2. **What is pseudo-Madelung's deformity?**
   Pseudo-Madelung's deformity may be secondary to infection or post trauma, with injury to radial growth plate.
3. **What are the genetic and bone dysplasia causes of this appearance?**
   Genetic disorders are Turner's syndrome, achondroplasia and Léri–Weill syndrome. Bone dysplasias associated with Madelung's deformity include multiple hereditary osteochondromatosis, Olliers disease, achondroplasia, multiple epiphyseal dysplasias and the mucopolysaccharidoses (e.g. Hurler and Morquio syndromes).
4. **What is the treatment?**
   Surgical correction of the bony deformity and ligamentous thickening can be performed.

Key points
- Female predominance. Idiopathic Madelung's deformity predominantly affects young girls around puberty. Severe non-traumatic Madelung's disease is rare in males.

- Madelung's deformity is defined as volar/ulnar angulation of the distal radius, dorsal prominence of the distal ulna and volar displacement of the wrist.
- Radiologically, there is shortening and curving of the radius, a widened distal radioulnar joint, complete dorsal dislocation of the distal ulna and a triangular configuration of the carpal bones.
- There is thickening of the radiolunate and Vickers ligaments.
- The goal of surgery is to alleviate and relieve pain, correct the cosmetic deformity and improve the range of motion, which is limited in patients with Madelung's deformity.

Further reading
Felman AH, Kirkpatrick JA. Madelung's deformity: observations in 17 patients. *Radiology* 1969; **93**: 1037–42.

Kim HK. Madelung deformity with Vickers ligament. *Pediatr Radiol* 2009; **39**: 1251.

Watt AJ, Chung KC. Generalized skeletal abnormalities. *Hand Clin* 2009; **25**: 265–76.

Paediatric Case 21

RACHANA SHUKLA

Clinical history
A neonate presents with respiratory distress.

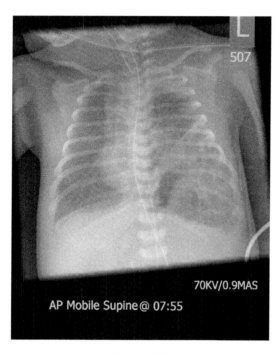

Figure 6.21

Model answer

This is a frontal radiograph of the chest in a neonate (Figure 6.21). There are multiple loops of bowel in the left lower chest with mediastinal shift to the right. There is associated compressive atelectasis of the lower part of the left lung. Endotracheal tube and nasogastric tube are correctly positioned. The tip of the UAC is visible at T9. The tip of the UVC is just visible at the edge of the film and it appears to be located at L2. Appearances are consistent with a left-sided diaphragmatic hernia. The UVC needs to be repositioned as well.

I would like to inform the referring paediatrician immediately, as urgent transfer to a specialist paediatric surgery unit will be required after repositioning the UVC.

Questions

1. **What are the different types of congenital diaphragmatic hernia that you are aware of?**
   - The commonest type of congenital diaphragmatic hernia is the Bochdalek hernia, which is a posterolateral defect, commoner on the left side.
   - The Morgagni hernia is a parasternal or retrosternal anterior diaphragmatic hernia.
   - The peritoneopericardial hernia is due to a defect in the central tendon of the diaphragm.
2. **What are the complications associated with congenital diaphragmatic hernia?**
   In utero, pulmonary hypoplasia can result from compression of the lungs. This can result in perinatal death. Gut volvulus as well as malrotation are also associated with congenital diaphragmatic hernia.
3. **Is congenital diaphragmatic hernia associated with any other abnormalities?**
   Yes, it is commonly associated with cardiac, gastrointestinal, genitourinary, skeletal and neural anomalies.

Key points

- Affects 1 in 2000 births.
- The severity of lung hypoplasia and pulmonary hypertension determines the probability of survival.
- The distal airways continue to develop until eight years of age.
- Because the development of the pulmonary vasculature follows airway development, this is affected.
- Ultrasound is the main imaging modality for prenatal diagnosis of congenital diaphragmatic hernia.

Further reading

Roessingh AS, Dinh-Xuan AT. Congenital diaphragmatic hernia: current status and review of the literature. *Eur J Pediatr* 2009; **168**: 393–406.

Slovis TL, Bulas D. Congenital and acquired lesions (mostly causing respiratory distress) of the neonatal lung and thorax. In Slovis TL, ed., *Caffey's Pediatric Diagnostic Imaging*, 11th edn. Philadelphia, PA: Elsevier, 2007.

Taylor GA, Atalabi OM, Estroff JA. Imaging of congenital diaphragmatic hernias. *Pediatr Radiol* 2009; **39**: 1–16.

Paediatric Case 22

RACHANA SHUKLA

Clinical history

A premature neonate presents with respiratory distress.

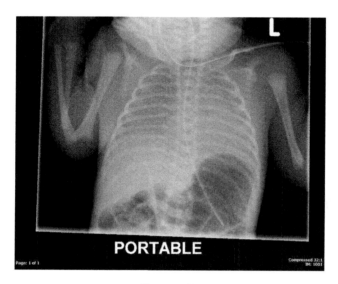

Figure 6.22

Model answer

The frontal chest radiograph (Figure 6.22) reveals poor pulmonary aeration with a granular appearance to both lungs, as well as bilateral air bronchograms. There is associated obscuration of the heart borders. The findings are suggestive of respiratory distress syndrome of the newborn. Differential diagnoses include transient tachypnoea of the newborn, severe neonatal pneumonia and pulmonary oedema. No pneumothorax or pneumomediastinum. The nasogastric tube passes into the stomach. The umbilical arterial catheter is projected at T10. The umbilical vein catheter is malpositioned, with its tip projected over the liver. This finding suggests that the catheter may have passed into the portal venous system rather than the IVC. Intrahepatic perforation of the vessel wall is another possibility. Therefore, the catheter needs to be repositioned or removed, preferably under image guidance.

Questions

1. **What would be the possible complication of this malpositioned UVC?**
   The neonate may develop portal vein thrombosis.
2. **How do you differentiate respiratory distress syndrome of the newborn from the other possible differential diagnoses?**
   Clinical history is important and could guide diagnosis. RDS occurs within eight hours of birth. Uncomplicated RDS is not associated with a pleural effusion. This is in contrast to heart failure and pneumonia, where pleural effusions are common. The airspace opacification of transient tachypnoea of the newborn is, as its name implies, transient and disappears spontaneously.

3. What are the complications of RDS?

Short-term complications include respiratory failure, pneumothorax and pneumo-mediastinum. The most important long-term complication is chronic lung disease, which may lead to long-term pulmonary morbidity.

Key points

- Respiratory distress syndrome (RDS) is common in premature infants, but it is not exclusive to preterm infants.
- RDS is of unknown aetiology and associated with maternal diabetes, maternal complications of pregnancy and perinatal fetal distress.
- RDS is characterized histologically by diffuse alveolar collapse.
- Transient tachypnoea of the newborn is thought to be due to incomplete resorption of fluid from the newborn lungs and usually presents within a few hours of birth.
- The risk factors for transient tachypnoea of the newborn are: caesarean section, male sex, maternal diabetes, macrosomia and family history of asthma.
- Bronchopulmonary dysplasia is the result of inflammation and scarring, which is most often due to the treatment of RDS with oxygen and positive pressure ventilation.
- Due to improvements in the treatment of RDS, there has been a reduction in the severity of diagnosed bronchopulmonary dysplasia. Conversely, the prevalence of bronchopulmonary dysplasia has increased because of improved survival.

Further reading

Guglani L, Lakshminrushimha S, Ryan RM. Transient tachypnea of the newborn. *Pediatr Rev* 2008; **29**: e59–65.

Leonidas JC. Miscellaneous conditions of the gastrointestinal and hepatobiliary systems. In Kuhn JP, Slovis TL, Haller JO, eds., *Caffey's Pediatric Diagnostic Imaging*, 10th edn. Philadelphia, PA: Mosby, 2003; 183.

Paediatric Case 23

RACHANA SHUKLA

Clinical history
Newborn infant with reduced oxygen saturation. Paediatrician finds it difficult to pass a nasogastric tube into the stomach.

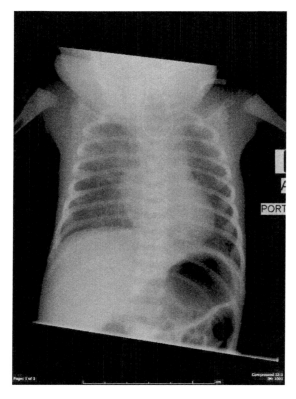

Figure 6.23

Model answer
AP chest radiograph in a neonate (Figure 6.23). The nasogastric tube is coiled in the upper chest. The stomach contains gas and is correctly located under the left hemi-diaphragm. The lungs are clear. Cardiac outline is normal. In view of the given clinical history of inability to pass a nasogastric tube, oesophageal atresia with a distal tracheo-oesophageal fistula is the most likely diagnosis. Urgent referral to paediatric surgery would be indicated for surgical repair, as the patient is at risk of aspiration pneumonia. The patient should have an echocardiogram and ultrasound examination to screen for associated abnormalities prior to surgery.

Questions
1. **What are the types of tracheo-oesophageal fistula that you know about?**
   There are four types of tracheo-oesophageal fistula:
   - oesophageal atresia with distal tracheo-oesophageal fistula

- H-type tracheo-oesophageal fistula
- oesophageal atresia with proximal fistula
- oesophageal atresia with proximal and distal fistula

Oesophageal atresia may also occur without a tracheo-oesophageal fistula.

2. **How would you investigate a tracheo-oesophageal fistula in the presence of a patent oesophagus?**

   A tubogram may be performed – instillation of contrast through a nasogastric tube, gradually withdrawing the tube under fluoroscopic guidance.

3. **What are the complications of surgical repair?**

   Oesophageal leak, strictures, oesophageal stenosis. The long-term complications of surgery are oesophageal dysmotility, gastro-oesophageal reflux, tracheomalacia, rib fusions, scoliosis.

4. **Can you name any abnormalities associated with tracheo-oesophageal fistula/ oesophageal atresia?**

   The so-called VACTERL abnormalities: vertebral, anorectal, cardiac, tracheo-oesophageal, renal, limb.

Key points

- Oesophageal atresia is the most common congenital oesophageal malformation. It is slightly more common in boys.
- Oesophageal atresia is also associated with trisomy 13, 18 and 21.
- A barium or water-soluble fluoroscopic study is performed if the patient has oesophageal atresia with a question on the presence of a proximal tracheo-oesphageal fistula.

Further reading

Fordham LA. Imaging of the esophagus in children. *Radiol Clin North Am* 2005; **43**: 283–302.

Schlesinger A, Parker B. Congenital esophageal malformations. In Kuhn JP, Slovis TL, Haller JO, eds., *Caffey's Pediatric Diagnostic Imaging*, 10th edn. Philadelphia, PA: Mosby, 2003; 1550–3.

Paediatric Case 24

RACHANA SHUKLA

Clinical history
A 3-year-old boy presents with left-sided chest pain and cough.

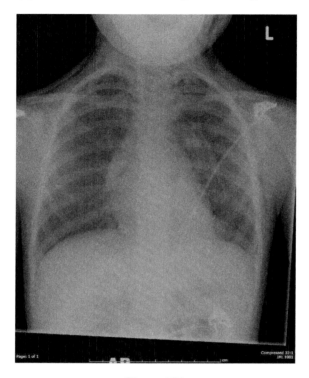

Figure 6.24

Model answer
Frontal radiograph of the chest in a child (Figure 6.24). There is evidence of thymic elevation on the left side with abnormal curvilinear lucencies in the left paramediastinal region consistent with a pneumomediastinum. Subcutaneous emphysema is present in the soft tissues of the neck bilaterally. No pneumothorax is visible. I would like to obtain additional clinical information from the clinicians in order to elicit the possible underlying causes of these findings.

Questions
1. **How will you distinguish between a medial pneumothorax and a pneumo-mediastinum?**
   A lateral decubitus chest radiograph may be useful for distinction, since gas in the pleural space moves freely unless the patient has a long-standing loculated pneumothorax. A CT would also help make the distinction if clinical concerns are present.

Key points
• A pneumothorax usually accompanies a pneumomediastinum.

- The causes of a pneumomediastinum are similar to the causes of a pneumothorax. They are:
  - spontaneous
  - trauma: penetrating and non-penetrating
  - iatrogenic: mechanical ventilation
  - underlying pulmonary disease: asthma and chronic obstructive airways disease
- The imaging feature of a pneumomediastinum is a linear lucent line between soft tissue planes, for example between the mediastinal pleura and heart.
- The 'continuous diaphragm line' occurs because when air tracks into the extrapleural space there is relative contrast between the soft tissue plane of the extrapleural space, air and the diaphragm.

Further reading

Binkovitz L, Binkovitz I, Kuhn J. Mediastinum. In Slovis TL, ed., *Caffey's Pediatric Diagnostic Imaging*, 11th edn. Philadelphia, PA: Elsevier, 2007.

Paediatric Case 25

RACHANA SHUKLA

Clinical history

A 14-year-old boy presents with right upper quadrant pain and high temperature. He also has a cough.

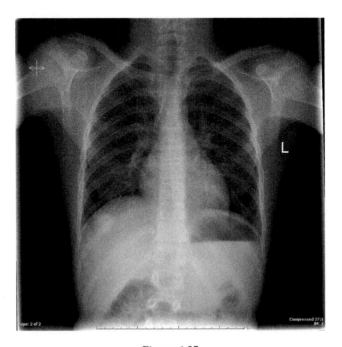

Figure 6.25

Model answer

The frontal chest radiograph (Figure 6.25) reveals a round opacity in the right sub-diaphragmatic region. Given the age of the child and the acute symptoms, the most likely diagnosis is round pneumonia involving the lung in the costophrenic recess. I would like to do a lateral chest radiograph for confirmation. The patient should be treated for pneumonia. A repeat chest radiograph should be arranged in four weeks (or sooner if there is no clinical improvement). Primary or secondary lung tumour would need to be considered if the lesion persists after treatment.

Questions

1. **What is the commonest causative organism in round pneumonia?**
   Streptococcus pneumoniae.
2. **Where is the predominant location for round pneumonia?**
   They predominantly occur in the lower lobes.

Key points

- Round pneumonia usually occurs in children, but it can occur in adults.
- It is less common after adolescence.
- *Streptococcus pneumoniae* is the most common cause of bacterial pneumonia, and respiratory syncytial virus is the most common cause of viral pneumonia.
- Infants younger than three months would require intravenous antibiotics, as there is a high risk of sepsis.

Further reading

Adler B, Effmann EL. Pneumonia and pulmonary infection. In Slovis TL, ed., *Caffey's Pediatric Diagnostic Imaging*, 11th edn. Philadelphia, PA: Elsevier, 2007.

Kim YW, Donnelly LF. Round pneumonia: imaging findings in a large series of children. *Pediatr Radiol* 2007; **37**: 1235–40.

Lichenstein R, Suggs AH, Campbell J. Pediatric pneumonia. *Emerg Med Clin North Am* 2003; **21**: 437–51.

Nuclear medicine Case 1

IAIN D. LYBURN

Clinical history
68-year-old man. Back pain for four weeks. Previous coronary artery bypass grafting (CABG). Report the whole-body views first.

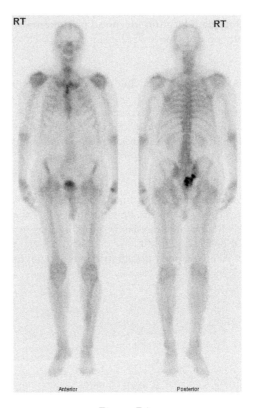

Figure 7.1a

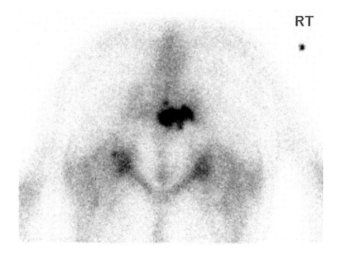

RT

Figure 7.1b

Model answer
Anterior and posterior views of a whole-body technetium-99m methylene diphos-phonate (^{99m}Tc-MDP) planar bone scan (Figure 7.1a). The increased uptake in the ster-num most likely relates to the previous CABG. The bladder contains physiologically excreted tracer that is obscuring pathological uptake in the sacrum on the anterior view. On the posterior image there is uptake projected over the inferior aspect of the right sacroiliac joint/sacrum.

An additional squat view or pelvic inlet view has been obtained (Figure 7.1b). This shows intense uptake related to the right sacral body and right sacral ala. The appear-ances are highly suggestive of a metastasis. Correlation with a plain radiograph of the pelvis is suggested.

Questions
1. **What should be the time interval between injection of the isotope and image acquisition when assessing the skeleton for metastases?**
   A minimum of two hours should elapse between injection and imaging. Better-quality studies are obtained by waiting for up to five hours, so that background soft tissue activity has further reduced.

Key points
- Tumours from the following organs are most likely to metastasize to bone:
  - prostate
  - breast
  - lung
  - colon
  - stomach
  - bladder
  - thyroid
  - kidney

Nuclear medicine Case 1

553

Further reading

Naddaf SY, Collier BD, Elgazzar AH, Khalil MM. Technical errors in planar bone scanning. *J Nucl Med Technol* 2004; **32**: 148–53.

O'Connor MK, Brown ML, Hung JC, Hayostek RJ. The art of bone scintigraphy: technical aspects. *J Nucl Med* 1991; **32**: 2332–41.

Schaberg J, Gainor BJ. A profile of metastatic carcinoma of the spine. *Spine* 1985; **10**: 19–20.

Nuclear medicine Case 2

IAIN D. LYBURN

Clinical history
57-year-old man. No further history.

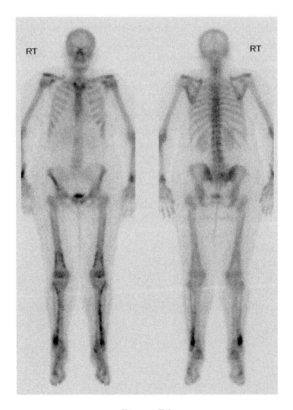

Figure 7.2

Model answer
Anterior and posterior views of a whole-body technetium-99m methylene diphosphonate (^{99m}Tc-MDP) planar bone scan (Figure 7.2). There is symmetrical increased uptake along the tibias, fibulas and distal femurs. The appearances are suggestive of hypertrophic osteoarthropathy (HOA). Correlation with plain radiographs of the

lower limbs to assess for the presence of a periosteal reaction is required. The patient will require a chest radiograph and a staging CT scan of the chest. The most likely cause of HOA is an underlying bronchogenic malignancy.

Questions

What are the causes of hypertrophic osteoarthropathy (HOA)?

Most cases (> 95%) of HOA are secondary; there is an association with several chronic conditions:

- pulmonary disease: bronchogenic carcinoma/pulmonary metastases, mesothelioma, pleural fibroma, chronic infection, cystic fibrosis, interstitial fibrosis
- cardiac disease: particularly conditions with left to right shunts
- extrathoracic disease: inflammatory bowel disease, liver disease, gastrointestinal tract malignancy

Primary HOA is rare. A third of cases are autosomal dominant. There is an association with pachydermoperiostitis.

Key points

- HOA leads to periosteal reactions of diaphyses and then metaphyses
- These appear smooth initially, becoming more irregular – 'onion-skin' configuration – with progression
- HOA usually involves distal femur, tibia/fibula and radius/ulna.

Further reading

Jajic Z, Jajic I, Nemcic T. Primary hypertrophic osteoarthropathy: clinical, radiologic, and scintigraphic characteristics. *Arch Med Res* 2001; **32**: 136–42.

Pineda C. Diagnostic imaging in hypertrophic osteoarthropathy. *Clin Exp Rheumatol* 1992; **10** (Suppl 7): 27–33.

Nuclear medicine Case 3

IAIN D. LYBURN

Clinical history

52-year-old woman. Deranged thyroid function tests.

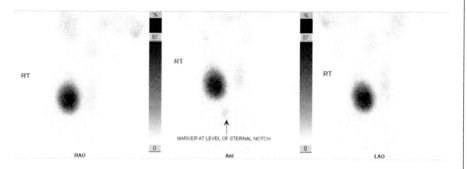

Figure 7.3

Model answer

Right anterior oblique, anterior and left anterior oblique views of a thyroid (^{99m}Tc pertechnetate) scan (Figure 7.3). There is a large focus of intense uptake in the right lobe of the thyroid gland and suppression of uptake in the remainder of the thyroid gland. The appearances are in keeping with thyrotoxicosis secondary to a large toxic adenoma. Ultrasound could be used to localize the lesion.

Questions

1. **What are some of the systemic symptoms this patient may be experiencing?**
   - Weight loss
   - Tachycardia
   - Palpitations
   - Heat intolerance
   - Amenorrhoea
2. **What is the risk of malignancy in toxic nodules?**
   - Less than 1%
3. **What agents may cause reduced uptake of ^{99m}Tc pertechnetate by the thyroid gland?**
   - Thyroid hormone
   - Thyroid blocking agents
   - Amiodarone
   - Iodinated intravenous contrast

Key points

- Thyrotoxicosis is most commonly caused by Graves' disease, subacute thyroiditis, toxic multinodular goitre and toxic adenoma.
- Graves' disease results in diffuse increased uptake of isotope by the thyroid gland. Toxic multinodular goitre demonstrates foci of variably increased uptake with suppression of uptake in normal glandular tissue. Toxic adenoma demonstrates focal increased uptake with suppression of the rest of the gland. Thyrotoxicosis due to subacute thyroiditis is associated with diffusely decreased uptake.

Further reading

Burch HB, Shakir F, Fitzsimmons TR, Jaques DP, Shriver CD. Diagnosis and management of the autonomously functioning thyroid nodule: the Walter Reed Army Medical Center experience, 1975–1996. *Thyroid* 1998; **8**: 871–80.

Pacini F, Burroni L, Ciuoli C, Di Cairano G, Guarino E. Management of thyroid nodules: a clinicopathological, evidence based approach. *Eur J Nucl Med Mol Imaging* 2004; **31**: 1443–9.

Nuclear medicine Case 4

IAIN D. LYBURN

Clinical history
32-year-old woman. Abdominal pain.

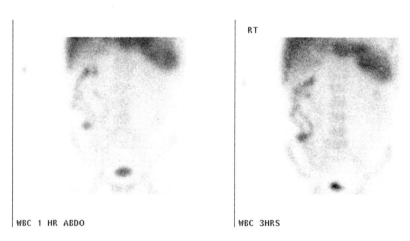

Figure 7.4

Model answer
Anterior abdominal views of a ^{99m}Tc hexamethylpropyleneamine oxime (HMPAO) leukocyte scan with images acquired at one and three hours post injection (Figure 7.4). There is increased uptake in the right side of the abdomen on both images that has a curvilinear configuration. The appearances are most likely due to inflammatory bowel disease. The increased uptake appears to originate from small bowel, suggestive of Crohn's disease. The patient should be referred to a gastroenterologist.

Questions
1. **What is the significance of bowel uptake on the one-hour image?**
   Uptake at one hour is almost always abnormal; uptake on the later images may be non-specific due to unbound ^{99m}Tc excretion.
2. **What is the significance of the uptake in the pelvis?**
   Renal and bladder activity in ^{99m}Tc hexamethylpropyleneamine oxime (HMPAO) white cell scanning is normal. Renal tract activity is not normally seen in ^{111}indium-labelled white cell imaging.
3. **What are some of the other pathological causes of ^{99m}Tc HMPAO uptake in bowel?**
   - Infection: enteritis, pseudomembranous colitis and enteritis
   - Vasculitis: leukocyte infiltration into vasa vasorum
   - Malignancy: inflammatory reaction to cancer
   - Mesenteric ischaemia
   - Haemorrhage: intraluminal blood containing radiolabelled leukocytes
   - Graft versus host disease: enteritis within the first 100 days after bone marrow transplant

Key points

- In both ^{99m}Tc hexamethylpropyleneamine oxime (HMPAO) and ^{111}indium-labelled white cell scans, autologous neutrophils are labelled with the radioactive tracer prior to reinjection into the body.
- ^{99m}Tc-HMPAO-labelled white cell scans are useful in detecting bowel inflammation, and may provide an indication of severity.

Further reading

Sans M, Fuster D, Llach J, *et al*. Optimization of technetium-99m-HMPAO leukocyte scintigraphy in evaluation of active inflammation bowel disease. *Dig Dis Sci* 2000; **45**: 1828–35.

Malcolm PN, Bearcroft CP, Pratt PG, Rampton DS, Garvie NW. Technetium-99m hexamethylpropyleneamineoxime labelled leucocyte scanning in the initial diagnosis of Crohn's disease. *Br J Radiol* 1994; **67**: 964–8.

Nuclear medicine Case 5

IAIN D. LYBURN

Clinical history

63-year-old woman. Bone pain and renal colic.

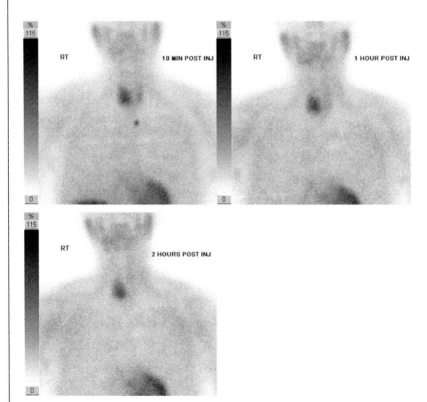

Figure 7.5a

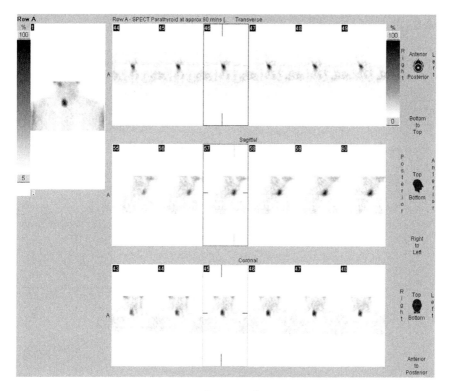

Figure 7.5b

Model answer

Parathyroid ^{99m}Tc sestamibi scan (Figures 7.5a, 7.5b). Anterior views acquired 10 minutes, one hour and two hours post injection and SPECT images in the transverse, coronal and sagittal planes acquired 90 minutes post injection. There is a large focus of intense uptake in the right side of the neck. On the later images there is relative washout of the uptake from the salivary glands and thyroid with focal retention in the right neck. The SPECT images localize the uptake to the posteroinferior part of the right lobe of the thyroid. The appearances are in keeping with a large right parathyroid adenoma. This lesion is most likely associated with hyperparathyroidism and hypercalcaemia.

Questions

1. **Why are delayed images acquired?**
   There is a slower washout of sestamibi from parathyroid adenomas than from the thyroid gland and background soft tissues. Therefore, an adenoma will become more conspicuous on delayed imaging.
2. **What endocrine neoplasias may be associated with parathyroid adenomas?**
   About 5% of cases are associated with multiple endocrine neoplasia (MEN) syndromes.
   - MEN-1
     - Parathyroid: hyperparathyroidism (~ 90% of patients)
     - Pancreatic islet cell tumours (~ 70% of patients)
     - Pituitary tumours (mainly prolactinomas) (~ 40% patients)
     - Adenomas and adenomatous hyperplasia of the thyroid and adrenal glands occur occasionally
   - MEN-2a
     - ~ 20% of patients have hyperparathyroidism, frequently involving multiple glands as either diffuse hyperplasia or multiple adenomas

- ○ Almost all patients have medullary thyroid carcinoma
- ○ Phaeochromocytoma (~50% of patients)

Key points
- Preoperative sestamibi localization of a parathyroid adenoma aids the surgeon in locating the gland.
- A nuclear medicine parathyroid scan may also aid identification of an ectopic parathyroid gland that cannot be visualized on ultrasound.

Further reading

O'Doherty MJ, Kettle AG, Wells P, Collins RE, Coakley AJ. Parathyroid imaging with technetium 99m sestamibi: preoperative localization and tissue uptake studies. *J Nucl Med* 1992; **33**: 313–18.

Scarsbrook AF, Thakker RV, Wass JA, Gleeson FV, Phillips RR. Multiple endocrine neoplasia: spectrum of radiologic appearances and discussion of a multitechnique imaging approach. *Radiographics* 2006; **26**: 433–51.

Nuclear medicine Case 6

IAIN D. LYBURN

Clinical history
63-year-old woman. Staging of a right lung upper lobe non-small-cell lung cancer.

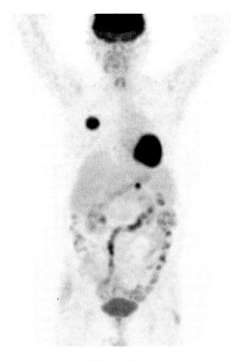

Figure 7.6a

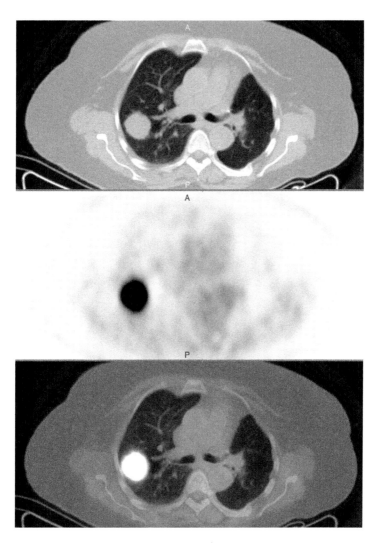

Figure 7.6b

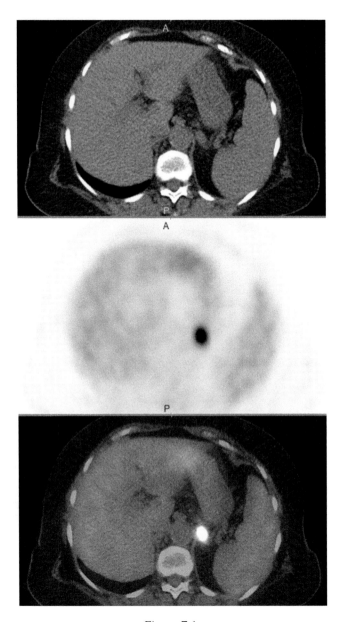

Figure 7.6c

Model answer

I am presented with various images from an ^{18}F fluorodeoxyglucose (^{18}F-FDG) PET-CT study (Figures 7.6a–7.6c). There is intense uptake in a spiculated mass in the upper lobe of the right lung due to the known lung tumour. Intense focal uptake within a soft tissue nodule in the left adrenal gland is suggestive of a metastasis.

There is physiological uptake of FDG in the brain and myocardium. The uptake in the bowel is likely physiological: the multiplanar images should be scrutinized to assess for any areas of focal uptake which may be equivocal or suspicious for a synchronous mucosal gastrointestinal tract malignancy. Physiologically excreted tracer is present in the urinary tract.

Questions

1. **Are there any non-malignant causes of uptake in a lung parenchymal mass?**
   Yes. These include:
   - Infection: bacterial pneumonia and other infections due to typical and atypical organisms
   - Inflammation due to:
     - non-infective granulomatous disease such as sarcoidosis
     - systemic vasculitis such as Wegener's granulomatosis
     - post-radiotherapy fibrosis
2. **What are the commonest sites of extrathoracic metastases from non-small-cell lung cancer?**
   - Skeleton
   - Liver
   - Adrenal gland
   - Brain
3. **Are there any malignancies that are not particularly FDG-avid?**
   - Yes, alveolar cell carcinoma.

Key points

- FDG, a glucose analogue, is not specific for malignancy. Malignant lesions tend to have a greater FDG avidity (higher standardized uptake values, SUV) than non-neoplastic lesions.
- The use of FDG is based on increased dependence of tumour (and inflammatory tissue) cells on glycolysis. Unlike 'normal' glucose, FDG cannot be metabolized and accumulates in cells, thus offering an indication of cellular glucose uptake.

Further reading

Bruzzi JF, Munden RF. PET/CT imaging of lung cancer. *J Thorac Imaging* 2006; **21**: 123–36.

Metintas M, Ak G, Akcayir IA, *et al*. Detecting extrathoracic metastases in patients with non-small cell lung cancer: is routine scanning necessary? *Lung Cancer* 2007; **58**: 59–67.

Nuclear medicine Case 7

IAIN D. LYBURN

Clinical history
58-year-old man. No history.

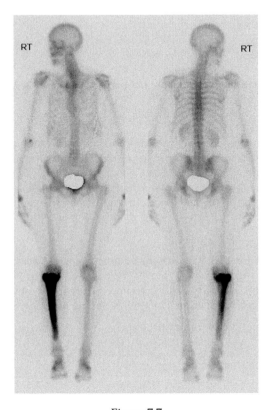

Figure 7.7

Model answer
Anterior and posterior views of a whole-body technetium-99m methylene diphos-phonate (^{99m}Tc-MDP) planar bone scan (Figure 7.7). There is diffuse increased uptake in the right tibia extending from the knee to just above the ankle. The affected bone appears expanded. The appearances are in keeping with Paget's disease of the bone. Radiographic and clinical correlation is required for further characterization of disease as well as for the detection of the complications of Paget's disease.

Questions
1. **What findings may a plain radiograph of the right tibia show?**
   - Thickening of the cortex.
   - Accentuation of the trabecular pattern.
   - 'Candle flame' or 'blade of grass' pattern of lysis at the lower end of the diaphysis at the interface with normal bone.
   - General expansion of the bone with slight anterior curvature.

2. What are some of the complications/associations of Paget's disease of bone?
- Osseous weakening: 'banana fracture', i.e. tiny horizontal cortical infractions on convex surfaces of lower extremity long bones resulting in bowing.
- Pathological insufficiency fracture.
- Malignant transformation: osteosarcoma, fibrosarcoma or chondrosarcoma.
- Early-onset secondary osteoarthritis of adjacent joint.
- In extreme cases of polyostotic involvement, high-output congestive heart failure from markedly increased perfusion of the skeleton (very rare).
- Deafness: sensorineural from overgrowth of the bony canal of the internal auditory meatus; conductive from pagetic change in the ossicles.
- Optic atrophy from bony overgrowth of the optic canal.
- Obstructive hydrocephalus from flattening of the skull base (platybasia) and subsequent 'stretching' of the aqueduct of Sylvius.

Key points
- Paget's disease of the bone is a condition of unknown aetiology that has three distinct phases: the early lytic phase, the mixed phase, and the late cold phase. The characteristic coarse thickened trabecula pattern in Paget's disease is seen in the mixed and late phases.
- Paget's disease is usually asymptomatic, although pain and pathological fractures can occur. Sarcomatous degeneration occurs in less than 1%.
- A radioisotope bone scan is more sensitive than plain radiography in the diagnosis of Paget's disease and allows the detection of disease affecting many bones.

Further reading
Fogelman I, Carr D, Boyle IT. The role of bone scanning in Paget's disease. *Metab Bone Dis Relat Res* 1981; **3**: 243–54.
Smith SE, Murphey MD, Motamedi K, *et al*. From the archives of the AFIP. Radiologic spectrum of Paget disease of bone and its complications with pathologic correlation. *Radiographics* 2002; **22**: 1191–216.

Nuclear medicine Case 8

IAIN D. LYBURN

Clinical history

54-year-old man. Wrist pain. Report the nuclear medicine scan first.

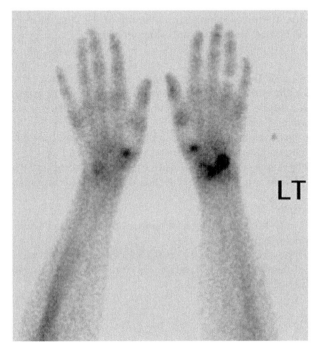

Figure 7.8a

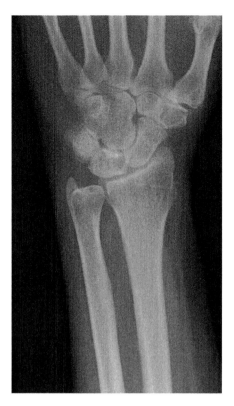

Figure 7.8b

Model answer

DP view of a technetium-99m methylene diphosphonate (^{99m}Tc-MDP) planar bone scan of the hands and wrists (Figure 7.8a). There is increased uptake in both first carpometacarpal joints consistent with degenerative change. There is also intense uptake within the proximal central aspect of the left carpus. The findings are non-specific and the differential diagnoses include degenerative change, infection, inflammatory arthropathy, avascular necrosis and fracture. Radiographic correlation is required to aid diagnosis.

The plain radiograph (Figure 7.8b) demonstrates ill-defined sclerosis with central lucency within the lunate. The appearances are in keeping with osteonecrosis of the lunate (Kienböck's disease). A possible radiological differential diagnosis is osteoid osteoma of the lunate, although this would be unusual in a 54-year-old.

Questions

1. **Which other bones are most frequently affected by osteonecrosis?**
   - Femoral head
   - Humeral head
   - Tarsal navicular
   - Talus
   - Scaphoid
   - Metatarsal head
2. **What are the causes of osteonecrosis?**
   - Trauma
   - Haematological disorders: haemoglobinopathies and sickle cell disease
   - Cytotoxics and steroids

- Radiotherapy
- Idiopathic

3. Is there a specific association with osteonecrosis of the lunate?

Yes, negative ulnar variance. About a quarter of the general population have negative ulnar variance; about three-quarters of individuals with Kienböck's disease have negative ulnar variance. Trauma is associated with Kienböck's disease.

Key points

- The radioisotope bone scan is sensitive but not specific for Kienböck's disease.
- The radiological appearance of Kienböck's disease has been classified by Lichtman into four stages:
  stage 1: normal radiograph
  stage 2: sclerosis of lunate
  stage 3: collapse of lunate
  stage 4: degenerative changes around lunate

Further reading

Hashizume H, Asahara H, Nishida K, Inoue H, Konishiike T. Histopathology of Kienbock's disease: correlation with magnetic resonance and other imaging techniques. *J Hand Surg Br* 1996; **21**: 89–93.

Mohammed A, Ryan P, Lewis M, *et al.* Registration bone scan in the evaluation of wrist pain. *J Hand Surg Br* 1997; **22**: 161–6.

Nuclear medicine Case 9

IAIN D. LYBURN

Clinical history

52-year-old woman. Deranged thyroid function tests.

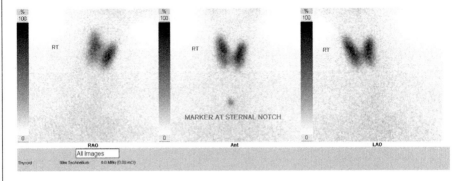

Figure 7.9

Model answer

Right anterior oblique, anterior and left anterior oblique views of a thyroid (^{99m}Tc pertechnetate) scan (Figure 7.9). There is a diffuse homogeneous increased uptake in the thyroid gland, with smooth contours. There is high target to background activity and no salivary gland uptake. The appearances are typical of thyrotoxicosis secondary to Graves' disease.

Questions
1. **What is Graves' disease?**
   Graves' disease is an autoimmune disorder. Circulating IgG antibodies bind to and activate the thyrotropin receptor. Thyrotropin receptor activation increases thyroid hormone production and stimulates follicular hypertrophy and hyperplasia, causing thyroid enlargement.
2. **What proportion of cases of hyperthyroidism does Graves' disease account for?**
   Up to 80%.
3. **What would you expect an ultrasound of the thyroid gland to show?**
   - Greyscale ultrasound would demonstrate a homogeneous echotexture without focal nodularity.
   - Colour Doppler would demonstrate generalized increased vascularity.

Key points
- Graves' disease is associated with other autoimmune conditions.
- Uptake of radioisotope tracer can be used to predict response to radioiodine treatment.
- Proptosis associated with Graves' disease can be imaged using either CT or MRI to provide an objective baseline measurement to aid assessment of disease progression.

Further reading
Brent GA. Graves' disease. *N Engl J Med* 2008; **358**: 2594–605.
Cappelli C, Pirola I, De Martino E, *et al.* The role of imaging in Graves' disease: a cost-effectiveness analysis. *Eur J Radiol* 2008; **65**: 99–103.

Nuclear medicine Case 10

IAIN D. LYBURN

Clinical history
72-year-old man. Back pain.

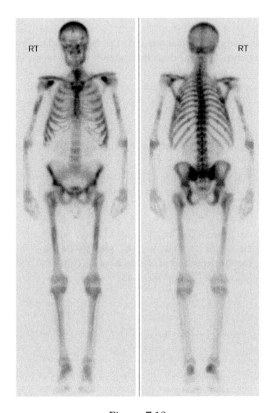

Figure 7.10

Model answer
Anterior and posterior views of a whole-body technetium-99m methylene diphos-phonate (^{99m}Tc-MDP) planar bone scan (Figure 7.10). There is diffuse heterogeneous uptake throughout the axial and appendicular skeleton, with marked contrast between the bone and soft tissues. There is minimal soft tissue activity, with virtually absent urinary tract activity. The appearances are consistent with a superscan due to diffuse metastatic bone disease. Correlation with plain radiographic findings is required. I would also like to compare with previous bone scans (if any) to assess dis-ease progression. Further management is dependent on the clinical picture.

Questions
1. **Diffuse bone metastases from which malignancies may give rise to a superscan?**
   - Prostate
   - Breast

- Lung
- Lymphoma

2. **What are the non-malignant causes of superscans?**
   - Metabolic bone disease – the pattern appears diffuse, involving the entire skeleton including the peripheral bones. (In metastatic disease the pattern follows the distribution of the red marrow – axial and proximal appendicular skeleton – and is usually heterogeneous. Also the calvarium is often spared, leading to the 'headless' bone scan appearance.)
     - hyperparathyroidism
     - osteomalacia
   - Paget's disease of bone.
   - Delayed imaging of a normal patient. Imaging at 5–6 hours post injection rather than 3–4 hours may result in sufficient soft tissue clearance to result in a 'false' superscan.

Key points
- A superscan is defined as a bone scan which demonstrates markedly increased skeletal radioisotope uptake relative to soft tissues, with absent or faint urinary tract activity.
- Always look for the kidneys in radioisotope bone scans.
- Apart from the causes mentioned above, renal failure is another cause for an absent kidney radioisotope uptake.

Further reading
Buckley O, O'Keeffe S, Geoghegan T, et al. ^{99m}Tc bone scintigraphy superscans: a review. *Nucl Med Commun* 2007; **28**: 521–7.

Love C, Din AS, Tomas MB, Kalapparambath TP, Palestro CJ. Radionuclide bone imaging: an illustrative review. *Radiographics* 2003; **23**: 341–58.

Nuclear medicine Case 11

IAIN D. LYBURN

Clinical history
43-year-old woman. No history.

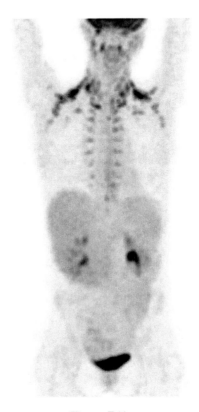

Figure 7.11a

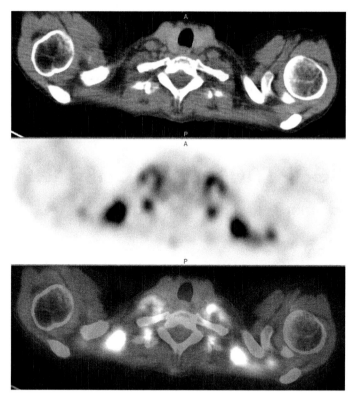

Figure 7.11b

Model answer

Maximum-intensity projection (MIP) anterior view of a half-body ^{18}F fluorodeoxy-glucose (^{18}F-FDG) PET-CT scan (Figure 7.11a). Integrated FDG-PET/CT selected axial series – CT, PET and fused PET/CT images through the supraclavicular fossae (Figure 7.11b). There is extensive uptake in the extracranial head and neck, supraclavicular fossae, axillae and paravertebral regions. The selected axial images demonstrate that the uptake is within fat between musculature. The appearances are in keeping with physiological uptake within brown adipose tissue, which represents a normal variant.

Questions

1. **What is brown adipose tissue/fat?**
   The human body contains two types of fat, white and brown. White fat stores energy. Brown fat generates heat in response to cold, and this activity may lead to increased FDG uptake, which can be very marked, mimicking or masking malignancy.

2. **In which situations is uptake within brown adipose tissue more likely?**
   Brown adipose tissue uptake is more common with colder temperatures. Many centres aim to keep patients warm with blankets and appropriate heating. In northern latitudes it is seen more frequently in the winter months. Brown adipose uptake is seen more frequently in young thinner patients.

Key points

- Apart from brown fat, other sites where physiological accumulation of FDG may occur include brain, myocardium, bowel (particularly colon) and skeletal muscle.

Further reading

Cohade C, Osman M, Pannu HK, Wahl RL. Uptake in the supraclavicular area fat ('USA-fat'): description on 18F-FDG PET/CT. *J Nucl Med* 2003; **44**: 170–6.

Yeung HW, Grewal RK, Gonen M, Schoder H, Larson SM. Patterns of (18)F-FDG uptake in adipose tissue and muscle: a potential source of false-positives for PET. *J Nucl Med* 2003; **44**: 1789–96.

Nuclear medicine Case 12

IAIN D. LYBURN

Clinical history

64-year-old woman. Deranged thyroid function tests. Possible solitary toxic nodule in the right lobe of the thyroid gland.

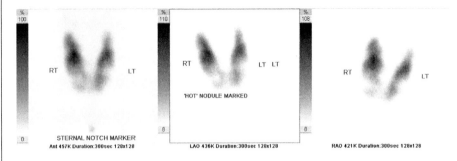

Figure 7.12

Model answer

Anterior, left anterior oblique and right anterior oblique views of a thyroid (^{99m}Tc pertechnetate) scan (Figure 7.12). There is heterogeneous increased uptake in the thyroid gland. Foci of increased uptake are present, most conspicuously in the interpolar aspect of the right lobe, but also in the left lobe.

Relatively photopenic areas most likely correspond to cystic degeneration. Uptake in the remainder of the thyroid gland is not suppressed. The appearances are in keeping with toxic multinodular goitre, rather than a toxic solitary nodule. The patient should have an ultrasound scan of the thyroid for further characterization.

Questions

1. **If your patient developed gradual dyspnoea, what would you suspect and how would you investigate it?**

   Retrosternal extension (which is reported in up to a third of cases).

   CT or MRI can assess the diameter of the trachea, site of airway compromise, inferior extension of the goitre and relationship to adjacent blood vessels/structures prior to surgical resection.

   Dyspnoea may occur suddenly due to acute rupture/haemorrhage of a nodule leading to tracheal compression, which requires urgent intervention.

Key points
- Toxic multinodular goitre is not an autoimmune disease.
- It is important to differentiate between a toxic multinodular goitre and Graves' disease, as treatment of the two condition differs, although this can sometimes be difficult.

Further reading
Cooper JC, Nakielny R, Talbot CH. The use of computed tomography in the evaluation of large multinodular goitres. *Ann R Coll Surg Engl* 1991; **73**: 32–5.

Smith JR, Oates E. Radionuclide imaging of the thyroid gland: patterns, pearls and pitfalls. *Clin Nucl Med* 2004; **29**: 181–93.

Nuclear medicine Case 13

IAIN D. LYBURN

Clinical history
7-year-old girl. Recurrent urinary tract infections.

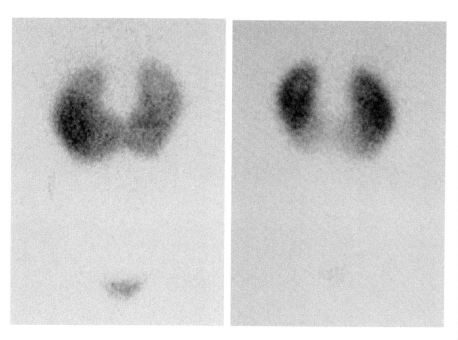

Figure 7.13a   Figure 7.13b

Model answer
Static anterior and posterior views from a technetium-99m dimercaptosuccinic acid (^{99m}Tc-DMSA) renal scan (Figures 7.13a, 7.13b). The orientation of the kidneys is abnormal, with medial orientation of the lower poles. The lower poles are connected by an isthmus of functioning renal parenchyma. No scarring evident. The configuration

is suggestive of a horseshoe kidney. Further investigation by ultrasound and mercaptoacetyltriglycine (MAG-3) may be useful for further anatomical and functional characterization as well as for the detection of complications.

Questions

Are there any complications of horseshoe kidneys?
- Yes. There are usually multiple renal arteries; the ureters arise anteriorly.
- Increased incidence of:
  - hydronephrosis and urinary stasis with infection and calculi formation, due to ureteropelvic junction (UPJ) obstruction as a result of the abnormal ureteric orientation
  - malignancy (Wilms' tumours up to four times more frequent)
  - traumatic injury due to positioning anterior to the spine
- There is an association with other congenital anomalies, and horseshoe kidney is found in up to 60% of cases of Turner's syndrome.

Key points

- Horseshoe kidney is the most common type of renal fusion anomaly. Fusion is between the upper poles in 10% of cases. The prevalence is approximately 1 in 500.
- Crossed ectopia (with or without fusion): the kidney is located on the contralateral side from which its ureter inserts into the bladder.
- 'Simple' ectopia (caudal ectopia): failure of complete embryonic ascent – pelvic, lumbar or abdominal.
- Thoracic kidney (cephalad ectopia): protrusion of the kidney above the level of the diaphragm into the posterior mediastinium.

Further reading

Glodny B, Petersen J, Hofmann KJ, *et al*. Kidney fusion anomalies revisited: clinical and radiological analysis of 209 cases of crossed fused ectopia and horseshoe kidney. *BJU Int* 2009; **103**: 224–35.

LaManna MM, Coll ME, Karafin LJ, Parker JA. The radionuclide diagnosis of horseshoe kidney. *Clin Nucl Med* 1985; **10**: 799–803.

Nuclear medicine Case 14

IAIN D. LYBURN

Clinical history
78-year-old woman. Low back pain.

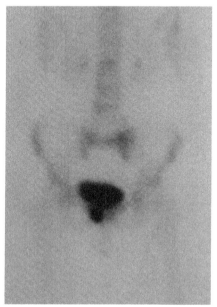
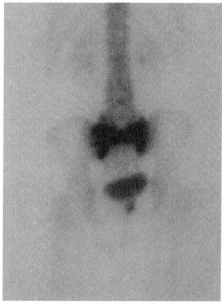

| Figure 7.14a | Figure 7.14b |

Model answer
Anterior and posterior views of a technetium-99m methylene diphosphonate (^{99m}Tc-MDP) planar bone scan centred on the pelvis (Figures 7.14a, 7.14b). There is increased uptake in the sacrum, with a butterfly or 'H' configuration (the 'Honda' sign). The appearances are in keeping with sacral insufficiency fractures. Correlation with a plain radiograph of the pelvis is suggested. The patient should have bone densitometry assessment. Any factors that may predispose to osteoporosis should be treated and malignancy (e.g. multiple myeloma) excluded.

Questions
1. **What are some of the main causes of pelvic insufficiency fractures?**
   - Post-radiotherapy osteonecrosis
   - Osteoporosis
   - Corticosteroid therapy
   - Rheumatoid arthritis
   - Paget's disease of bone
2. **Apart from in the sacrum, in which other bony regions around the pelvis may insufficiency fractures be seen?**
   - Pubic rami
   - Symphysis pubis

- Supra-acetabular region
- Femoral neck

Key points
- Stress fractures can be classified into two types:
    1. fatigue fracture, where normal bone is subjected to repeated abnormal stresses
    2. insufficiency fracture, where abnormal bone fractures when subjected to normal stress
- MDP radioisotope scanning is a sensitive modality for the diagnosis of stress fractures.

Further reading
Lyders EM, Whitlow CT, Baker MD, Morris PP. Imaging and treatment of sacral insufficiency fractures. *AJNR Am J Neuroradiol* 2010; **31**: 201–10.

Wat SY, Seshadri N, Markose G, Balan K. Clinical and scintigraphic evaluation of insufficiency fractures in the elderly. *Nucl Med Commun* 2007; **28**: 179–85.

Nuclear medicine Case 15

IAIN D. LYBURN

Clinical history
5-year-old girl. Persistent urinary tract infections.

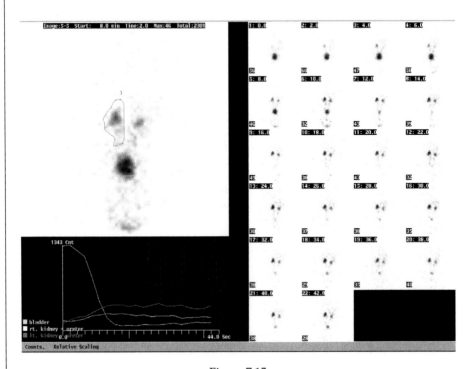

Figure 7.15

Model answer

Technetium-99m pertechnetate voiding cystourethrography (VCUG) study (Figure 7.15). Serial static images of the renal tract with background subtracted count profiles have been obtained. The count profile over the bladder falls rapidly, demonstrating satisfactory emptying.

There is increased activity over both renal pelves with micturition on the serial images. This is confirmed quantitatively by a rise in radioactivity with micturition demonstrated by the count profiles of the regions of interest in both kidneys.

The appearances are in keeping with bilateral vesicoureteric reflux. I would like to review the previous ultrasound and DMSA images. Plain abdominal radiographic examination is required if there is a suspicion of urolithiasis. A referral to the paediatricians/urologists is required. Further investigation is guided by the clinical picture.

Questions

1. **What are the causes of vesicoureteric reflux?**
   - Shortening or abnormal angulation of the intramural ureter; 80% of patients outgrow reflux by puberty. In these cases, reflux is thought to be due to anatomical changes at the ureterovesical junction due to growth
   - Ureterocele
   - Periureteric diverticulum
   - Bladder outlet obstruction
   - Neurogenic bladder
2. **What are the complications of vesicoureteric reflux?**
   - Renal scarring
   - Hypertension
   - Renal insufficiency
   - End-stage renal failure
3. **How is the IVU appearance of reflux categorized?**
   Vesicoureteric reflux may be graded as follows:
   - I Reflux into the ureter not reaching the renal pelvis
   - II Reflux reaching the renal pelvis; no calyceal blunting
   - III Mild calyceal blunting
   - IV Calyceal and ureteric dilatation
   - V Marked calyceal and ureteric dilatation; intrarenal reflux

Key points

- An indirect radioisotope cystogram involves the intravenous administration of tracer (usually MAG-3) followed by serial imaging of the urinary tract. This investigation has the advantage of being able to give a true indication of physiology. The disadvantage is that the child has to be toilet-trained.
- Direct radioisotope cystography is performed by instilling radioisotope, usually ^{99m}Tc pertechnetate, into the bladder (in a manner akin to MCUG).

Further reading

Boubaker A, Prior JO, Meuwly JY, Bischof-Delaloye A. Radionuclide investigations of the urinary tract in the era of multimodality imaging. *J Nucl Med* 2006; **47**: 1819–36.

Pollet JE, Sharpe PF, Smith RW. Radionuclide imaging for vesico-renal reflux using intravenous ^{99m}Tc-D.T.P.A. *Pediatr Radiol* 1979; **8**: 165–7.

Nuclear medicine Case 16

IAIN D. LYBURN

Clinical history
63-year-old woman. Hypercalcaemia.

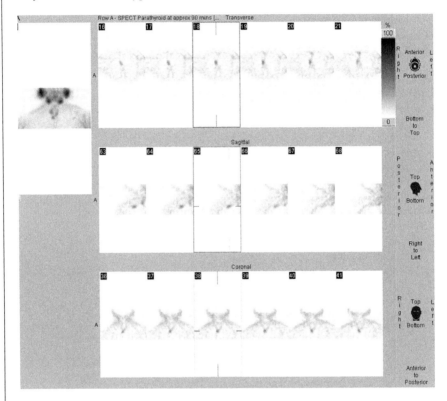

Figure 7.16a

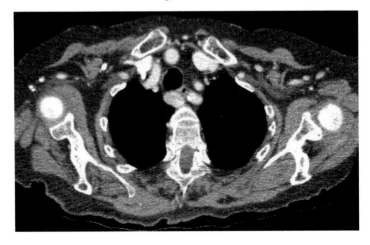

Figure 7.16b

Model answer

I am presented with a parathyroid sestamibi scan with images acquired at 90 minutes post injection (Figure 7.16a) as well as a single image from a contrast-enhanced axial CT of the thoracic inlet (Figure 7.16b). On the anterior view of the sestamibi scan, there is a focus of uptake in the centre of the neck just to the right of the midline, below the level of the thyroid isthmus. The SPECT images show this to lie in the posterior part of the superior mediastinum. The axial CT demonstrates an ovoid enhancing mass abutting the right side of the oesophagus that corresponds with the focus of increased uptake on the sestamibi scan.

The appearances are in keeping with an ectopic parathyroid adenoma, resulting in hyperparathyroidism.

Questions

1. **What proportion of solitary parathyroid adenomas is ectopic?**
   About 10%.
2. **What are the MR imaging appearances of a parathyroid adenoma?**
   A well-defined mass: T1WI hypointense and T2WI similar or of higher intensity than fat.

Key points

- The superior parathyroid glands arise from the fourth branchial complex. Ectopic parathyroid glands may be located around the carotid sheath, within or posterior to the thyroid gland and in the peritracheal region.
- The inferior parathyroid glands arise from the third branchial complex. Ectopic locations occur in the anterior mediastinum (including within the thymus).

Further reading

Palestro CJ, Tomas MB, Tronco GG. Radionuclide imaging of the parathyroid glands. *Semin Nucl Med* 2005; **35**: 266–76.

Smith JR, Oates MA. Radionuclide imaging of the parathyroid glands: patterns, pearls and pitfalls. *Radiographics* 2004; **24**: 1101–15.

Nuclear medicine Case 17

IAIN D. LYBURN

Clinical history
59-year-old woman. Memory loss.

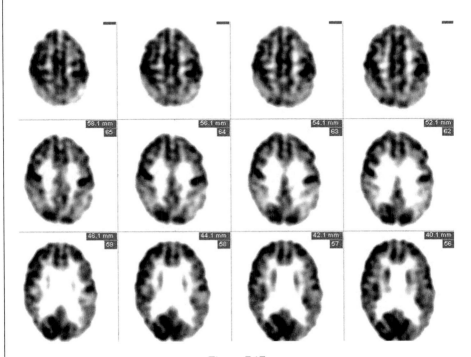

Figure 7.17

Model answer
These are selected axial images from a cranial ^{18}F fluorodeoxyglucose (^{18}F-FDG) PET scan (Figure 71.7). There is reduced uptake, reflecting hypometabolism, in both parietal regions. Uptake is normal in the motor-sensory cortex around the region of the central sulcus and the visual cortex. The appearances are suggestive of Alzheimer's disease.

Questions
1. **What other nuclear medicine imaging test can be used to assess this disease?**
   Tc-99m hexamethylpropyleneamine oxime (HMPAO) scan.
2. **If the patient had multi-infarct dementia, what would you expect the scan to show?**
   Multiple asymmetrical focal cortical and subcortical defects.
3. **Apart from evaluation of dementia, what are some of the other main clinical applications of FDG-PET in the brain?**
   - Detection of potential seizure focus.
   - Differentiation of recurrent tumour from post-radiation necrosis.

Key points

- The brain uses glucose as its primary source of energy. Therefore, FDG accumulates in healthy brain.

Further reading

Herholz, K, Schopphoff H, Schmidt M, *et al*. Direct comparison of spatially normalized PET and SPECT scans in Alzheimer's disease. *J Nucl Med* 2002; **43**: 21–6.

Van Heertum RL, Greenstein EA, Tikofsky RS. 2-deoxy-fluoroglucose-positron emission tomography imaging of the brain: current clinical applications with emphasis on dementias. *Semin Nucl Med* 2004; **34**: 300–12.

Nuclear medicine Case 18

IAIN D. LYBURN

Clinical history

73-year-old man. No history. Report the nuclear medicine scan first.

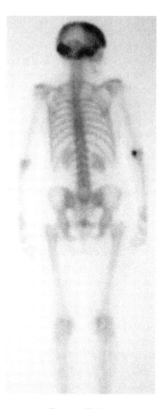

Figure 7.18a

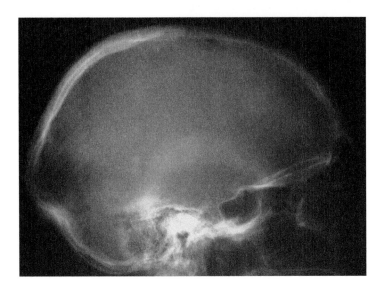

Figure 7.18b

Model answer

I am presented with the posterior view of a whole-body technetium-99m methylene diphosphonate (^{99m}Tc-MDP) planar bone scan (Figure 7.18a). There is increased uptake in the frontal, temporal and occipital regions. No other areas of increased uptake. The differential diagnoses include osteoporosis circumscripta and metastatic disease, although it would be unusual for a patient to present with only widespread skull metastasis in the latter. Plain radiographic correlation is required.

The plain lateral radiograph of the skull (Figure 7.18b) shows extensive well-defined radiolucent lesions in the frontal, temporal and occipital regions. The inner table of the skull is more severely affected. There is no associated sclerosis. The findings are characteristic for osteoporosis circumscripta, which is also known as the lytic phase of Paget's disease.

Questions

1. **What are some of the neurological complications of Paget's disease?**
   - Calvarial enlargement may lead to foraminal stenosis, leading to cranial nerve compression – absence of sense of smell, loss of pupillary reflexes, blindness, ptosis, extraocular muscle palsies, facial pain, tinnitus, dysphagia, trigeminal neuralgia and hearing loss have been reported.
   - Basilar invagination – vertebral column prolapse into the skull base with secondary stenosis at the level of the foramen magnum (up to 30% of patients with Paget's disease of the skull).
2. **Is the skull a common site for Paget's Disease?**
   Yes. The skull is frequently affected by the disease (reports vary from 29% to 65% of cases).
3. **Which other bones are frequently affected by this disease?**
   - The axial skeleton is most frequently involved:
     - pelvis
     - spine
   - The appendicular skeleton is less frequently affected:
     - proximal long bones, particularly the femur
     - shoulder girdle
     - other sites: ribs, patella, tibial tubercle, fibula, calcaneum, phalanges

Key points
- Osteoporosis circumscripta most commonly affects the frontal and occipital regions.
- More severe involvement of the inner table of the skull helps differentiate Paget's disease from fibrous dysplasia, which tends to affect the outer table.

Further reading
Mirra JM, Brien EW, Tehranzadeh J. Paget's disease of bone: review with emphasis on radiologic features, part II. *Skeletal Radiol* 1995; **24**: 173–84.

Smith SE, Murphey MD, Motamedi K, *et al*. From the archives of the AFIP: radiologic spectrum of Paget disease of bone and its complications with pathologic correlation. *Radiographics* 2002; **22**: 1191–216.

Nuclear medicine Case 19

IAIN D. LYBURN

Clinical history
7-year-old girl. Recurrent urinary tract infections.

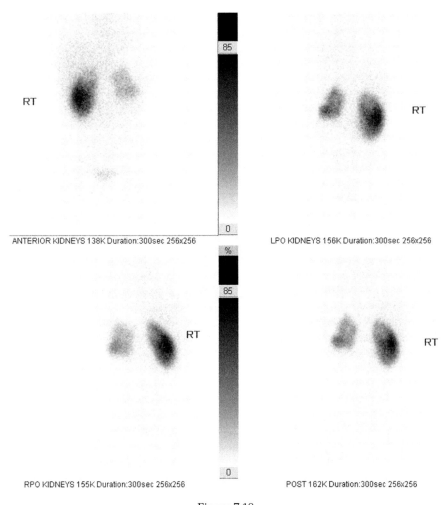

ANTERIOR KIDNEYS 138K Duration:300sec 256x256

LPO KIDNEYS 156K Duration:300sec 256x256

RPO KIDNEYS 155K Duration:300sec 256x256

POST 162K Duration:300sec 256x256

Figure 7.19

Model answer
Static anterior, left posterior oblique, right posterior oblique and posterior views from a technetium-99m dimercaptosuccinic acid (^{99m}Tc-DMSA) renal scan (Figure 7.19). There is extensive decreased uptake in the lower pole of the left kidney and patchy defects in both upper poles. The configuration is suggestive of bilateral renal scarring. Less likely differential diagnoses include cysts and renal tumours. Correlation with a renal tract ultrasound is suggested. The patient should be considered for investigation of ureteric reflux after the ultrasound.

Questions

1. **How does DMSA scanning compare with IVU and ultrasound for detecting renal cortical scars?**
   - DMSA detects four times as many lesions as IVU.
   - DMSA detects scars in about a third of kidneys reported as normal on ultrasound.
2. **What are the difficulties of scanning during an episode of infection?**
   Focal pyelonephritis can mimic a scar. The possibility of infection should be taken into account when interpreting the images. Defects due to infection without scarring are transient and will usually resolve within three months.

Key points

- Initial investigation of reflux in the paediatric population is almost always ultrasound.
- DMSA can detect renal scarring (e.g. post-pyelonephritis, reflux), give an indication of differential renal function, and assess renal parenchymal abnormalities.

Further reading

Rossleigh MA. Scintigraphic imaging in renal infections. *Q J Nucl Med Mol Imaging* 2009; **53**: 72–7.

Stokland E, Hellström M, Jakobsson B, Sixt R. Imaging of renal scarring. *Acta Paediatr Suppl* 1999; **88**: 13–21.

Nuclear medicine Case 20

IAIN D. LYBURN

Clinical history
43-year-old man. Non-Hodgkin's lymphoma was confirmed from left neck node biopsy. Scans before and after two cycles of chemotherapy.

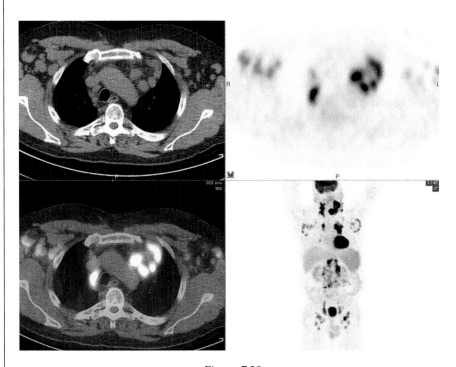

Figure 7.20a

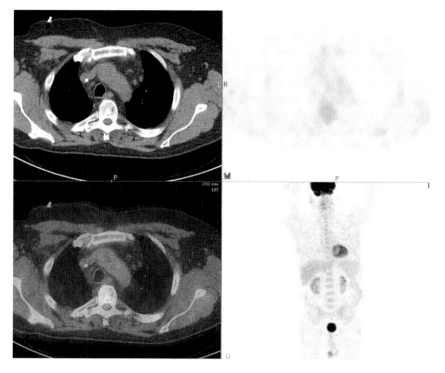

Figure 7.20b

Model answer

I am presented with selected CT, PET and fused ^{18}F fluorodeoxyglucose (^{18}F-FDG) axial images through the upper chest pre- and post-treatment along with the anterior maximum-intensity projection (MIP) views of these PET scans (Figures 7.20a, 7.20b). The pre-treatment MIP image shows uptake in both sides of the neck, axillae, medias-tinum, abdominal para-aortic, iliac and inguinal regions, consistent with lymphaden-opathy. The spleen is slightly enlarged and splenic uptake appears greater than that of liver. The selected axial image through the upper chest shows enlarged anterior mediastinal, right high paratracheal and bilateral axillary nodes that avidly take up FDG. The appearances are consistent with lymphoma involving nodes above and below the diaphragm along with the spleen.

There is physiological uptake of FDG in the brain and myocardium. Excreted tracer is present in the urinary tract.

The post-treatment MIP image shows no abnormal uptake of FDG. The selected axial image through the upper chest shows a reduction in the size of the nodes with no uptake of FDG. There is no increased splenic uptake. The appearances are consist-ent with a good response to treatment.

Questions

1. **Are all lymphomas FDG-avid?**

   No. The sensitivity and specificity of FDG-PET in lymphoma are about 90%. There is a high sensitivity in the three main classes of lymphoma in clinical practice: Hodgkin's disease, diffuse large B-cell and follicular non-Hodgkin's lymphomas. Some low-grade non-Hodgkin's lymphomas are not FDG-avid.

2. **Given the findings on the second scan, should the treatment be stopped?**

   No. The initial treatment regimen should be completed, because residual disease cannot be excluded.

Key points

- The following conditions cause increased FDG uptake in lymph nodes:
  - infection – typical and atypical microorganisms including tuberculosis
  - inflammation – including granulomatous conditions such as sarcoidosis
  - lymphoma and metastatic disease

Further reading

Isasi CR, Lu P, Blaufox MD. A metaanalysis of 18F-2-deoxy-2-fluoro-D-glucose positron emission tomography in the staging and restaging of patients with lymphoma *Cancer* 2005; **104**: 1066–74.

Seam P, Juweid ME, Cheson BD. The role of FDG-PET scans in patients with lymphoma. *Blood* 2007; **110**: 3507–16.

Acknowledgements

Iain Lyburn would like to acknowledge the help of Dr Ian Hagan and Dr Jes Green, who provided images for some of the cases in this section.

Index